Fourth Edition

Body Therapy & Facial Work

Electrical Treatments for Beauty Therapists

Mo Rosser

updated and edited by
Greta Couldridge & Sue Rosser

D1264728

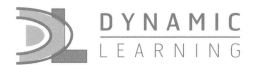

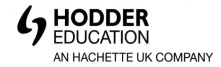

HODDER
EDUCATION
AN HACHETTE UK COMPANY

To Zachary, Joshua, Hannah and Isobel

In loving memory of their Granny

Photo credits: Figure 1.1 contains public sector information published by the Health and Safety Executive and licensed under the Open Government Licence v1.0; Figure 1.2 karam miri – Fotolia; Figure 1.4 (clockwise from top) Kamil Ćwiklewski – Fotolia; Figure 1.5 Science Photo Library/Alamy; Figure 2.5 DR P. MARAZZI/SCIENCE PHOTO LIBRARY; Figure 2.6 DR H.C.ROBINSON/SCIENCE PHOTO LIBRARY; Figure 2.7 Getty Images/Science Faction; Figure 2.8 Wellcome Photo Library; Figure 2.10 Science VU/Visuals Unlimited, Inc.; Figure 2.11 CUSTOM MEDICAL STOCK PHOTO/SCIENCE PHOTO LIBRARY; Figure 2.12 Hermes Morrison/Alamy; Figure 2.13 DAVID SCHARF/SCIENCE PHOTO LIBRARY; Figure 2.14 DR P. MARAZZI/SCIENCE PHOTO LIBRARY; Figure 2.15 Medical-on-Line/Alamy; Figure 2.16 SCIENCE PHOTO LIBRARY; Figure 2.17 DR P. MARAZZI/SCIENCE PHOTO LIBRARY; Figure 2.18 worldthroughthelens-medical/Alamy; Figure 2.20 © Phototake RM/docstock; Figure 2.22 Wellcome Photo Library; Figure 2.24 DR P. MARAZZI/SCIENCE PHOTO LIBRARY; Figure 2.26 DR P. MARAZZI/SCIENCE PHOTO LIBRARY; Figure 3.1 (from left) Paul Vinten/Alamy, Vladimir Sklyarov – Fotolia; Figure 3.2 John Warburton-Lee Photography/Alamy; Figure 3.7 (left) Spencer Grant/Alamy, (right) Solaria – Fotolia; Figure 3.8 © Mike Randolph/Radius Images/Corbis; Figure 3.9 Yuri Arcurs – Fotolia; Figure 3.10 DR P. MARAZZI/SCIENCE PHOTO LIBRARY; Figure 3.11 Science Photo Library/Alamy; Figure 3.12 Medical-on-Line/Alamy; Figure 3.13 JANE SHEMILT/SCIENCE PHOTO LIBRARY; Figure 3.14 olavs – Fotolia; Figure 3.15 DR H.C.ROBINSON/SCIENCE PHOTO LIBRARY; Figure 3.16 Medical-on-Line/Alamy; Figure 3.17 BSIP, GIRAND/SCIENCE PHOTO LIBRARY; Figure 3.22 (left) Nic Cleave/Alamy, (right) Nic Cleave/Alamy; Figure 3.30 Bubbles Photolibrary/Alamy; Figure 3.31 BIOPHOTO ASSOCIATES/SCIENCE PHOTO LIBRARY; Figure 3.36 amana images RF/Getty Images; Figure 3.37 Mark Fairey/Alamy; Figure 3.44 DR P. MARAZZI/SCIENCE PHOTO LIBRARY; Figure 3.45 Regis Martin/Alamy; photo on page 85 Nadezda Razvodovska – Fotolia; Figure 8.1 © Silhouette International; Figure 9.1 © Silhouette International; Figure 11.11a Kamil Ćwiklewski – Fotolia; Figure 11.11b Ruslan Olinchuk – Fotolia; Figure 11.12 BSIP SA/Alamy; Figure 11.13 John Lamb/The Image Bank/Getty Images; Figure 11.14 John Miller/Alamy; Figure 11.15 BIOPHOTO ASSOCIATES/SCIENCE PHOTO LIBRARY; Figure 11.16 RTimages/Alamy; Figure 11.17 © Fake Bake; Figure 11.18 Stockbyte/Getty Images; Figure 11.19 Martin Shields/Alamy; Figure 12.1 Stockbyte/Getty Images; Figure 12.2 Roger Bamber/Alamy; Figure 12.4 diego cervo – Fotolia; Figure 12.8 © Louise Van Heerden.

The following photos are © Greta Couldridge: photo on p. 1; Figures 3.4 and 3.5 (reproduced with kind permission by Guinot UK and Ireland); Figure 3.47 (reproduced with kind permission from Guinot UK and Ireland); Figures 11.8–11.9.

The following photos are © The Carlton Group: Figures 2.28–2.30; Figure 3.3; photo on page 99; Figures 5.1–5.3, 6.1–6.2, 6.5, 6.7–6.9, 7.1, 7.6–7.7, 8.4–8.5, 8.7–8.10, 8.12, 9.2, 9.13, 9.21, 9.24, 10.2 (top), 10.4, 10.6–10.7 and 11.3

The following photos are © House of Famuir: 6.3, 6.6, 7.5, 10.2 (bottom), 12.5–12.7, 12.10 and 12.11.

The following photos are © Paul Gill: Figures 1.4 (bottom), 2.27; photo on page 37; Figures 3.6, 5.5 and 7.8.

The following photos are © Andrew Callaghan: photos in Table 3.5; Figures 5.7 and 6.10.

Every effort has been made to trace and acknowledge the ownership of copyright material. The publishers apologise if any sources remain inadvertently unacknowledged and will be pleased to make suitable arrangements at the earliest opportunity.

Orders: please contact Bookpoint Ltd, 130 Milton Park, Abingdon, Oxon OX14 4SB. Telephone: +44 (0)1235 827720. Fax: +44 (0)1235 400454. Lines are open from 9.00a.m. to 5.00p.m., Monday to Saturday, with a 24-hour message-answering service. You can also order through our website www.hoddereducation.co.uk

> If you have any comments to make about this, or any of our other titles, please send them to educationenquiries@hodder.co.uk

British Library Cataloguing in Publication Data
A catalogue record for this title is available from the British Library

ISBN: 978 1 444 137 453

First Edition Published 1996
Second Edition Published 2004
Third Edition Published 2006
This Edition Published 2012

Impression number	10 9 8 7 6 5
Year	2017

Copyright © Greta Couldridge and Sue Rosser

Cover photo Blend Images/Getty Images

Illustrations by Barking Dog Art
Typeset by Datapage India Pvt Ltd

Printed in Dubai for Hodder Education, an Hachette UK company, Carmelite House, 50 Victoria Embankment, London EC4Y 0DZ.

Contents

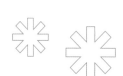

Acknowledgments

Before her death in 2006, Mo asked us to work together on rewrites and new editions of her books. This, the 4th edition of Body Therapy and Facial Work, is our second collaboration. It has been an enormous undertaking, and we are very proud of the finished book. Mo was an extremely conscientious and diligent person who dedicated herself to the pursuit of excellence in everything she did: a hard act to follow. Since the last edition there have been many developments in the industry and we wanted to present these changes in the same depth and detail as her earlier research. We have established a strong bond while working together on these books, which is one of the best outcomes of the project.

We couldn't have done it without the support and encouragement of our partners, Peter Thompson and John Bramley, and the patient tolerance of my daughter, Izzy.

We would like to express our grateful thanks to the following people for providing and checking information, for answering our many queries, and for their support and contribution: Gwyn Rosser, for his constant encouragement and particularly for advice on the science; Angela Barbagelata-Fabes, Chairman of the Carlton Group, for providing photographs and treatment information; Angela Sawicki, Trainer, the Carlton Group, who was most generous with her time and expertise; Vanessa Puttnick, Technical Director, The Equipment Centre, HBEC, who spent many a phone call advising and providing information; Janice Brown, Director, HOF Beauty, House of Famuir Ltd.; Pete Ayres, Manager, Overstone Park Leisure Club, for advice on spa pools; Julie Wilkins, BTEC Senior Standards Verifier (Beauty Therapy); Sally Roscoe, Manager, Luton Hoo Spa; Lorna Lawson, The Boutique Salon; Leah Jeltsch, Kingsley Health & Beauty Solarium; Adele Barnett, Head of School for Commercial Enterprise, Northampton College; Claire Hill, Course Leader for Level 3 Beauty Therapy at Northampton College; Wendy Woolnough, Owner of Kingsley Health & Beauty Solarium; Phil Wantling at Silhouette International for suppling photographs; and The Sunbed Association for allowing us to refer to their manual.

Thanks also to our models: Dominica Mimma Deufemia, Isabella Grafton, Janet Hargreaves, Samantha Scally, Eloise Robb and Paige Harding.

Sue Rosser and Greta Couldridge

Introduction

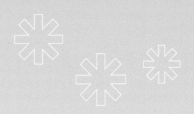

This book has been revised to meet the new standards and requirements of the various awarding bodies relating to electrical treatments for the face and body. It will provide you with the necessary underpinning knowledge to select appropriate treatments and the skills to operate the equipment safely. The information will explain the science relating to each treatment, the application technique and the effects. This detail will enable you to discuss and fully explain the selected treatment with each client and to carry out the procedure in a safe and effective manner.

Emphasis is placed on your responsibilities and the legal requirements under the Health, Safety and Hygiene Acts. These are very important issues, which must be adhered to in order to protect you, your clients and colleagues from injury and cross-infection.

In addition to having detailed knowledge and understanding of all the available treatments, you must be competent and have the professionalism, confidence and personality to deal with the broader aspects of your role. Guidance is provided for developing good communication skills and for dealing with a wide range of clients with differing personalities. Contra-indications and contra-actions are explained and advice given on client consultation, assessment, planning outcomes and selecting effective appropriate treatments. Consideration is given to the timing and costing of treatments, together with post-treatment observation, feedback and homecare advice.

The book is broadly divided into four sections.

Health, safety and hygiene issues

This section (Chapters 1 and 2) covers the legal requirements relating to health and safety in the workplace. It identifies potential hazards and risks and suggests ways of eliminating them. Information is provided on the role of the inspectorate, responsibilities of employers, managers, supervisors and employees under these Acts. This section offers guidance for legal and safe practice.

Ethics, planning, preparation and client consultation

This chapter (Chapter 3) deals with developing the highest standards of personal behaviour and projecting an efficient, professional and caring image. It includes consultation and assessment; preparation of self, the client, and the working area; dealing with and adapting to a wide range of clients; the recording of data and the importance of confidentiality; an explanation of contra-indications, contra-actions, feedback and aftercare.

Basic science

This chapter (Chapter 4) covers basic scientific principles, describes the different currents used in the treatments and explains the mode by which treatments are effective.

The application of individual treatments

This section (Chapters 5–12) includes the underpinning knowledge and skills instruction for each treatment. The information covers relevant scientific theory, the benefits, effects, contra-indications, dangers, safety precautions, treatment technique, contra-actions, feedback and recommendations.

The aim of the book is to provide you with comprehensive information which will facilitate your understanding of electrotherapy and enable you to practise effectively and safely. A summary is included in the text and questions are added at the end of each chapter.

The information will enable you to self-study and acquire an understanding of each electrical treatment. The step by step practical instructions provide the guidance necessary to carry out the treatments efficiently and safely to commercially acceptable standards and timescales.

Electrical treatments are effective with visually obvious results; they are therefore among the most popular treatments offered in beauty salons, spas, clinics, leisure centres, etc. As a competent therapist with a caring attitude, who maintains high ethical standards and projects a positive, professional image, you will always be in demand. You will establish an excellent reputation among colleagues and clients and will contribute to the efficiency and success of your place of work. A qualification in electrotherapy offers many opportunities for an exciting and rewarding career.

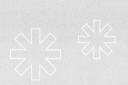

As you pursue this course of study and practice, the information provided in this book will enable you to:

- communicate effectively, pleasantly and professionally with colleagues and clients.

- acquire the knowledge and understanding of how and why electrical treatments work.

- assess the client's needs; select, advise and discuss the most suitable treatments.

- gain the skills necessary to perform electrical treatments safely and effectively on different types of client for a variety of conditions of the face and body.

Learning

Knowledge and understanding

You will require background knowledge to be competent in your work and to be able to explain the benefits and effects of the treatment to your clients.

Health and safety legislation

You must understand the health, safety and welfare requirements related to your work. These will enable you to practise safely and protect yourself, colleagues and clients from harm. The relevant health, safety and welfare issues are discussed in the next chapter together with local authority regulations. These are legal requirements and are concerned with identifying and rectifying the hazards and risks in your place of work.

Remember that as a therapist you carry the responsibility of ensuring your own safety and the safety and welfare of the clients and others who come to the workplace. In these days of litigation you may well be sued if anyone sustains an injury or is harmed due to your negligence. Therefore it is vital that all safety requirements are adhered to and accurate records kept of all risk assessments or incidents that occur.

Without doubt, treatments using electrical equipment pose the greatest risks of any treatments in beauty therapy. It is therefore crucial that you fully understand and learn all the safety issues related to the equipment, the practices and the precautions necessary to avoid any problems. You must also learn important emergency procedures such as fire drill and first aid.

It is very important that you maintain the highest standards of hygiene and cleanliness. If you consistently maintain high standards, this will become normal practice. However, if you allow your standards to slip you will find it difficult to raise them and you will be a danger to the clients and a liability in the workplace. Throughout the working day, the highest standards of hygiene must be practised to prevent the spread of diseases and to protect staff, clients and others from cross-infection and infestation.

Hygiene relates to your own personal appearance and hygiene practices, such as a freshly laundered overall; neat appearance; short, well-manicured nails; minimal jewellery; frequent bathing; hand washing before touching the client and after each treatment. It includes salon hygiene, such as a clean, well-ventilated, adequately lit workplace; clean, boil-washed linen, robes and towels for each client; clean couch roll and clean disinfected equipment; prompt and safe disposal of waste into covered waste bins. It also covers client hygiene, such as taking a shower before treatment; cleansing the areas of the body that are to be treated; checking for and dealing with any contra-indications.

You will require background knowledge and clear understanding to be competent in your work and to be able to explain the effects and benefits of the treatment to your clients.

Best practice · B

Use your time in training to consolidate your knowledge and clarify any areas of confusion. *Always ask* for further explanation if you are unclear about anything.

Communication

You must be able to communicate effectively and pleasantly with all types of people. You must recognise the importance of carrying out and recording a detailed client consultation and obtaining a signed consent form before starting the treatment. You must be able to create the right conditions and prepare the room and the client for treatment. Appropriate body language, tone of voice and a friendly manner are vital for developing a rapport with clients. It is this rapport that will ensure repeat business and recommendation.

Best practice B

Establishing client trust through good communication also helps with aftercare sales of products to maximise the benefit of the treatment.

Anatomy and physiology

A knowledge of the structure and function of the body is necessary, as this will enable you to identify the structures you are working over and understand the effects produced on the body systems.

Activities

It will help you to learn this subject if you try to visualise the tissues underneath your hands as you examine and cleanse the area. Work with a partner and take it in turns to work over different parts of the body, talking as you work as follows:

○ Your hands are in contact with the skin: what is the skin composed of?

○ Identify the different skin type and conditions.

○ Under the skin is the subcutaneous layer: what is it made of?

○ Under the subcutaneous layer lie the muscles. Can you name them and give their actions?

○ Under the muscles lie the bones connected at joints. Can you name the bones and the joints?

Test yourself frequently so that it becomes second nature to visualise anatomical features as you work. For example, label a cross-section through the skin; label muscles and bones; picture where the lymph nodes are located.

During assessment you may be required to give the name, the position and the action of certain superficial muscles. These are covered in this book, together with the name and location of the lymph nodes.

It is not the purpose of this book to cover detailed anatomy, but some topics are revised to help you understand the treatments. Detailed anatomy is covered in *Body Massage 3rd edition* by Mo Rosser, Greta Couldridge and Sue Rosser (Hodder Education, 2012).

Equipment

You must ensure that you are familiar with all equipment that you use:

○ Always read the manufacturer's instructions. Ensure that you understand all the detail. If you do not, contact the company and ask for an explanation.

Remember

There is such a vast range of equipment available now. Machines which look similar may have very different operating instructions. Whenever you encounter a new machine, check the manufacturer's instructions.

○ Pay particular attention to all the safety features.

○ Check the machine before each use; it must be clean and in sound condition.

○ Check that the cable and leads have no breaks in the insulation; there should be no exposed wires.

○ Ensure that the cable is not trailing over the floor or working area.

○ Check that the cable is firmly held at the plug end and in the machine; check that the terminals are safely and securely engaged in their correct sockets.

○ Identify the type of current produced.

○ Ensure that you are familiar with all the controls and connections.

○ Ensure that you fully understand what is happening when you make any adjustment to any of the controls.

○ Test the current on yourself before applying it to the client.

○ Ensure that all the intensity controls are at zero before switching on.

○ Clean the equipment according to manufacturer's instructions after use.

Guide to study

Some of you will find study and learning easy and pleasurable. It is always exciting to learn new things, particularly if the course is one you have chosen and success means that there will be an interesting and rewarding career ahead. Others may find study difficult, especially if there has been a long gap in the learning process or there is little prior knowledge of the subject matter. The material in this book has been carefully organised so that you can learn one step at a time. I hope that you find it interesting and easy to follow.

Many of you will have established your own way of study but those of you who find it difficult may find the following pointers helpful:

- Prepare for study, preferably in a quiet place. Have some paper and a pen beside you.
- Select a small piece of text. Read it through from beginning to the end; this will give you an idea of what it's all about.
- Take one or two paragraphs at a time and read them through several times until you really understand the detail.
- Write down the important points and the definitions that you must know.
- Now close the book and try and remember the detail. Test yourself mentally then write down the main facts.
- Move on to the next section and repeat the above process. Do this until you reach the end of your selected text.
- Turn to the summary at the end of the chapter. Do you remember all that is written here?

The questions are multiple-choice and oral questions. You may wish to study these with a partner so that you can test each other. Now try and answer the questions; answers to the multiple-choice questions are provided at the back of the book.

Activity (A)

When you are studying the text, select small chunks, read these several times, write your own notes on key points, use the summaries, ask yourself questions and answer them.

Assessment

Different awarding bodies will have different ways of assessing whether you are competent to practice. Any assessment is an opportunity for you to show how able you are. You will provide evidence of this ability to the assessor or examiner, who will judge your performance against the requirements of the awarding body.

Do not be apprehensive when you come to be assessed. Providing you have worked consistently you will have gained the skills and knowledge required to succeed. This book has been designed to help you achieve your goals.

Best practice (B)

It is a good idea to obtain a copy of the requirements of your awarding body at the start of your course. This will enable you to put your learning into context and keep a check on your progress. If you know where you are going you are more able to help yourself get there.

During training, develop the habit of reflecting on:

- what you have learnt
- your performance of techniques
- feedback from others about your skills.

Following this reflection, establish a plan for self-development.

Here are some career profiles of beauty therapy professionals to inspire you.

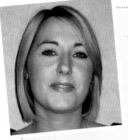

Sally Roscoe

Sally Roscoe manages a busy hotel-based spa. Her travels around Australia inspired her interest in complementary and holistic therapies and resulted in her gaining an HND in Complementary Therapies. She started her career focussing on the holistic side, offering treatments including reiki, acupuncture and crystal therapy. She enjoyed the environment and, being open to new ideas, was keen to learn different techniques.

Sally feels that a conscientious, caring and diligent approach is essential to being a therapist. She says: "Giving a high standard of treatment is an art – you find many mediocre therapists in the industry and it is difficult to find a high calibre of therapist." As an employer, she wants staff who always strive to be the best.

Sally has kept on developing her skills, gaining numerous product house qualifications. She has enjoyed working in a busy spa and finds client feedback very rewarding. She describes being part of a team as a fun environment in which to work. In addition to this she has a teaching qualification and now gets enormous satisfaction from instilling her attitudes to the industry in others. She says: "I have a passion for training and love identifying where people need developing and helping them progress in their career. I find it very satisfying to see therapists grow into senior positions and know that you have helped them reach that point."

Sally advises anyone seeking a career in the beauty industry that it has to be a passion; you must have a strong work ethic and be prepared to work anti-social hours or you won't succeed. She recommends learning as many skills as you can to broaden your appeal to employers and clients.

Her excellent advice to students of beauty therapy is to try to get work experience, perhaps as a receptionist in salon or spa, while you are training. This will give you valuable insight and will make you more interesting to potential employers in a competitive market.

Lorna Lawson

Lorna Lawson now runs her own salon. She started in the industry 1995 when her mother's career in hairdressing inspired her to study Hair and Beauty as a combined course. She cites her early industry experience at a health farm as giving her a lot of varied experience, but describes the setting as rather a conveyor belt of clients. The downside to this, she says, is that you don't really get to know clients and build up a relationship with them.

Lorna believes that a sense of humour is one of the main qualities required to work in this industry! She also lists good communication skills; a professional approach; sensitivity and understanding and being a good listener as vital to providing your client with a thorough and satisfying experience.

As with any profession, there are downsides. Lorna finds it frustrating when clients do not turn up as it upsets planning and, of course, you lose income. She also has to use her diplomatic skills when clients think they know best; but she gets a real sense of satisfaction from proving them wrong!

Lorna's advice to those aspiring to a career in the industry is excellent: "Practise, practise, practise. Always strive to be the best you can be and always be willing to learn new things to keep up with this ever-changing industry."

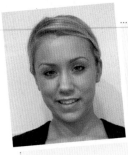

Leah Jelsch

Career profile

Leah Jelsch works full-time at Kingsley Health and Beauty Solarium. Having studied Beauty Therapy at college and gained a Level 1 qualification, a period of work experience at Kingsley inspired Leah to further her study of Beauty Therapy. She did this part-time while continuing to work, gaining qualifications at Levels 2 and 3.

Leah also feels that taking opportunities to train in specific techniques and specialised treatments is an important ongoing part of the work of a beauty therapist, and has continued to add to the range of treatments she is able to offer clients.

Leah highlights the importance of personal presentation and people skills as being key to success as a therapist. This includes the obvious - manners, patience and good listening skills - but also a willingness to help and work as part of a team.

Job satisfaction when clients start to see positive results is one of the most positive aspects of Leah's work. She loves carrying out treatments and also likes the fact that it is possible to work anywhere in the world with these skills. The downsides include mundane tasks such as cleaning treatment rooms and washing towels, as well as the long and sometimes anti-social hours.

Leah's advice to students is that you must be prepared to put in the hard work. It can be physically and mentally draining, but is a very rewarding career. Remember to think commercially - time is money.

'If you know where you are going, you are more able to help yourself get there.'

Section 1: Underpinning knowledge

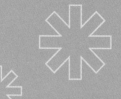

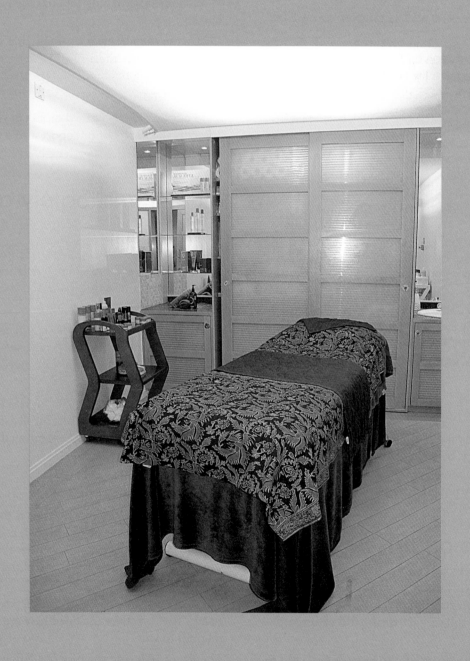

1 Health, safety and welfare

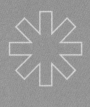

Objectives

After you have studied this chapter you will be able to:

▌ distinguish between hazard and risk

▌ explain the legal requirements under the Health and Safety at Work Act

▌ explain the role of the Health and Safety Executive (HSE)

▌ differentiate between health, safety and welfare issues in the workplace

▌ explain the safety considerations related to hazardous substances

▌ explain the safety considerations related to electrical equipment

▌ explain the importance of reporting injuries, diseases and dangerous occurrences

▌ describe the requirements relating to First Aid regulations

▌ describe the correct techniques for lifting

▌ explain safety and preventative measures relating to fire in the workplace

▌ carry out risk assessments in the workplace.

Health and safety is about preventing any person sustaining injury, being harmed in any way or becoming ill at work. It involves following correct, safe procedures and taking every possible precaution to protect everyone in the workplace.

Hazards and risks

Health and safety laws and regulations apply to you and everyone working with you. These include employers, managers, supervisors, employees, and self-employed, full or part-time, paid or unpaid workers.

Health and safety issues refer to hazards and risks in the workplace and how to eliminate them.

Definitions

Hazard means anything that has the potential to cause harm.

Risk is the chance, great or small, that someone will be harmed by the hazard.

> **Be aware**
> Do not ignore any hazard or risk in your workplace. Rectify the problem or report it to a senior person who can.

Health and Safety at Work Act 1974

This is the main legislation covering health and safety in the workplace; other safety regulations and codes of practice come under this main Act.

This Act states that:

Employers/managers have a legal duty to ensure, so far as is reasonably practicable, the health, safety and welfare of all persons at work, that is all employees and other persons on the premises, such as clients.

The Health and Safety Executive (HSE) provides information and publications on all aspects of health and safety regulations, implementing directives from the European Commission.

> **Learning point**
> The European Commission (EC) is the executive body of the European Union (EU) and is responsible for proposing legislation, implementing decisions and the general day-to-day running of the EU.

These cover a wide range of health, safety and welfare issues. The directives included here are those most relevant to you.

The Act of 1974 and the new regulations mean that employers must, by law, provide a safe working environment for all members of the workforce, including those with disabilities and other persons using their premises.

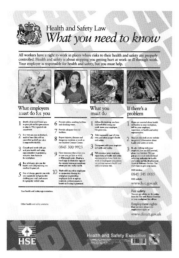

△ **Figure 1.1** Health and Safety Law – what you need to know (Source: Health and Safety Executive)

Maintaining health and safety in the workplace

As an *employer* you are required to:

○ provide a safe working environment; you must recognise hazards or problems, and take the appropriate actions to minimise or eliminate them

○ have a written health and safety policy that sets out how these issues are managed

○ assess the risks that may arise from work activities

○ record the findings of the risk assessment

○ consult with employees regarding health and safety issues

○ provide health and safety information, training and supervision for all employees.

○ keep a record of any problems that have been identified and rectified.

In the workplace

If you are renting premises you may also need to liaise with your landlord over health and safety issues.

The Health and Safety Executive (HSE)

This is a body of people appointed to enforce health and safety law. Inspectors from the HSE or from your

Local Authority have the statutory right to inspect your workplace at any time, with or without prior notice. During the visit the inspector will be looking at the premises, the working environment and the work practices. They will check that you are complying with health and safety law and will assess whether there are any hazards or risks to the health, safety or welfare of anyone on the premises.

The inspector can:

○ inspect all aspects relating to health, safety and welfare

○ take photographs

○ ask questions or talk to anyone in the workplace

○ investigate any complaint

○ offer guidance and advice.

The inspector will ensure that you, as an employer, have arrangements in place for consulting with, training and informing all staff on all matters relating to health, safety and welfare. All staff will be given the opportunity to speak to the inspector privately should they wish to do so. The inspector will provide you with information and highlight areas of concern. They will also explain why enforcement action is to be taken.

If a breach of the law is found, the inspector will decide what action to take. The action will depend on the severity of the problem.

Actions that may be taken by HSE inspectors include:

○ **Informal notice:** If the problem is a minor one, the inspector may simply explain what must be done to comply with the law. If asked, they will confirm any advice in writing.

○ **Improvement notice**: If the problem is more serious, the inspector may issue an improvement notice. This will state what needs to be done and the time limit by which it must be done. At least 21 days must be allowed for corrective action to be taken.

○ **Prohibition notice:** If the problem poses a serious risk, the inspector may give notice to stop the activity immediately and not allow it to be resumed until corrective action is taken. The notice will explain why such action is necessary.

○ **Prosecution:** A failure to act upon an improvement or prohibition notice may result in prosecution. The courts have the power to impose unlimited fines and, in some severe cases, imprisonment.

As an employer, you have the right of appeal to an industrial tribunal when an improvement or prohibition notice is served should you disagree with it, or feel that it is unjust. The instructions on how to appeal appear on the back of the notice.

As an *employee* you are required to:

○ take reasonable care to avoid harm to yourself or to others by your behaviour or working practices

○ co-operate with, and help your employer to meet the statutory requirements

○ refrain from misusing or interfering with anything provided to protect the health, safety and welfare of all persons as required by the Act.

To comply with these requirements you must:

○ not put yourself or others at risk by your actions

○ abide by the rules and regulations of the workplace

○ know who is responsible for what in the workplace and to whom you should report problems

○ adopt good working practices and follow correct procedures

○ be alert to any hazard that may pose a risk to yourself or to others and promptly take the appropriate action to minimise or eliminate the risk

○ be competent in selecting appropriate treatments and in administering them correctly and safely to the clients

In the workplace

If you are unable to, or unsure of how to deal quickly with a hazard (for example spillages, slippery surfaces or boxes obstructing a fire door) then you must report the situation to someone else immediately. Seek advice from a supervisor or someone qualified to deal with the situation.

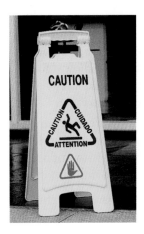

△ **Figure 1.2** Hazards

○ follow the correct technique for all treatments, understand the effects, and be alert to contra-indications and contra-actions

○ adopt high professional standards of dress and appearance

○ maintain the highest standards of personal and workplace hygiene

○ report faulty equipment to the person responsible for dealing with these issues

○ not ignore any hazard or risk; make sure that corrective action is taken

○ report any problems that you have identified and rectified.

In the workplace

At a staff meeting, be prepared to discuss issues of health and safety with all other workers, as shared knowledge makes for a safer working environment.

Health, safety and welfare

The Workplace (Health, Safety and Welfare) Regulations (1992) (as amended)

This regulation covers health, safety and welfare in the workplace.

A 'workplace' means any place where people are employed or are self-employed. It includes outdoor areas, such as paths.

Health issues under these regulations

Adequate ventilation

Premises must be well ventilated: removing stale air and drawing in fresh clean air without draughts.

Comfortable working temperature

It is difficult to select the temperature to suit everybody: around 16°C is recommended. The temperature should be comfortable for working but the client will usually be inactive and may feel cold: make sure that they are also warm enough.

Adequate lighting

Lighting must be adequate to enable people to work and move around safely. It should be suitable for the treatment in progress. Where soft lighting is desirable it must be bright enough to see the machine controls clearly and to operate safely.

Cleanliness and hygiene

Premises must be cleaned regularly to the highest standard. Floors, furniture and fittings should be washed and disinfected where possible. Walls and ceilings should be kept free from dust and cobwebs. All towels and linen used should be washed after each client.

In the workplace

Towels and linen should be washed at a minimum of 60°C, although there are now environmentally friendly products available that claim to reduce the need for high temperatures. They contain stain-removing enzymes. If a client has an infectious condition like head-lice or scabies, however, boil washing will be necessary.

Best practice B

Place used towels in a covered bin to maintain a hygienic and tidy work area.

Waste

Waste must be stored in suitable, covered bins and disposed of in accordance with regulations.

In the workplace

Under the Environmental Protection Act 1990 and the Controlled Waste Regulations 1992, materials contaminated by body fluids are categorised as Group A clinical waste. Such waste must be disposed of in yellow refuse sacks, which must be sealed when they are three-quarters full. A registered waste carrier will then collect these sacks.

Adequate space for working

The working area (containing a couch, trolley, chair, stools and waste bin) should be large enough for you and the client to move around in easily, without having to negotiate obstacles.

Safety issues under these regulations

Maintenance of equipment

Everything in the workplace, the equipment and systems, should be maintained in efficient working order. If a fault occurs in any machine or other equipment, it must be taken out of use immediately. It must be clearly labelled 'FAULTY, OUT OF USE' and stored away from the working area. The fault must be reported and the appropriate action taken to repair it.

Floors and traffic routes

Floors should be sound and even, with a non-slippery surface, and they must be kept free of obstacles. Any spillages, such as water, oil and powder should be wiped up immediately because they will make the floor slippery, which may result in someone slipping and falling. Doors should be wide enough for easy access and exit. Stairs should be sound and well lit. A handrail should be provided on at least one side of the stairs.

Falls and falling objects

Every effort must be made to prevent anyone falling on the premises. Stable, even, non-slip floors will help. Leads should not trail across the floor but should lie along the wall. Stools and bins should be stored under couches. Other equipment must not be left around but must be stored correctly.

Every effort must be made to prevent objects falling and injuring people. Storage shelves must be checked regularly and examined for any damage that may weaken them. Objects should be stored and stacked safely in such a way that they are not likely to fall. Shelves should not be overloaded and should have maximum load notices.

Windows

These should be clean, and open easily. Ensure that they can be seen clearly, so that people will not walk into them.

Sanitary conveniences

Toilets and washing facilities should be available to all persons. These rooms should be cleaned and disinfected regularly, well lit and ventilated. There should be hot and cold running water; soap, preferably in a dispenser; and drying facilities such as paper towels, or dry air machines to prevent the spread of micro-organisms.

Welfare issues under these regulations

Drinking water

An adequate supply of fresh drinking water must be provided: either direct mains water, a chilled water dispenser or bottled water.

Changing rooms

These rooms must be clean, suitable and secure, where outer garments can be removed and uniforms put on.

Changing rooms are also desirable for clients, although the treatment area may be used if privacy for the user can be ensured.

Facilities for resting and eating

Food and drink should not be consumed in the treatment areas. A suitable room should be allocated for eating, and furnished appropriately.

Safety considerations when dealing with hazardous substances

The Control of Substances Hazardous to Health (COSHH) Regulations (2002) (as amended)

This law requires you, as an employer, to control exposure to hazardous substances to prevent ill health. It protects everyone in the workplace from exposure to hazardous substances.

Hazardous substances found in the workplace include:

○ cleaning agents
○ disinfectants
○ massage products – oils, creams, lotions, gels and talcum powder.

Hazardous substances can enter the body via many routes, for example:

○ broken or damaged skin
○ eyes and ears
○ nose and mouth
○ hair follicles.

Substances hazardous to health may cause the following:

○ skin burn
○ skin allergic reaction, such as dermatitis
○ skin irritation
○ irritation of nasal passages and lungs or allergies to products, especially fine powder or dust, resulting in the development of asthma

○ breathing difficulties
○ nausea and vomiting if swallowed
○ eye damage.

COSHH requires you to:

○ *assess* the risk from exposure to hazardous substances to anyone using your workplace. You will need to examine all the substances stored and used in your place of work and identify the ones that could cause damage or injury. You will need to consider any risks that these substances present to people's health.

○ *decide* what precautions need to be taken. Check the manufacturer's advice on use, storage and disposal. Read the information carefully. Consider whether the substance can enter the body or damage any part of the body.

○ *control* or reduce the exposure to hazardous substances. Consider the use of other, safer, products. Store all products safely, away from heat, direct sunlight and damp conditions. Label them clearly to reduce any errors in handling. Wear gloves when

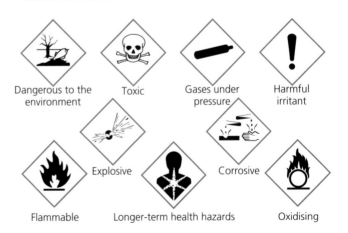

△ **Figure 1.3** The nine hazard symbols

handling hazardous substances and do not smoke, eat or drink during this process. Take care when handling and using fine powders such as talc; avoid releasing the fine particles into the air and avoid inhaling any powders (also protect your client). Replace lids as soon as possible to avoid over-exposure to the substance. Check end date on the packaging. Always refer to manufacturer's instructions when using or disposing of hazardous substances.

○ *ensure* that control measures are in place and regularly monitored for effectiveness. Keep records of all control measures and any tests or problems arising.

○ *prepare* procedures to deal with accidents, incidents and emergencies. Immediate steps must be taken to minimise the harmful effects and damage. These procedures should be clearly written and placed in a prominent and accessible place.

○ *train* and supervise all staff. Ensure that all employees understand the risks from all the hazardous substances they have to deal with. Inform them of the rules and regulations for using, storing and transporting or disposing of hazardous substances.

In the workplace

Compile a file containing all MSDSs and COSHH assessments and store where everyone can access the information.

○ *ensure* that all employees understand the importance of reporting any problems or shortcomings when dealing with hazardous substances.

Activity

Consider any hazardous substances in the workplace. These will include any fine powders such as talcum powder, oils, creams or lotions, cleaning agents etc. Fill in a COSHH risk assessment, including all possible risks from each substance.

Best practice B

Health and safety of staff and clients should underlie everything in the workplace. A regular meeting should always include an agenda item allowing all staff to report and discuss health and safety issues, and matters arising should be dealt with swiftly.

Learning point

Many organisations, including the HSE, use a formula to calculate the level of risk. This involves comparing the likelihood of the risk occurring with the impact of the risk. You can find useful tools on the internet or by contacting the HSE.

Safety considerations when using electrical equipment

The Provision and Use of Work Equipment Regulations (PUWER) (1998) (as amended)

Together with the Electricity at Work Regulations 1989, the PUWER regulations require that all equipment provided for use at work is:

○ suitable and safe for the intended use

○ inspected regularly by a competent person and maintained in a safe condition

○ used only by those who are fully informed, trained and competent in their use.

Learning point

Portable appliance testing (PAT testing) should be carried out by suitably competent individuals who are able to use and interpret the findings of the specialised testing equipment. Faulty equipment is best dealt with through the manufacturers.

In the workplace

How regularly PAT testing is done is dependent on a variety of factors, such as how frequently equipment is used, the type of equipment and the construction of the equipment. Refer to the manufacturers' guidelines.

Be aware

The checking of equipment should never be overlooked. It is a requirement of Public Liability Insurance that equipment used is fit for purpose. Failure to notice faulty equipment could result in a claim against you for negligence.

▽ **Table 1.1** Sample COSHH Risk Assessment

Organisation:					Recorded by: Date:				
What is the hazard?	Indicate the people at risk	Describe the possible risk	Assessment of the level of risk: High Med Low	What controls do you have in place?	What further actions need to be taken?	By whom	By when (agree specific date)	Review date (agree specific date)	Comments
Disinfectant	Therapist and other staff	Skin irritation	Medium	Use of gloves	Training in correct usage and procedure in case of accidental spillage				
	Therapist and other staff	Eye irritation	Low	First aid box equipped with eye bath	Training in emergency procedure				
	Therapist and client	Loss of effectiveness if stored for a long time/ incorrectly, leading to contamination and cross-infection	Medium	MSDS forms. Appropriate labelling and dating of decanted solution, including hazard symbols	Training in handling of hazardous substances, including appropriate dilutions				

Hazards and risks associated with electrical equipment

You may use many different types of electrical equipment to treat clients. It is therefore very important that you understand, and are able to assess, the hazards and risks associated with their use and know what action to take to eliminate or minimise them.

The main hazards and risks are:

H. exposed parts of the leads, wiring or cables

R. contact with these will result in shock or/and burns, which may prove fatal

H. faulty equipment

R. contact will cause electric shock

H. faults in the wiring or overloading the circuit

R. may cause fires resulting in injury, or even death if the fire is severe

H. water in the area where electrical equipment is used or working with wet hands

R. will result in electric shock

H. trailing leads and cables across the floor

R. will trip people up and may result in injury

H. loose-fitting bulbs

R. may fall on clients, causing burns, or fall on linen and towels, causing fires

H. loose angle-poise joints on lamps

R. lamp may fall onto client, causing burns, or fall on linen and towels, causing a fire

H. positioning lamps directly over clients

R. falling or exploding bulbs may cause burns and injure the client.

See page 15 for more information on risk assessments.

Activity

When you have set up your work area for an electro-therapy treatment, carry out a risk assessment using the form on page 16.

Precautions and responsibilities when using electrical equipment

○ Arrange regular testing of electrical equipment – this is required by law.

○ Ensure that people using electrical equipment are trained and competent to do so.

○ Follow the correct procedures when using electrical equipment.

○ Purchase equipment from a reputable dealer who will provide an after-sales service.

○ Ensure that all equipment is regularly maintained and in a safe condition for use.

○ Examine leads and cables regularly to ensure that they are without splits or breaks that may expose bare wires.

○ Use proper connectors to join wire and flexes; do not use insulating tape.

○ Examine all connections making sure that they are secure.

○ Ensure that the cable is firmly clamped into the plug to make certain that the wires, particularly the earth wire, cannot be pulled out of the terminal.

○ Do not overload the circuit by using multiple adaptors. Report any overloading of the circuit to appropriate person.

○ Plug the machine into a near and accessible identified socket so that it can be switched off or disconnected easily in an emergency.

○ Keep electrical equipment away from water. Do not touch any electrical part with wet hands.

○ Ensure that flexes and cables do not trail over the working area but are fixed along the wall.

○ Examine all equipment regularly, especially portable machines, as they are subjected to wear and tear.

○ Remove faulty equipment from the working area and label clearly 'FAULTY: DO NOT USE' and inform the appropriate person.

○ Keep a dated record of when checks were carried out, including all findings and maintenance.

Electric shock

Mild electric shock may be caused by a sudden surge of current. This feels like a sudden tingle and although unpleasant, is rarely serious. The main causes are:

○ intensity controls not at zero when the machine is switched on

○ terminals pushed into the sockets when the intensity is turned up

○ pads moved with the intensity turned up

○ intensity control turned up and down too quickly

○ current discharging through a metal contact.

However, severe electric shock can occur through accidental contact with exposed parts of electrical equipment, appliances and wires.

Be aware

Direct contact with an electrical current can be fatal.

Definition

An *electric shock* is an injury to the body when a person is exposed to an electric current.

An *electric current* can pass easily through the body because the body is a good conductor of electricity. There are three main ways in which the body sustains injury:

a cardiac arrest due to the effect of the current on the heart

b muscle and tissue destruction as the current passes through the body

c thermal burns of the tissues from contact with the current.

The symptoms may include: skin burns, weakness,

muscle pain and contraction, heart arrhythmias, cardiac arrest, respiratory failure and unconsciousness.

Action

It is vitally important to act quickly. *Do not touch the person.* Ensure that you are safe, then if possible, switch off the source of electricity at the socket switch. Call for help. If the current cannot be turned off, use a wooden broom or chair to push the person away from the source of the current. *Do not use a wet or metal object.* Check the person's airway, breathing and pulse. Stay with the person until the first-aider or ambulance arrives.

Personal Protective Equipment (PPE) Regulations 2002

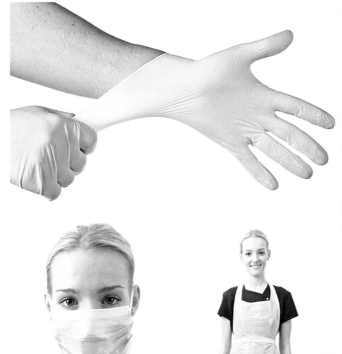

△ Figure 1.4 PPE

Under these regulations you are required to use or wear PPE at work if there is any risk to your health and safety. PPE must be identified through risk assessment, together with the type and grade of the equipment and clothing to be provided.

Be aware

When buying PPE, ensure that it has the mark 'CE'. This means it conforms to minimum safety requirements.

Be aware

Employers must provide appropriate PPE. *Employees* must use PPE as instructed.

Be aware

When using a micro-lance during treatment, wear protective disposable surgical gloves to prevent the risk of cross-infection, as there is a possibility you will come into contact with body fluids.

Be aware

Gloves that contain latex may cause an allergic reaction to you and your clients. Latex is a natural product extracted from tropical rubber trees. Reactions include sneezing, inflammation and anaphylactic shock, which can be fatal. Choose gloves with nitrile or PVC.

Learning point

An allergic reaction is being hypersensitive to a substance (allergen) to which most people show no reaction. The body responds by producing histamine in the skin.

Reporting health and safety issues

Reporting of Injuries, Diseases and Dangerous Occurrences Regulations (RIDDOR) (1995)

RIDDOR places a legal duty on employers, the self-employed and those in control of premises to report work-related incidents. These incidents must be reported to the Health and Safety Executive (HSE) or your Local Authority (LA).

If you inform the Incident Contact Centre (ICC), they will report and forward the information to the correct enforcing authority on your behalf.

See this website for more information: www.riddor.gov.uk

By law, the following incidents must be reported:

○ deaths

○ major injuries or poisonings

○ any accident where the person injured is away from work for more than three days

○ injuries where members of the public are taken to hospital

○ diseases contracted at work

○ dangerous occurrences that did not result in reportable injury but might have done.

First aid at work

The Health and Safety (First Aid) Regulations (1981) (as amended)

These regulations require you, as an employer, to provide adequate and appropriate equipment, facilities and personnel to enable first aid to be given to employees and others if they are injured or become ill at work.

First aid is the immediate treatment administered when any person suffers an injury or becomes ill at work. The minimum first-aid provision at any workplace includes:

○ a suitably stocked first-aid box placed in a precise, easily accessible and clearly labelled site

○ an appointed person to take charge of first aid arrangements.

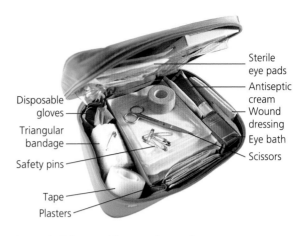

Disposable gloves

Triangular bandage

Safety pins

Tape

Plasters

Sterile eye pads

Antiseptic cream

Wound dressing

Eye bath

Scissors

△ **Figure1.5** First aid box and sample contents

The duties of the designated first-aider include:

○ taking charge and administering appropriate treatment, if able, when someone is injured or falls ill

○ calling an ambulance if required, depending on the seriousness of the injury

○ taking responsibility for the contents of the first-aid box and restocking as required.

The duties of the appointed person are limited to:

○ calling an ambulance if required, depending on the seriousness of the injury

○ taking responsibility for the contents of the first-aid box and restocking as required.

All employees must be informed of the arrangements for first aid. Notices situated in clearly visible places must inform them of who the appointed person and/or the designated first-aider is, where they can be found, and where the first-aid box is located.

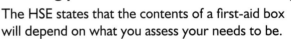

Accident records

You must record the details of reportable injuries, diseases and dangerous occurrences, with the following headings:

○ Date

○ Time

○ Persons involved and their details

○ Overview of the incident.

Be aware !

As these records will include personal details you must ensure they are kept securely to comply with the Data Protection Act.

In the workplace

If you employ more than ten staff you are legally required to keep an accident book.

Best practice B

Logging accidents, however small, will help you to continually assess and improve your workplace practices.

Manual handling

The Manual Handling Operations Regulations (1992) (as amended)

This regulation requires you, as an employer, to assess the risk to employees when lifting or handling heavy goods and to provide training in safe techniques.

Many of the injuries reported each year to the HSE and LAs are the result of manual handling, i.e. lifting, transporting or supporting loads by hand or bodily force. The accidents primarily cause back injuries but hands, arms and feet may also be injured. These injuries may build up over time as a result of repetitive movements, or may be caused by a single instance of poor-lifting technique or an attempt to manage too heavy a load. You may be required to receive, check and handle deliveries and transport them to the stock room,

or to move couches in the workplace. It is therefore essential that you are able to assess the risk and protect yourself from injury.

Before lifting or moving anything, assess the risk, as follows:

○ How heavy is the load?

○ Can you reduce the load?

○ Do you have to lift it off the floor – this produces the greatest risk?

○ Can you get assistance from another person?

○ How far do you have to move it?

○ Can you rest it halfway on a chair or table to ease the effort?

Manual lifting techniques

○ Feet apart on either side of the load for a balanced stable base.

○ Good posture; maintain natural curves.

○ Tuck chin in, keep a straight back, lower and bend the knees.

○ Take a firm grip.

○ Keep the arms into the sides; hold the load close to the body. If you hold it away from the body, this increases the leverage and risk of injury.

○ Lift smoothly; do not jerk or twist the body as you lift. Move the feet and place the load in position.

○ Do not twist the trunk when placing the load down.

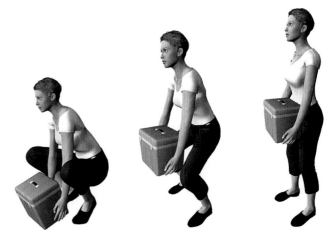

△ **Figure 1.6** Manual lifting technique

Fire precautions
Regulatory Reform (Fire Safety) Order 2005

This requires you, as an employer, to ensure that safety measures are in place to prevent and deal with the outbreak of fire in the workplace. You must assess the fire risks, keep a written record and inform all employees of the findings. The following precautions and measures must be in place.

Be aware

This order replaces *The Fire Precautions (Workplace) Regulations 1997.*

- A detailed fire risk assessment (see below).
- Smoke alarms or other fire detection equipment must be fitted, checked regularly and maintained in good working order.
- Fire-fighting equipment must be in good working order and suitable for the type of fire.
- Fire-fighting equipment must be clearly visible and easily accessible.
- Fire doors should be fitted if the risk of fire is assessed as high.
- A means of escape must be provided and marked Fire Exit.
- Doors should be left unlocked and kept free of obstruction for quick escape.
- All employees must be kept informed and trained in fire procedures.
- Notices for fire procedures and evacuation should be clear and prominently displayed.

Fire risk assessment

- Identify possible dangers and risks: possible sources of ignition; sources of fuel; sources of oxygen.
- Identify who is at risk: know how many people are on the premises at all times; be aware of people who may be particularly at risk, e.g. those who have poor mobility or impaired vision.

- Minimise risk from fire as far as possible: remove fire hazards; establish fire precautions.
- Plan: establish evacuation procedures and prepare an emergency plan.
- Train: ensure all staff know procedures and discuss them at staff meetings.
- Record: Using a risk-assessment form (similar to Table 1.3), keep a note of the findings, procedures and actions taken. Keep in an easily accessible place.
- Review: have regular updates and checks.

All members of staff should ensure that they receive training in fire drill and fire evacuation procedures.

Fire evacuation procedures must be practised regularly.

All staff should know:

- how to recognise the fire or smoke alarm
- who to report to and how to raise the alarm
- how to contact the emergency services or inform the person who is responsible for doing this
- the exact position of the fire-fighting equipment and how to use it should the fire be small and easy to control
- the colour coding on the fire extinguishers and what type of fire they are suitable for (read the instructions on each one and, if you are unsure of any detail, ask the supervisor or the person responsible)
- where the exit doors and exit routes are and in what order the workplace is to be evacuated (depending on location of fire)
- what and how checks are to be made on the numbers of staff and clients or others to ensure that everyone is safe
- how to contain the fire and limit the damage by closing any doors other than exit doors, closing windows, switching off electrical equipment and using a fire blanket to smother the fire. *Note: These actions must only be taken if it is safe to do so and would not put yourself or anyone else at risk.*

Fire is a hazard in any place of work and it is very important that you familiarise yourself with the fire procedures and evacuation drill in the workplace. If a fire occurs you will need to act very quickly; it is therefore very important to know exactly what to do to ensure your own safety and the safety of others. Knowing exactly what procedure to take beforehand will enable you to act promptly.

▽ **Table 1.2** Types of fire extinguishers, their uses and colour coding

Type of extinguisher	Colour	Example	Uses	Comments
Dry powder	Blue marking	**Powder**	Safe to use on paper, wood, plastic and flammable liquids and gases	*Do not* use in enclosed spaces
Carbon dioxide	Black marking	**Carbon dioxide**	Electrical equipment and liquid fires	
Water	Red marking	**Water**	Paper, wood, plastic, fabrics and furniture	*Do not* use on electrical fires
Foam	Cream marking	**Foam**	Paper, wood, plastic and flammable liquids	*Do not* use on electrical fires

Activity (A)

Identify anything that may be a fire hazard in your workplace and take every precaution to avoid risk to yourself and others. It is also useful to do this in the home.

Activity (A)

Draw a plan of the position of all the fire-fighting equipment in your workplace. Label each piece, state its colour coding and the type of fire it is suitable for.

Risk assessment

You may be required to carry out a risk assessment in your workplace to ensure that everything possible is in place to prevent anyone being harmed or contracting illness.

Best practice B

It is a legal requirement to keep a written record of the risk assessment if there are five or more employees but it is good practice to do so even if there are fewer employees.

Consider the following:

○ safe maintenance, care and use of equipment
○ the safe use, handling and storage of hazardous substances
○ safe and hygienic working practices
○ personal hygiene and hygiene in the workplace
○ adequate procedures for dealing with emergencies such as fire, electric shock
○ appropriate temperature, ventilation, noise levels, etc.

Risk assessment procedure

○ Identify possible hazards that pose a risk of harm to anyone on the premises.
○ Identify who is at risk: clients, staff, visitors, etc.
○ Identify what the risk is; i.e. what might happen as a result of the hazard.
○ Assess the level of risk; low, medium or high.
○ Check the controls and procedures already in place.
○ Plan for any changes or updates to those controls and procedures.
○ Identify a person responsible for further actions.
○ Train: ensure all staff know procedures and discuss them at staff meetings.
○ Record using risk assessment forms and keep in an easily accessible place.
○ Review: have regular updates and checks.

Examples of risks in a salon

High risk:

○ unsafe equipment
○ uneven and cluttered floor space
○ electrical equipment (units, cables, sockets, leads, plugs)
○ substances and materials
○ unhygienic practices
○ unsafe behaviour
○ unsafe storage
○ unsafe practices.

Low risk:

○ spillages
○ breakages
○ environmental factors.

Local authority requirements

The Local Government (Miscellaneous Provisions) Act (1982)

Be aware !

Local Authorities vary in their requirements. Check with your own LA for details of legislation.

Local Authorities issue licences and register businesses offering certain treatments. They also issue regulations with which, by law, you must comply. Before setting up a business you must contact your Local Authority to ensure that you comply with the exact requirements. When you meet all the requirements you will be issued with a Certificate of Registration. These by-laws are mainly concerned with issues of hygiene and safety as explained in this text. Environmental Health officers have the right under this law to inspect your business and can issue fines or withdraw your registration if you are not complying with the regulations.

▽ **Table 1.3** Sample risk assessment form

Organisation:						Recorded by: Date:				
What is the hazard?	**Indicate the people at risk**	**Describe the possible risk**	**Assess-ment of the level of risk:** **High** **Med** **Low**	**What controls do you have in place?**	**What further actions need to be taken?**	**By whom**	**By when (agree spe-cific date)**	**Review date (agree spe-cific date)**	**Comments**
Positioning infrared lamp di-rectly over client	Client and therapist	Lamp falling on client and causing burns	Medium	Manu-facturer's instructions available in central file.	Regular staff meeting agenda item regarding all aspects of health and safety and electrical equipment.				
		Bulb exploding and caus-ing burns or other injury	Low	Training in appropri-ate use of equipment.					
				Checking equipment for loose angle poise joints and dents to reflectors.					
				Clear procedures for report-ing faulty equipment.	Regular staff training and updates on use of equipment.				

QUESTIONS

Multiple-choice questions

1. Which of the following is the main legislation covering health and safety in the workplace?
   a The Local Government (Miscellaneous Provisions) Act 1982.
   b Health and Safety at Work Act 1974.
   c Health and Safety Executive.
   d The Workplace (Health, Safety and Welfare) Regulations 1992.

2. If materials are contaminated by body fluids how should you dispose of them?
   a Place in a black refuse sack for the recycling advisors to collect.
   b Place in a sturdy box and add to the general waste.
   c Place in a yellow refuse sack for the registered waste carrier to collect.
   d Place in a blue polythene bag and take it to the doctors' surgery or pharmacist.

3. A product that has a hazardous warning symbol, with a skull and crossbones on it, shows the substance is:
   a an irritant
   b toxic
   c corrosive
   d an oxidising agent.

4. The Health and Safety Executive is the:
   a person responsible for carrying out a risk assessment
   b person responsible for health and safety in the workplace
   c local authority under the (Miscellaneous Provisions) Act 1982
   d body of people appointed to enforce health and safety law.

5. What is risk assessment?
   a A requirement for employers to assess only the most likely serious dangers to employees.
   b Mathematical formulae used to assess danger in the workplace.
   c A legal requirement for an employer to assess the dangers of harming employees and clients.
   d A review to assess workplace polices and procedures.

6. An improvement notice can be:
   a imposed on an employer by the Health and Safety Executive, requiring the employer to improve a specified system of work
   b given to an employee by a Health and Safety representative from a trade union
   c given as a warning to an employee following a disciplinary hearing by their manager
   d imposed on an employer who does not follow employment laws when recruiting staff.

7. Regular testing of electrical equipment is:
   a best practice
   b required by law
   c a recommendation of the HSE
   d a requirement of the local council.

8. A carbon dioxide fire extinguisher is for use on:
   a paper
   b flammable liquid
   c wood
   d electrical equipment.

9. The mark 'CE' on personal protective equipment means it:
   a conforms to minimum safety requirements
   b has been through a sterilisation process
   c contains substances that may cause an allergic reaction
   d is reuseable and therefore good for the environment.

10. When lifting a heavy box you should:
    a keep the legs straight and bend your back
    b bend the knees and keep your arms out to the side
    c place feet on either side of the load and bend your knees
    d hold the load away from your body and tuck your chin in.

2 Hygiene

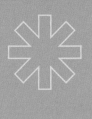

Objectives

After you have studied this chapter you will be able to:

▮ distinguish between infection and infestation

▮ distinguish between natural immunity and artificial immunity

▮ list the ways in which micro-organisms enter the body or may be transmitted

▮ differentiate between bacteria, viruses, fungi and diseases caused by each

▮ explain the methods used in control of micro-organisms

▮ describe the factors to be considered in maintaining high standards of hygiene in the workplace.

Hygiene deals with the precautions and procedures necessary for maintaining health and preventing the spread of disease. In the workplace, the highest priority must be given to preventing infection, cross-infection and infestation. You carry a heavy responsibility for protecting yourself, other staff and the clients from the risk of contamination by micro-organisms that cause disease.

Definitions:

An *infection* or infectious disease is caused by micro-organisms invading the body. The symptoms and severity of the illness will depend on the type of invading micro-organism and the part of the body that is affected.

An *infestation* is the invasion of the body by animal parasites such as lice, fleas etc; they may live in or on the body. Some parasites merely cause itchy irritation, while others cause serious illness.

Micro-organisms

There are many different types of micro-organisms (microbes) present in the environment. The main groups that may be present in your workplace include:

○ bacteria

○ viruses

○ fungi.

Micro-organisms entering the body do not always produce disease, as the immune system is stimulated to protect the body. However, if the invading organisms are in large enough numbers to overcome the immune system then disease and illness will occur. Disease will also occur if the body has little immunity to the invading microbe or if the immune system has itself been damaged by disease, as in acquired immunodeficiency syndrome (AIDS). If the body's defences are overcome then the microbes will cause damage or destruction of the cells. Some microbes release toxins that destroy the cells, while others multiply and directly destroy them. The various micro-organisms produce a wide variety of diseases, each one showing particular symptoms. When the immune system fails to contain a disease, drugs are necessary to treat the infections. Antibacterial or antibiotic drugs are used to treat bacterial infections. Antiviral drugs are used to treat viral infections, antifungal drugs to treat fungal and yeast infections.

Ways in which the body resists infection

Non-specific resistance

○ Unbroken skin forms a physical barrier.

○ Mucous membranes, mucus, hairs and cilia help to trap and filter microbes.

○ Saliva washes microbes from teeth and mouth.

○ Tears wash microbes from the eyes.

○ Urine washes microbes from the urethra.

○ Faeces remove microbes from the bowel.

○ The acidic pH of the skin limits growth of bacteria.

○ Sebum produces an oily film, which protects the skin.

○ Gastric juices destroy bacteria in the stomach.

○ Various antimicrobial substances are produced by the body in response to infection (e.g. interferon).

○ Macrophages and granulocytes ingest and destroy micro-organisms by a process of phagocytosis.

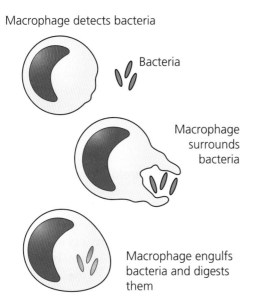

Macrophage detects bacteria

Bacteria

Macrophage surrounds bacteria

Macrophage engulfs bacteria and digests them

△ **Figure 2.1** Phagocytosis

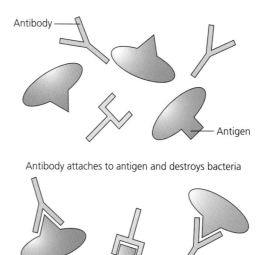

Antibody

Antigen

Antibody attaches to antigen and destroys bacteria

△ **Figure 2.2** The antibody defence system

Specific resistance (immunity)

The body also produces specific antibodies to destroy a particular antigen. An *antigen* is a substance that is harmful to the body. An *antibody* is a specialised protein that identifies and neutralises antigens.

This specific resistance to disease is known as *immunity*. Disease will occur if the body has little immunity to the invading microbes, or if the immune system has itself been damaged, as happens with the Human Immunodeficiency Virus (HIV).

> **Learning point** Ⓛ
>
> HIV is a virus that weakens the body's immune system leaving it susceptible to many diseases. AIDS is the final stage of HIV infection.

Immunity is gained as a result of the body coming into contact with an antigen and producing T-cells or antibodies to control it. Immunity may be acquired naturally or artificially.

> **Learning point** Ⓛ
>
> T-cells are lymphocytes located in the thymus gland that destroy foreign cells.

Natural active immunity

This is obtained when a person comes into contact with a particular microbe and produces antibodies or T-cells to repel and control it. These antibodies remain in the body to control future infection. Many infectious diseases occur only once in a lifetime as immunity is lifelong while others may recur as immunity may last for only a few years.

Natural passive immunity

This involves the transfer of antibodies from an immunised donor to a recipient. Immunity may be passed from mother to baby via the placenta or mother's milk.

Artificial active immunity

Artificial immunity can be provided by the use of vaccines. These are prepared from altered or diluted forms of the organism. Once they are introduced into the body, they stimulate the immune system in the same way as an infection, but are not strong enough to cause the disease.

Artificial passive immunity

Another type of immunisation relies on transferring antibodies from someone who has recovered from that particular disease. The transfer is made via a serum containing the antibodies.

Invasion

Micro-organisms enter the body via many routes:

○ through broken or damaged skin

○ through orifices, such as the nose, mouth, anus, vagina and urethra

○ through the eyes and ears

○ into hair follicles

○ into the blood stream via bloodsucking insects such as mosquitoes and lice.

Some micro-organisms produce immediate symptoms, while others can lie dormant for a long time and attack when the body's immune system is low.

Transmission

Micro-organisms are transmitted in many ways:

○ By droplet infection: an infected person coughing and sneezing or spitting will expel organisms into the air where they may be inhaled by others.

○ By handling contaminated articles, such as clothing, towels and equipment, when micro-organisms may be transmitted to the handler.

○ Dirty surfaces or dusty atmospheres will contain micro-organisms, which may be inhaled or may enter via the eyes or ears.

○ Organisms present in faeces and urine may be transferred to others if the hands are not thoroughly washed after visiting the toilet.

○ Food may become contaminated by handling with unwashed hands and also by flies carrying contamination from excreta and rubbish. Water may become contaminated and then organisms will be transmitted to humans through drinking the water or eating foods washed with it.

○ Through contact with animals.

○ Through direct contact with others, for example kissing, hand contact or touching.

○ Organisms may be spread through intermediary hosts, such as fleas and bloodsucking insects.

○ Sexual intercourse can spread certain organisms that produce diseases.

○ Contaminated blood, if transmitted to another person, can cause serious and, sometimes, fatal illness. Organisms can be transmitted through blood transfusion, infected needles or micro-lances or at any time when the blood of the carrier (infected person) enters the body of the recipient. Hepatitis B and HIV are transmitted in this way, and great care must be taken in the workplace to avoid any contact with blood. Any blood spots should be dealt with by wearing gloves, wiping the area with cotton wool or tissue and disposing of these in a yellow refuse sack.

Be aware

Micro-lances must be carefully disposed of into a sharps container.

○ Infection can be caused by the spread of certain organisms within one's own body. These organisms may be harmless in one part of the body, but will produce inflammation in another; for example certain organisms in the intestine are harmless, but if they invade the bladder they produce cystitis.

The conditions required for the growth of micro-organisms include:

○ a food supply

○ a water supply or moisture

○ warmth (pathogenic bacteria favour body temperature of 37°C)

○ dark conditions.

Learning point

Low temperatures found in the refrigerator or freezer will prevent growth of bacteria but will not destroy them.

○ oxygen is required by some bacteria for aerobic respiration but others are anaerobic and survive without oxygen

Learning point

Strong ultra violet light (UVL) will kill bacteria.

○ slightly alkaline conditions.

Learning point

The acidity of the skin's acid mantle, helps to protect against growth of bacteria.

Bacteria

Bacteria are single-cell organisms, varying in size from 0.2µm to 2.0µm in diameter. They are found everywhere in the environment but can only be seen through an optical microscope. Many bacteria are harmless and may be useful to humans – these are called *non-pathogenic bacteria*. Some are used in the production of food such as cheese and yoghurt. Others help to dispose of unwanted organic material such as the breakdown of sewage, rendering it harmless. Some bacteria in the human intestine help to synthesise vitamins K and B_2.

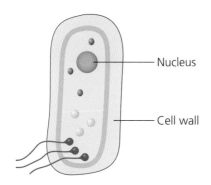

△ **Figure 2.3** A bacterium

Bacteria are the simplest of living organisms, composed of a single cell with cytoplasm surrounded by a protective cell membrane but devoid of organelles.

Some bacteria have whip-like projections on the surface of the cell, called flagella: these enable the bacteria to move around. Bacteria may be aerobic, requiring oxygen to sustain life, or they may be anaerobic, able to survive without oxygen.

The aerobic variety is found invading surface tissues of the skin and mucous membranes of the respiratory tract. The anaerobic variety is found in the bowel or deep wounds. Some bacteria develop into spores; these can lie dormant for long periods of time and become active when conditions are suitable. Spores develop a hard, thick outer shell that protects the contents and makes them very difficult to destroy. They are more resistant to heat and disinfectants; higher temperatures and strong chemical disinfectants are required to kill spores.

Bacteria cause disease by producing toxins or poisons that are harmful to body cells. They grow and multiply if the conditions are right.

Types of bacterium

There are three types of bacterium: cocci, bacilli and spirochete.

Bacteria are classified according to their shape:

a   *Cocci*: these spherical-shaped bacteria may form clusters known as staphylococci, or chains known as streptococci, or pairs known as diplococci. They can cause a wide variety of conditions such as boils, carbuncles, impetigo, sore throat, meningitis, pneumonia etc.

b   *Bacilli*: these rod-shaped bacteria cause serious illness, such as diphtheria, tuberculosis, and typhoid fever.

c   *Spirochetes*: these spiral- or curved-shaped bacteria include spirillium and vibros and cause venereal disease, such as syphilis, and serious disease such as cholera.

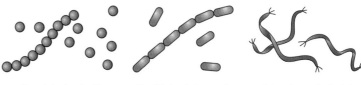

Cocci (spherical)   Bacilli (rod-shaped)   Spirochete (spirals)

△ **Figure 2.4** Three types of bacterium: a) cocci, b) bacilli and c) spirochete

The body protects itself against bacterial infection by several methods. It produces:

○ antitoxins, which neutralise toxins produced by the bacteria

○ large numbers of white cells, macrophages and granulocytes, which circulate in the blood and which engulf and destroy bacteria

○ antibodies, which attack and destroy the bacteria.

The discovery of penicillin and development of other antibiotics and antibacterials mean that bacterial infections can usually be brought under control. Antibiotics must be used in adequate doses for at least five days. Some antibiotics kill the bacteria directly while others prevent multiplication of the bacteria.

Bacteria grow and multiply if the conditions are right. These are:

○ a food supply

○ a water supply or moisture

○ warmth; pathogenic bacteria favour a body temperature of 37°C (Note: low temperatures found in the refrigerator or freezer will limit the growth of bacteria, but will not destroy them.)

○ dark conditions; strong ultraviolet light will kill bacteria

○ oxygen is required by some bacteria for aerobic respiration, but others are anaerobic and survive without oxygen

○ slightly alkaline conditions: the acidity of the skin (acid mantle), helps to protect against the growth of bacteria.

Bacterial infections of the skin

These include impetigo, conjunctivitis, furuncles and carbuncles.

Impetigo

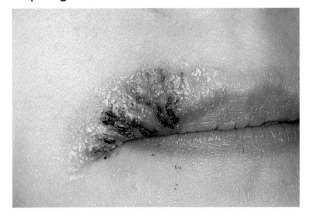

△ **Figure 2.5** Impetigo

This is a highly contagious bacterial infection of the skin. Usually located around the mouth, it begins as an itchy red patch that develops into pustules and further into flaky crusts. It is usually found in children, but adults may also be affected. This condition should be medically treated.

Conjunctivitis

This is an inflammation of the conjunctiva; the thin membrane that covers the white of the eye and inside of the eyelids.

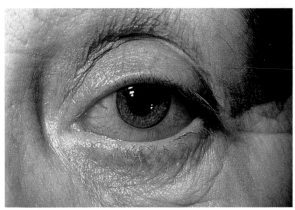

△ **Figure 2.6** Conjunctivitis

Furuncle (boil)

This is an abscess under the skin filled with pus, which is caused by bacteria entering the skin, usually through a hair follicle. Boils can be painful and should be medically treated.

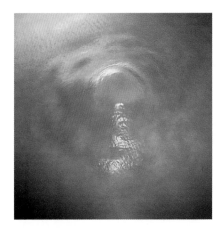

△ **Figure 2.7** Furuncle

Carbuncle

This is a collection of boils, which can be very painful and must be referred for medical treatment.

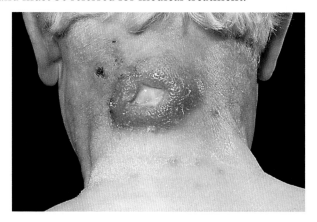

△ **Figure 2.8** Carbuncle

Viruses

Viruses are the smallest known infective particles: smaller than bacteria, they can only be seen through an electron microscope. They are between 0.1μm and 0.2μm in size, and vary in shape from spheres, cubes or rods.

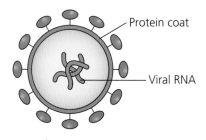

Protein coat

Viral RNA

△ **Figure 2.9** A virus

They consist of a core of nucleic acid, ribonucleic acid (RNA) or deoxyribonucleic acid (DNA), enclosed in a protein shell or capsid. Viruses cannot metabolise or reproduce: they are parasitic, living inside a host cell. Once inside a host cell, a virus causes the host cell to make copies of the virus. Eventually, the host cell is destroyed and hundreds of new viruses released that attack other cells. After the virus enters the host cell there is a period of incubation when the host cells show no sign of disease. Many cycles of viral spread occur and more and more host cells are affected; eventually typical signs and symptoms of the disease occur. By the time the symptoms appear, the viruses are so numerous that antiviral drugs have limited effect. The body protects itself against viral infection by producing specific antibodies. These will also provide future immunity to some diseases; immunity can be produced artificially to combat some viral infections.

Body cells also produce interferons, which interfere with the multiplication of viruses. Antiviral drugs are now available, some of which prevent the multiplication of viruses while others alter the DNA within the cell, preventing the virus from using it. In this way, the spread of infection is halted.

> **Learning point**
>
> Interferons are proteins produced in host cells and released to fight pathogens.

Viral diseases include the common cold, influenza, poliomyelitis, mumps, hepatitis and acquired immune deficiency syndrome (AIDS).

Viral infections of the skin

These include herpes simplex, herpes zoster and warts.

Herpes simplex

This is caused by a virus living in the skin, usually of the lips, when it is often referred to as a cold sore. It produces an eruption around the mouth that starts as an itchy red patch and develops into vesicles or a weeping blister, which then form a crust. It is very contagious. Do not treat the face of a client with cold sores to avoid cross-infection.

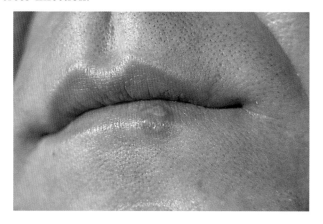

△ **Figure 2.10** Herpes simplex

Herpes zoster

This is caused by the same virus that causes chicken pox. Most people have chicken pox during childhood and the virus lies dormant in the body. In adulthood it can be reactivated and cause shingles. It infects the nerve and the area of skin that the nerve supplies. Symptoms include a tingling sensation, followed by pain and a rash usually around the chest, abdomen or face.

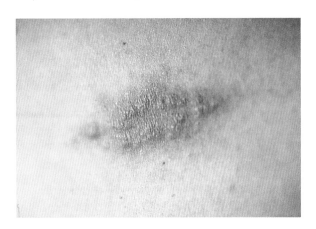

△ **Figure 2.11** Herpes zoster (shingles)

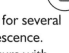

Learning point

If you have not had chicken pox, then you cannot catch shingles, but you can catch chicken pox from a person who has shingles.

Warts

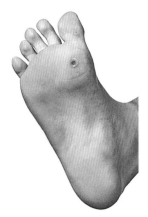

△ **Figure 2.12** Verrucae (plantar warts)

These are caused by a virus that causes rapid cell division. Common warts are raised with a rough surface and are usually found on the hands. Plantar warts (verrucae) are found on the soles of the feet and grow inwards. They are painful upon pressure and should be referred for medical treatment. Warts are very contagious: avoid touching them and avoid working on clients if you have a wart.

Hepatitis and HIV

The two most serious viral infections that could be transmitted between clients or staff and clients in the workplace are hepatitis B and HIV, both of which are carried in the blood. Minute amounts of blood or organic material can carry infection; it may not be visible to the naked eye. The correct hygiene procedures must be followed to prevent any possibility of infection (see page 29).

Hepatitis – inflammation of the liver

Hepatitis is caused by viruses or by amoebae. There are many forms of the disease, each having similar symptoms but contracted by different viruses, namely: hepatitis A virus, hepatitis B virus and hepatitis non-A and non-B.

The symptoms of hepatitis include:

○ fever

○ loss of appetite

○ nausea and vomiting

○ jaundice (yellow colouring of the skin and whites of the eyes)

○ pain in the abdomen with tenderness over the liver

○ dark urine.

Learning point

People who contract hepatitis feel very ill for several months and need a long period of convalescence. Most recover eventually. Death rarely occurs with hepatitis A but is more common with hepatitis B.

Hepatitis A virus

The hepatitis A virus has a short incubation period of around three weeks. It is contracted through faecal contact due to poor sanitation and poor personal hygiene. It may be contracted by UK residents travelling abroad where faecal–oral contamination is likely and waste disposal may be basic with open sewers, etc. The virus may have already been passed on before the sufferer realises that they are infected, as it is most contagious during the incubation period. It does not cause any lasting damage to the liver.

Hepatitis B virus

This has a long incubation period – around three months. It is transmitted through breaks in the skin or by punctures with contaminated equipment. It may also be transmitted sexually or following transfusion with contaminated blood. Highly infectious mothers usually pass it on to their babies. The virus is detected in blood, saliva, semen and body fluids. High-risk groups are: drug abusers, homosexuals and renal dialysis patients.

The disease is most contagious during the incubation period when a carrier may not be showing any symptoms. There are thousands of symptomless carriers worldwide. Hepatitis B can cause lasting chronic liver damage, which may result in death.

The particular risk to you and your clients is the transmission of this disease when using a micro-lance or on any occasion where blood contamination is likely. Blood, tissue fluid and skin debris may be carried on the micro-lance and transmitted from one client to another or to you by accidental stabs or scratches.

Disposable sterile micro-lances must always be used to prevent the spread of this disease. Used micro-lances should be very carefully handled and disposed of in a sharps container. Hepatitis B is a particularly resistant virus. Sterilisation using the autoclave and the use of disinfectants, such as hypochlorite solutions (bleach), are the most effective methods of control.

Hepatitis non-A and non-B

These have an incubation period of around one month and are distinct from hepatitis A and B but produce very similar symptoms. They may be contracted from contaminated food and water or blood transfusions. They can cause inflammation of the liver, followed by cirrhosis (scarring of the liver).

Human Immunodeficiency Virus (HIV)

HIV is the virus that causes Acquired Immune Deficiency Syndrome (AIDS). AIDS was first reported in the New England Medical Journal in 1981 and by the end of that year the first case was reported in the United Kingdom. It is a disease that affects both male and female homosexuals and heterosexuals.

In 1983 scientists in the United States of America and France isolated the HIV virus. This virus attacks a group of cells called T4 or the T-helper cells that play a part in coordinating the action of the immune system.

Following infection with HIV, there may be no immediate symptoms and the incubation period may be up to eight years. There are many thousands of symptomless carriers worldwide. The first symptoms are usually fatigue, fever, swollen glands and headaches. After a few weeks these symptoms may disappear.

Some time later the next stage of the disease appears when the glands of the neck, armpit and groin become chronically swollen. During this time the helper T-cells, which play a key role in antibody production, diminish in number until eventually the body's immune system is destroyed. The body is then defenceless against a wide variety of diseases, which include pneumonia, tuberculosis, thrush and Karposi's sarcoma (a deadly skin cancer which produces purple-brownish marks on the skin). The heart, liver and brain may also become affected, leading to dementia and death.

This virus has been located in:

○ blood

○ semen

○ vaginal fluid

○ tears

○ saliva

○ cerebro-spinal fluid.

However, to be transmitted the virus must be present in large numbers and these are found only in blood, semen and vaginal secretions.

Ways in which HIV is transmitted include:

○ sexual intercourse with an infected person male to male, male to female or female to male

○ through blood exchange from open bleeding cuts and wounds; from contaminated needles or other con-taminated instruments piercing the skin

○ infected mothers pass it to their babies through the placenta, during birth or through breast feeding.

No cure has been found to date and preventative measures must be taken to avoid spread of the disease. The virus is quite fragile outside the body and can be destroyed by:

○ autoclaving all contaminated instruments

○ washing towels, dishes etc. at 56°C for ten minutes

○ disinfecting surfaces and cleaning up blood, vomit and urine with hypochlorite solutions (bleach).

Fungi

Fungi are larger than bacteria: they may be unicellular, as in yeasts, or multicellular, as in moulds. The cells contain nuclei and other cell components but do not contain chlorophyll. They obtain their food by secreting enzymes through the cell walls: this digests any organic matter, which is then absorbed as liquid food. Fungi may be saprophytes, which obtain food from dead organic matter, or they may be parasites, which live off plants, animals or humans, feeding off skin and mucous membranes and producing diseases. They reproduce by forming spores. The unicellular fungi and spores are not visible to the naked eye but the filamentous fungi-forming mycelia are visible (e.g. moulds and mildews).

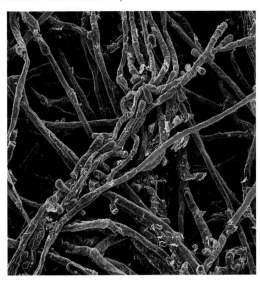

△ **Figure 2.13** Fungi

Fungi require similar conditions to bacteria for growth:

○ a food supply
○ damp, moist conditions
○ warmth
○ oxygen, although some survive for a short time without.

Diseases caused by fungi

Ringworm

This affects different parts of the body and is named according to the part affected.

Tinea pedis (athlete's foot)

This affects the skin around and between the toes, forming red, itchy, scaly patches on the soles and between the toes. The skin may become sore, soggy and white. It is highly contagious. Do not treat the feet and ensure they are covered when treating other areas.

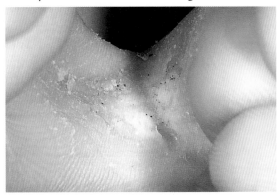

△ **Figure 2.14** Tinea pedis

Tinea corporis

This infects the skin all over the body. Red, round, scaly patches that spread outwards can appear anywhere on the body. Advise the client to seek medical advice.

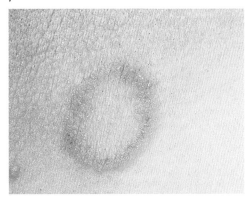

△ **Figure 2.15** Tinea corporis

Tinea capitis

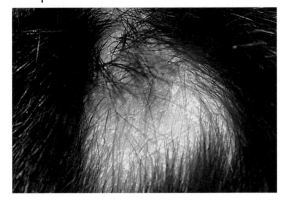

△ **Figure 2.16** Tinea capitis

This infects the scalp and the hair shaft as it emerges from the scalp, causing greyish, scaly areas with short, broken hairs.

Tinea unguium

This usually affects the toe nails. Symptoms include thickened and discoloured nail plate with yellow or white streaks. The nails soften and crumble and in some cases become detached from the nail bed.

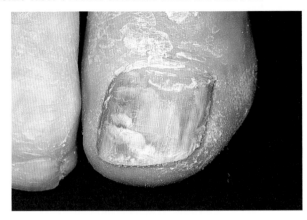

△ **Figure 2.17** Tinea unguium

Thrush

This is caused by the fungus candida albicans. Symptoms include itching, erythema and pain.

More serious internal fungal infections, those of the lungs and heart, can be fatal.

Once a fungal infection invades the body and grow, antifungal drugs are required to control it, as the condition will rarely improve without drugs. Some antifungal drugs are applied to the areas, while others are taken by mouth. They destroy the fungal cell wall and the cell dies.

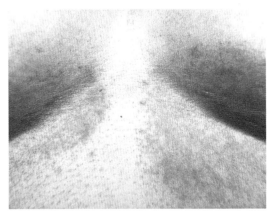

△ **Figure 2.18** Candida albicans

Animal parasites

Parasites are living organisms that live in or on another living organism and derive their food supply from that host. The parasites you are most likely to encounter in the workplace are called ectoparasites. These live outside the host, e.g. lice, fleas.

Learning point

Endoparasites live inside the host, e.g. tapeworms or threadworms, roundworms and flukes.

The presence of any parasite on the body is known as an infestation.

Ectoparasites

Head lice (Pediculus capitis)

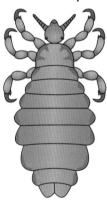

△ **Figure 2.19** Head louse

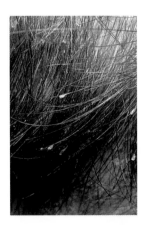

△ **Figure 2.20** Head lice

The head louse is an insect found on the human scalp. It obtains its nourishment by piercing the skin and sucking blood. The adult female is slightly larger than the male, about 2–3 mm long and 1 mm wide. The female lays white, shiny, oval-shaped eggs called nits, which are cemented to the hair close to the scalp. They take approximately one week to mature and can reproduce in another week. The life cycle of a louse lasts 4–5 weeks, during which time the female will lay around 300 eggs. They cause intense itching, and secondary infections may result due to scratching. Lice and nits may be killed by using special shampoos or lotions containing insecticide and combing out with a fine-tooth comb.

Body lice (*Pediculus corporis*)

These are similar to but larger than head lice. They obtain nutrients by sucking blood and laying eggs in underclothing. The crab louse is smaller and is found in pubic and underarm hair. Treatment is by insecticidal shampoo. Fabrics that have been in contact (clothing, towels, etc.) must be washed in insecticidal soap and boil-washed.

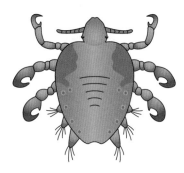

△ **Figure 2.21** Body louse

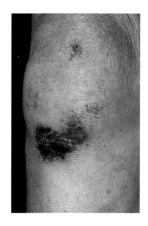

△ **Figure 2.22** Body lice

Itch mites (Sarcoptes scabiei)

This is a tiny animal that burrows into the skin, producing a condition called scabies. It has 8 legs and is around 0.3 mm long and 0.2 mm wide. The fertilised female burrows into the skin forming dark lines about 1 cm long. She lays around 60 eggs in the burrows, which hatch in 4–8 days. The burrows are seen between the fingers, on the front of the wrists and forearms and may be on male genitalia. They cause intense irritation, vesicles, papules and pustules. They are easily passed from person to person. Medical opinion should be sought and any clothing, towels etc. that have come into contact with the infected client must be burned.

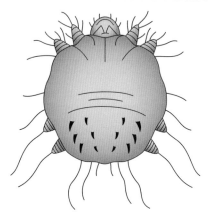

△ **Figure 2.23** Itch mite

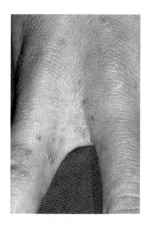

△ **Figure 2.24** Scabies

Fleas

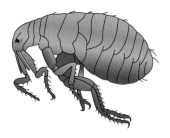

◁ **Figure 2.25** A flea

The flea is an insect with three pairs of legs that enable it to jump long distances from host to host. It obtains nourishment by biting and sucking the blood of the host. The bites cause red spots that are usually found in groups. They are intensely itchy. Fleas lay eggs in dust, carpets or furniture. They can be eliminated by spraying with insecticides, washing clothing and bedding and thorough cleaning of soft furnishings.

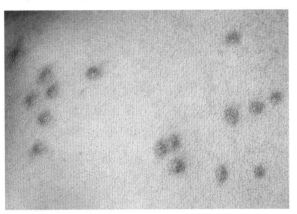

△ Figure 2.26 Fleas

Learning point

Fleas are responsible for carrying plague infections.

Methods of controlling micro-organisms

The process of controlling micro-organisms in the workplace is your responsibility and must be taken seriously. Correct hygiene procedures must be adopted as a matter of routine. Instruments must always be cleaned after use and then sterilised or disinfected.

Various words are used to explain hygiene procedures. Their meaning must be clearly understood so that the appropriate methods are selected.

Sterilisation and disinfection

While it is impossible to create a perfectly sterile environment in the workplace, every effort must be made to limit the growth and to destroy micro-organisms by practising high standards of hygiene. You and your clients must be protected from cross-infection.

Most treatments require you to touch the client, therefore every precaution must be taken to prevent cross-infection from one to the other. Your hands must be washed using bactericidal lotions and the client's skin must be cleaned by them taking a shower, or by wiping over the area using suitable cleansing products for facial and body treatments. Any small cuts and abrasions on your hands or on the client's skin must be covered with waterproof plaster. If there is any danger of blood seepage, the treatment should not be carried out.

Learning point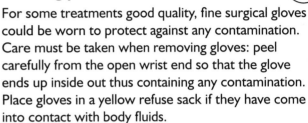

For some treatments good quality, fine surgical gloves could be worn to protect against any contamination. Care must be taken when removing gloves: peel carefully from the open wrist end so that the glove ends up inside out thus containing any contamination. Place gloves in a yellow refuse sack if they have come into contact with body fluids.

Be aware !

There have been situations where therapists and clients have experienced an allergic reaction to surgical gloves that contain latex. Ensure you have in stock an alternative product for example nitrile or PVC.

Extreme care must be taken when carrying out procedures that pierce the skin. In certain procedures, such as using a micro-lance, it is necessary to pierce the skin, but other procedures may result in blood loss due to accidental piercing of the skin.

Be aware !

All blood spills must be dealt with immediately because serious diseases such as HIV and hepatitis can be transmitted via blood contamination.

Learning point L

Disposable equipment should always be used if it is economically viable. Reusable equipment should be sterilised, if suitable; or otherwise must be disinfected.

Cleaning of equipment

All equipment must be thoroughly clean before being sterilised or disinfected. The equipment should be thoroughly soaked, washed and scrubbed with a hard brush in water and detergent. Care must be taken to reach

▽ **Table 2.1** Definitions of hygiene procedures

Term	Definition
Antibiotic	An organic chemical substance, which in dilute solution can destroy or inhibit the growth of bacteria and some other micro-organisms. They are used to treat infectious diseases in humans, animals and plants.
Antiseptic	A chemical agent that destroys or inhibits the growth of micro-organisms on living tissues, thus limiting or preventing the harmful results of infection (usually used on wounds, sores or skin cleansing).
Aseptic methods	Procedures adopted for creating conditions for avoiding infection.
Bactericide	A chemical agent that, under defined conditions, is capable of killing bacteria, but not necessarily the spores.
Bacteriostat/fungistat	Chemical agents that, under defined conditions, are capable of inhibiting the multiplication of bacteria/fungi.
Biocide, fungicide, virucide, sporicide	The destruction of bacteria, fungi, viruses and spores. Biocides kill everything.
Disinfectant	A chemical agent that destroys micro-organisms but not spores (usually used on articles, implements, surfaces, drains, etc.).
Sanitation	The establishment of conditions favourable to health and preventing the spread of disease.
Sterilisation	The total destruction or removal of all living micro-organisms and their spores.

the more inaccessible parts so that all matter is removed. Finally, they should be rinsed thoroughly under running water.

This procedure is very important for the following reasons:

○ To remove dirt and all organic matter which may be left on equipment.
○ To remove all infective matter.
○ To remove all grease or oil, which forms a barrier and interferes with the sterilising or disinfecting process, reducing its effectiveness.
○ To remove all dirt and organic matter, which would harden, forming a permanent coating on the equipment. This would interfere with sterilising or disinfecting and would cause deterioration of certain instruments.

Sterilisation

Sterilisation is the best procedure for small instruments and should be a major consideration when purchasing equipment. You should check with the manufacturer that the materials are suitable for the chosen method of sterilisation.

Be aware

Instruments made of stainless steel and certain plastics are suitable, although sharp edges may be blunted by exposure to heat.

There are two main methods of sterilisation available: by radiation and by heat.

Sterilisation by radiation

Two types of rays are used: gamma radiation and ultraviolet radiation.

○ Gamma radiation is only suitable for use on a large scale. Equipment to be sterilised is pre-packed and exposed to radiation. Colour change indicators are used in the packages to show that sterilisation has been achieved. There is little temperature rise so it is particularly useful for heat-sensitive materials. Disposable needles and micro-lances are usually sterilised in this way. It has the advantage that materials can be pre-packed before sterilisation.

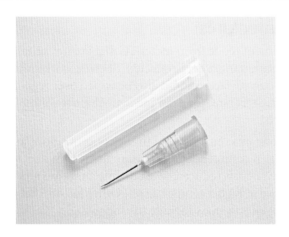

△ **Figure 2.27** Micro-lance

○ Ultraviolet radiation is no longer recommended for sterilisation. It will destroy bacteria, but spores are resistant. It is also difficult to ensure penetration of the rays and equipment requires turning to ensure irradiation of all surfaces. Ultraviolet cabinets are frequently found in the workplace and although they must not be used as sterilisers, they can be used for storing equipment after it has been sterilised.

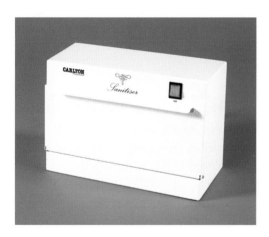

△ **Figure 2.28** Germicidal UVL cabinet designed to sanitise but not sterilise

Sterilisation by heat

Two methods can be used:

○ moist heat

○ dry heat.

With all methods of heat sterilisation, the combination of correct temperature and time of exposure are necessary for sterility to be achieved. For moist heat, the pressure in the steriliser is also important. The sterilisation process can be broken up into four time factors:

○ heating up time – the time taken for the steriliser to reach the sterilising temperature.

○ heat penetration time – the time taken for all parts of the load to reach the sterilising temperature.

○ holding time – the time required to sterilise the load at the selected temperature.

○ safety time – an addition of 50 per cent to the holding time to ensure that resistant spores are destroyed.

Both methods are suitable for use in the workplace as small models are manufactured for sterilising small instruments.

Autoclaves (pressure vessels) are used for moist heat.

> **!**
> **Be aware**
> The process of boiling water is no longer considered as a method of sterilisation as spores will survive at this temperature. It is now considered to be a process of disinfecting.

Glass bead sterilisers are used for dry heat sterilisation.

Moist heat

The autoclave is a vessel that boils water under pressure so that higher temperatures can be reached. It sterilises by steam under pressure. Water boils at atmospheric pressure at 100°C, but if the pressure is increased, then the temperature at which the water boils is raised. The autoclave is a closed vessel, constructed to withstand high pressure so that the temperature of the water and steam will reach the 100–150°C needed for sterilisation. Air must be eliminated from the vessel in order to achieve the pressure/temperature, relationship. Timing will depend on the temperature set, usually three minutes at 134°C. However, always refer to manufacturer's instructions for specific information.

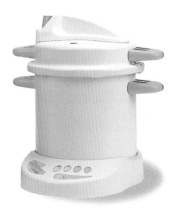

△ **Figure 2.29** An autoclave

Very large autoclaves are manufactured for commercial and hospital use. For use in the workplace, smaller, simple automatic autoclaves are now manufactured for small-scale sterilisation. The required volume of water is placed in the steriliser. Equipment to be sterilised is placed in dishes or on racks within the autoclave.

The items must be loaded with care to avoid trapping large bubbles of air, which could interfere with pressure, temperature and timing relationships:

○ Small dishes and vessels should be placed on their side and not inverted.
○ Instruments should be positioned so that steam can contact all surfaces; they should not be placed in bundles.

Once the steriliser is switched on, the cycle is automatically controlled.

Colour-change indicators are available to ensure that sterilising conditions have been reached.

Dry heat

Glass bead sterilisers are suitable for very small equipment, for example tweezers (read the manufacturer's instructions). They are made of an electrically heated box, covered by an insulating case. The box is filled with tiny glass beads. The temperature can range from 190–300°C, and the sterilising times will vary accordingly; be sure to follow the instructions on the model.

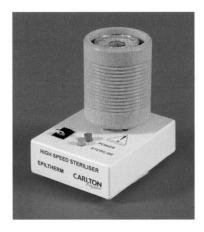

△ **Figure 2.30** Glass bead steriliser

These have the disadvantages that they are only suitable for small objects and these cannot be fully immersed. Therefore, a small part outside the beads will remain unsterilised.

Disinfectants

Equipment made from materials that are not suitable for sterilisation must be disinfected. Shelves, work surfaces and other surfaces should also be wiped over regularly with disinfectant, for example hypochlorite solutions (bleach).

Disinfectants must be used in the concentrations and timings recommended. If they are further diluted, their effectiveness is reduced. Most disinfectants are more effective at higher temperatures. Other factors that may reduce effectiveness include the following:

○ the presence of organic matter, such as dead skin, dried blood or vomit. As previously stated, all equipment should be cleaned before disinfection.
○ Some disinfectants are inactivated by hard water, while others are inactivated by soaps.
○ Effectiveness is progressively diminished with age. Store only for the recommended time; do not use after expiry date.

> **Be aware** !
> Disinfectants, if incorrectly stored, used and diluted, can themselves become infected and be a source of infection.

Hygiene in the workplace

This is your responsibility and must be taken very seriously. As well as protecting the client from the risk of infection, you need to protect yourself.

Great care must be taken when handling unsterilised sharps and instruments to avoid cuts and stabs, which may result in infection. Great care must also be taken when handling disinfectants. These are strong chemicals capable of destroying micro-organisms, but they can also cause damage to the handler, producing burns, etc. When handling these substances, rubber gloves should always be worn, and care taken not to splash the skin, eyes, nose or mouth. Any drops on these areas must be thoroughly rinsed off immediately with cold water. Always refer to manufacturer's instructions.

The following guidelines should be followed to establish high standards of practice and hygiene in the workplace.

○ You should wash your hands before and after treatment using a product such as an antibacterial soap. Dry with a disposable towel or hot air dryer.

In the workplace

A convenient method to cleanse your hands during treatment without disturbing the client is to have an antibacterial hand gel on your trolley.

○ The client's skin should be cleansed before treatment using suitable products or wipes. Any cuts must be covered with waterproof plasters.

○ Disposable instruments and equipment should be used whenever possible.

○ All metal instruments should be washed and sterilised, if suitable, using one of the following methods:

  ○ dry heat, glass bead sterilisation – this is useful for tweezers and other small instruments. However, it is important to remember that any part of the instrument that is not immersed remains unsterilised.

  ○ moist heat, autoclave– this is the best method for all equipment made of suitable materials.

Metal instruments not suitable for the autoclave must be disinfected in a product that does not cause rusting.

○ All equipment that is unsuitable for sterilisation must be washed and disinfected. Immerse for the directed time in a suitable product.

○ Equipment made from other materials should be cleaned as follows:

○ Working surfaces should be wiped down frequently during the day with a disinfectant. Chairs, stools, couches and trolleys should also be cleaned in this way at the end of the day.

○ A plentiful supply of good quality towels should be available for covering the couch and for client use. These should be boil-washed after each client. Disposable paper sheets should be used to protect the couch cover.

○ Commodities should be chosen with care. Creams and lotions in tubes or narrow-necked bottles have a smaller surface to be contaminated than wide-necked jars.

○ Always use a new clean spatula to remove creams or lotions; do not return any contaminated article back to the product.

○ The stock cupboard should be clean, neat and tidy. Commodities should be clearly labelled showing the use-by date, which should not be exceeded.

○ Covered bins with plastic liners should be easily reached. All waste should be immediately disposed of. The waste bins should be emptied and disinfected every night and clean liners inserted.

○ Blood spills must be dealt with immediately. Wearing rubber gloves, wipe over the surface to remove the blood before disinfecting it with a hypochlorite

▽ Table 2.2 Cleaning other equipment

Equipment/Material	Example	Suggestion for cleaning
Vacuum suction (VS) (glass and perspex)		Wash thoroughly with hot water and detergent using a small brush to reach inaccessible parts, rinse, dry and store in a sanitiser. Or: check with manufacturer if the items are suitable for autoclaving as the heat may cause deterioration.
High frequency electrodes (glass, metal rod)		Keep the metal contact dry. Wipe over with a disinfecting solution. When dry, place in a sanitiser.

(Continued)

(Continued)

Equipment/ Material	Example	Suggestion for cleaning
Rubber pads (EMS and galvanic)		Keep the metal contact dry. Wipe pads with warm soapy water. Avoid scrubbing the carbon facing; rinse carefully and dry thoroughly.
Straps (EMS and galvanic)		Wash straps in warm soapy water regularly.
Sponge covers (galvanic)		Wash in hot soapy water, rinse and dry.

solution (bleach). Refer to the label on the bottle for details of appropriate dilution. General guidance is a 1:10 solution, but household bleach does not have a standard concentration. Any cloth or paper towel used for cleaning body fluid spills must be placed in a yellow refuse sack.

○ A special sharps container should be available for disposal of micro-lances, etc., which have penetrated the skin and a yellow refuse sack for cotton wool, tissues and materials contaminated with body fluids. Special arrangements for the collection and

subsequent disposal of these containers and sacks can be organised by contacting your local authority to find out information on registered waste carriers in your area.

○ A first-aid box should be positioned in an obvious, easily accessible place.

○ Toilet facilities should be easily accessible. These should be well ventilated and disinfected at least once a day. Sanitary ware and floors can be cleaned using an appropriate solution.

SUMMARY

- If micro-organisms invade the body in sufficient numbers to overcome the immune system, they will cause disease.
- Micro-organisms that infect the body are bacteria, viruses and fungi.

Immunity

- **Natural immunity** is acquired by previous contact with a disease (the antibodies remain in the body) or acquired via the placenta or milk from the mother.
- **Artificial immunity** is acquired from vaccines introduced into the body, which stimulate the immune system to produce antibodies, or may be acquired by the transfer of antibodies from a person who has recovered from the disease.

Micro-organisms

- **Bacteria:** single-cell organisms, non-pathogenic or pathogenic – cocci, bacilli, spirochetes; diseases: boils, impetigo, sore throat, meningitis, pneumonia, typhoid fever, syphilis, cholera.
- **Viruses:** multiply and destroy the host cells; diseases: colds, influenza, poliomyelitis, mumps, chickenpox, herpes simplex and zoster, warts, hepatitis, HIV.
  - Hepatitis and HIV are found in semen, saliva and blood.
  - Ways of transmitting a virus: through blood transfusion, drug users sharing needles, the transfer of blood from an infected person into a cut or puncture of the skin, infected women can pass it to the foetus.

- **Fungi:** yeasts and moulds; diseases: tinea of various parts of body, thrush, fungal infections of organs such as heart and lungs.
- **Parasites** live in or on another living organism: **Ectoparasites** live outside host (e.g. lice and fleas).

Sterilisation and disinfection

- **Sterilisation** is the total destruction of microbes and spores.
- Methods of sterilisation in the workplace:
  - Autoclave.
  - Glass bead steriliser – small articles only.
- **Disinfecting:** the use of a chemical agent that destroys microbes but not spores.

Multiple-choice questions

1. Which of the following conditions is required for the growth of micro-organisms?
   a Slightly alkaline conditions.
   b Ultraviolet light.
   c Low temperature.
   d Dry environment.

2. Macrophages:
   a neutralise toxins produced by microbes
   b produce T-cells
   c secrete antibodies
   d engulf and destroy microbes.

3. Hepatitis B is transmitted:
   a by droplet infection
   b through contaminated blood
   c by handling contaminated articles
   d through contact with animals.

4. Tinea corporis is recognised by:
   a a rash, usually around the chest and abdomen
   b red, round scaly patches that spread outwards
   c itchy, inflamed, weeping and crusting skin
   d large red patches covered by thick silvery white scales.

5. Which of these is a bacterial infection of the skin?
   a Herpes simples.
   b Verruca.
   c Impetigo.
   d Tinea corporis.

6. Which of the following lives inside a host cell?
   a Bacteria.
   b Ectoparasite.
   c Fungus.
   d Virus.

7. An autoclave is used to:
   a sterilise equipment
   b sanitise equipment
   c store sterilised equipment
   d disinfect equipment.

8. Micro-lances should be disposed of:
   a in a yellow refuse sack
   b in an empty box and placed in the general waste
   c in a sharps container
   d wrapped in tissue, placed in a box and taken to the pharmacy.

9. Which substance found in surgical gloves may cause an allergic reaction?
   a PVC.
   b Latex.
   c Vinyl.
   d Nitrile.

10. The parasite that causes intense irritation, with vesicles, papules and pustules usually found between the fingers and on the wrist is called the:
    a threadworm
    b flea
    c itch mite
    d body louse.

Section 2: Ethics, consultation and care of the client

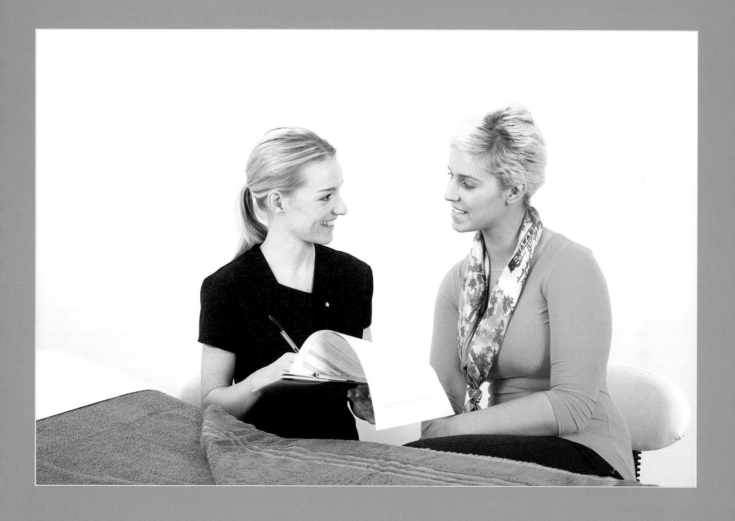

3 Ethics, planning, preparation and client consultation

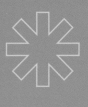

Objectives

After you have studied this chapter you will be able to:

▌ list the factors that contribute to professional behaviour

▌ prepare the working area, trolley and yourself

▌ explain the importance of client consultation

▌ list the essential information which must be recorded on the client consultation

▌ explain the importance of, and the procedures involved in, observation and assessment of the client's condition

▌ explain the contra-indications to treatment

▌ explain why the evaluation of a treatment is important

▌ recommend appropriate homecare and aftercare advice

▌ explain the purpose of reflecting on your own performance and carry out a self-evaluation.

Professional conduct and ethics

Professional conduct and ethics refers to the standards, moral principles and conduct of behaviour of an individual or professional group. You must undergo a course of reputable training to acquire the understanding and skills necessary to carry out safe and effective treatment. In addition, you must consider your standard of behaviour in relation to colleagues, clients and the general public.

In the workplace

There are various professional associations that you can join, which offer members direct benefits such as professional insurance deals, training opportunities, networking and access to websites; as well as indirect benefits, such as giving clients and employers confidence in you. Members of these associations agree to abide by a code of conduct, by-laws and disciplinary procedures in order to ensure the safety and well-being of their clients.

A high standard of professional conduct will gain the confidence of clients and establish an excellent reputation, which is the basis for success. Abide by the following code of practices:

○ Look professional: be clean, neat and tidy.

○ Be punctual; keep to appointment times; do not cancel appointments at the last minute.

○ Be discreet and refrain from gossip. Remember that clients often confide personal problems during consultation. These facts and all personal details must be treated with the utmost confidentiality. Do not repeat information or gossip to colleagues or others.

In the workplace

Always be aware of who can overhear your own conversations, for example during breaks or standing at reception. You must present a professional image at *all* times. Clients want to feel that their privacy will be respected, or they will take their custom elsewhere.

○ Be loyal to your employer, colleagues and clients. Create a friendly, but not over-familiar working relationship with everyone.

○ Be honest and reliable: this will gain the trust of others and establish a high reputation. Do not make false claims for treatments, but explain the benefits fairly.

○ Speak correctly and politely to everyone. Do not use improper language. Consider the manner in which you speak on the telephone. Be competent, helpful and pleasant.

In the workplace

Remember to address clients tactfully, particularly if you notice a condition that should be referred to a medical professional. You must not cause undue alarm. Be sensitive to their reaction.

○ Be courteous at all times. There may be difficult clients to deal with: learn to handle tricky situations with tact and diplomacy.

○ Always practise the highest standards of personal hygiene and hygiene in the workplace.

○ Do your utmost to deliver the most effective treatment suited to the needs of the client.

○ Organise yourself and your working practices to ensure a smooth-running, efficient service for the benefit of all concerned.

○ Know and abide by legal requirements and local authority by-laws, rules and regulations.

○ Keep up to date with new theories, techniques and treatments. Attend courses on a regular basis and keep in touch with other professionals in your field.

Best practice   **B**

Continuing Professional Development (CPD) is the mark of a true professional. For many of the professional associations it is a requirement for membership. However, even if you are not a member of a professional body, it is vital to maintaining the highest possible standards of knowledge and skill, which will enhance your earning power.

Insurance

If you are an employee working in a salon, always check at the interview stage if your employer has insurance that will cover you should a client take legal action against you. Find out exactly what you will be covered for.

Employers' Liability Insurance

Businesses are required by law to have this insurance with cover of at least £5,000,000. Employers have overall responsibility for health and safety in the workplace. If an employee is injured or becomes ill due to the fault of the employer, the employee could sue the business.

Public Liability Insurance

This covers your business if a client has an accident or their property is damaged while on your premises, or during a visit to their premises. The policy will cover the costs of defending you and paying for any damages or compensation for which you may be liable, to the maximum amount stated in the policy.

Professional Indemnity Insurance

This covers you should a client make a claim against you for negligence, defamation or breach of confidentiality, if it is linked to a professional service or advice. The

policy will cover the cost of defending you and paying out for damages or compensation for which you are liable, to the maximum amount stated in the policy. Professional Associations offer this type of insurance so it is worth investigating what is on offer. The rate is usually favourable as they can liaise with companies on behalf of their members for the best deal.

Be aware   **!**

If you are self-employed you are strongly advised to have both Public Liability and Professional Indemnity insurance. The former protects you for accidents and damage to property, the latter protects you for negligence when carrying out a treatment.

Planning the working day

The efficiency and smooth running of any organisation will depend on good planning. You must work out an overall plan for the working day, which will depend on the type and number of appointments booked, and you must plan for each individual treatment. Working methodically and developing a good routine while allowing a degree of flexibility will contribute to the efficiency of the workplace and enhance its reputation.

○ Arrive early for work, allowing plenty of preparation time before the first appointment.

○ Change from outdoor clothes into your uniform in the changing room. Check your appearance.

○ Prepare the working area.

○ Check the machines for cleanliness and safety.

○ Prepare the couch using clean linen, then cover.

○ Check and prepare other treatment areas and facilities such as the sunbed, sauna, steam and spa pool.

○ Check the cloakroom, toilets and laundry cupboard, etc. Ensure that everything meets the requirements of the health and safety legislation.

○ Organise the reception area making sure that everything is in pristine order.

○ Check the appointment book and prepare consultation records.

○ Read the notes on the consultation record or computer for the regular clients or prepare new consultation records for new clients.

○ Behave in a responsible manner at all times; be friendly and supportive to other staff and offer help as required.

Preparation of the environment and working area

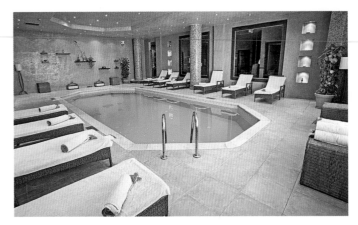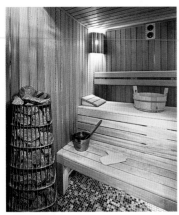

△ **Figure 3.1** Treatment areas

Ensure that the working area affords the client total privacy to change and receive treatment without being overlooked by others. The area may be a curtained section in a salon, an individual walled cubicle or treatment room. You should ensure there is enough space to walk around the couch and work from all sides and that there is room for a trolley with products, the equipment and a stool.

Environment

The atmosphere created in the working environment should be quiet and calming. The area must be private, warm, well ventilated and free from distracting noises. Lighting should be soft and diffused, not directed from above and shining in the client's face. The client must be positioned in a comfortable, well-supported position and must feel safe and secure.

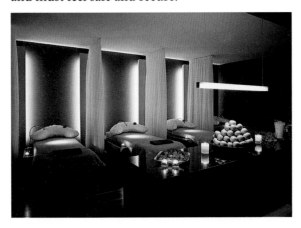

△ **Figure 3.2** Creating a suitable ambience

The following factors affect the client's experience of the treatment and should be addressed before the client arrives.

Always check that the client is comfortable and make adjustments where necessary and where it is possible.

Besides these physical factors, other things contribute to the atmosphere of the workplace. Any tensions between colleagues will be picked up by the client. Personal presentation, attitude and body language will all impact on the client's confidence. The look and presentation of the workplace also affects the client's first impressions.

○ The environment should be warm, well ventilated and draught-free.

○ It should be quiet, peaceful and free from distracting noise. Soft relaxing music may be played, but check with the client – some clients prefer quiet.

○ The lighting should be soft and diffuse, not directed from above and shining into the client's face.

○ The colour scheme should be pale but warming, using pastel rather than harsh, bold colours.

○ The area must be spotlessly clean and tidy.

○ Items required during the treatment must be neatly arranged on the trolley shelf and protected with clean paper tissue or a small sheet.

○ A plentiful supply of clean, laundered towels and linen should be to hand.

○ Extra pillows, small support pillows or rolled towels should also be to hand.

○ A lined bin with lid should be to hand for disposal of waste.

○ Toilet facilities for the client should be accessible and regularly cleaned. A hand basin or sink should be available for washing your hands. Disposable towels or hot air dryers should be used to dry the hands. These must all be scrupulously clean.

▽ **Table 3.1** Factors affecting the client experience

Lighting	Too bright	Too dim	Ideal
Lighting is an easy and immediate way to affect environment and mood.	Client won't relax.	Health and safety – you or your client could trip.	Soft lighting, e.g. from uplighters or wall lights. Dimmer switches. Corner lighting with uplighting shades. Softly coloured shades. Directional lamps. All these will encourage the client to relax and will be beneficial for body electrical muscle stimulation (EMS) and galvanic treatments after you have positioned the pads and turned up the intensity dials. Also for facial treatments after applying the mask.
	Could cause headaches.	You may not be able to see the dials on the machine.	
	Could cause eye strain.	Could cause eye strain.	
	Could cause temporary blind spots.	Could cause sense of claustrophobia.	
	Atmosphere is spoilt.	Could make client feel insecure.	
Temperature	**Too hot**	**Too cold**	**Ideal**
	You will get hot and sweaty.	Your hands will be cold, making the client tense.	Room temperature should be maintained at around 21°C. Thermostatically controlled heating is desirable. Additional blankets, or a heated blanket or towels or a lightweight duvet should be available. Appropriate medium should be warmed in your hands before applying to the client's skin.
	Could cause fatigue or feeling of faintness.	Could make concentration difficult.	
	Saps your energy.	Misdirects your energy.	
	Client will sweat, making the skin moist and difficult to treat.	Client will not want to undress.	
	Client will feel sticky and uncomfortable.	Will cause dissatisfaction.	
	Vaso-dilation will cause erythema.	Vaso-constriction will cause client's skin to go pale and feel cold.	
	Could cause agitation and irritation and prevent relaxation.	Could cause agitation and irritation and prevent relaxation.	

(Continued)

(Continued)

Ventilation	Too stuffy	Too draughty	Ideal
	Causes headaches.	Client will not want to undress.	Windows that can be opened and closed are desirable.
	Build up of CO_2 causes feelings of lethargy and lightheadedness.	Effects as for **'Too cold'** above.	Natural ventilation is best but air conditioning is an alternative.
	Could cause agitation and irritation and prevent relaxation.		Free-standing fans can aid flow of air but they can be hazardous.

Sound	Too quiet	Too loud	Ideal
	No sound can cause you and the client to feel self-conscious.	Will cause irritation and prevent relaxation. This can also occur if the client doesn't like the music.	Select appropriate music for the treatment, for example soothing music for relaxation.
	Emphasises bodily noises which can cause embarrassment.		Music should be in the background and should enhance the mood.
	Can prevent relaxation.		
Aroma			A pleasant but not overpowering aroma is conducive to relaxation, such as subtle oils, which can sit in containers over a heat source.

Selection of a couch

Selecting and purchasing a couch can be difficult as there is a wide choice available. Selection is often based on the cost of the couch, but there are other important points to bear in mind when buying. Consider the following points:

○ It must be wide enough for the clients to turn over easily and to feel safe and secure.

○ It must be long enough to support the length of the body.

○ It must be robust, secure and firm. It must not move or rock, nor grate or squeak as this will disturb the client and prevent relaxation.

○ It must be at the correct height for working. If it is too high you will have to stretch to reach certain

areas and you will not be able to use body weight correctly to apply the required pressure, for example during a gyratory vibrator treatment. If it is too low, you will have to bend over too much. This will cause shoulder and back problems. When standing upright next to the couch with the arms by the side, the couch should be just below the level of the wrist.

○ The covering should be of smooth, washable material that is easy to wipe over and keep clean.

○ If you need a couch that you can move from room to room or take on home visits, then select the portable folding variety. Ensure that the legs are sturdy and that the hinges are secure and firm. Apply pressure sideways and to the top and bottom to test whether it shakes or rocks – it should remain firm.

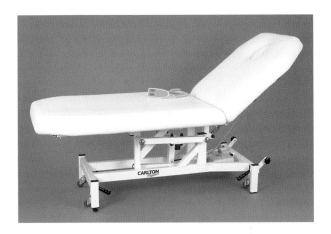

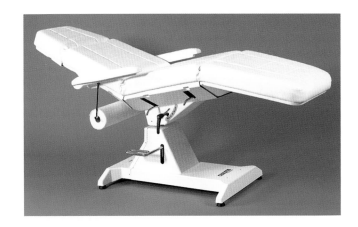

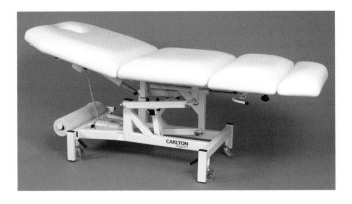

△ **Figure 3.3** A range of couches

If you are using the couch for a variety of treatments, select from the multi-purpose varieties. The most useful couches are the adjustable height hydraulic varieties, but these are expensive and may be outside your budget. However, they are ideal for any treatment as the height can be adjusted to accommodate all types of client such as small and thin, or large and obese. Some couches have a hole for the face to make positioning and breathing easier when lying prone.

Preparation of treatment couch

Prepare the couch before the client arrives:

○ Cover the entire surface with a towelling or cotton sheet – the fitted types are best as they stay neat and tidy.

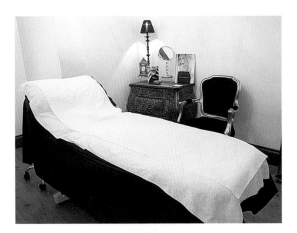

△ **Figure 3.4** Prepared couch

In the workplace

Cosset the client during cold spells with a heated under- or over-blanket and a duvet to keep them warm and relaxed.

○ Next, cover this with a large bath towel or cotton sheet. This must be removed and boil-washed after each client and a clean one reapplied.

○ Use one or two pillows for the head. Cover these with pillow slips and then a towel.

○ Fold one small and one large towel and place them at the foot of the couch. These will be used to cover the client as required.

○ Place extra pillows, large and small, on the trolley for use if extra support is required during the treatment.

○ Make sure that the couch is at the correct height. A couch that is too high will result in a strain on the arms, neck and shoulders; a couch that is too low will result in back strain.

Preparation of the trolley

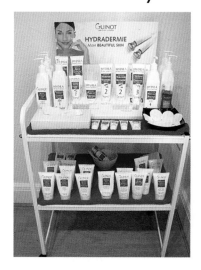

△ **Figure 3.5** Prepared trolley

○ Select a trolley with a hard, smooth surface, free of cracks and easy to clean. Ensure that it is robust and sturdy so that it cannot be pushed over. Wheels are an advantage as the trolley may be pulled or pushed into a convenient position.

○ Place the trolley near the treatment couch so that all items will be to hand when required. Ensure that the trolley is large enough to safely support the equipment.

○ The trolley and electrical equipment should be placed on your dominant side, on the right if you are right-handed and on the left if you are left-handed. This avoids reaching over the client to adjust the controls or continually changing the electrode from one hand to the other, especially during facial work.

○ Wipe the shelves with disinfectant of the correct dilution.

○ Cover the shelves with paper sheets – fold under all edges for neatness.

○ Position the machine on the trolley unless it is free standing and arrange products and bowls neatly. Always place products in the same order to ensure that they are easy to identify and reach when needed.

○ A lined bin with a lid may be placed by the side of the trolley. This is to avoid the risk of contamination of equipment and products.

○ Cover the shelf and equipment and products with a clean paper sheet when not in use. This will protect items from dust and dirt.

○ At the end of each day strip the trolley down, wipe the shelves with a disinfecting solution, clean the lids and rims of bottles and jars and wash the bowls. Then either store these in a cupboard ready for use the following day or re-lay the trolley and cover.

Equipment and products for face and body:

- magnifying lamp
- cleansing products for face and body
- exfoliants
- massage media
- moisturisers
- body lotion
- containers: for cotton wool, tissues, cotton buds, spatulas
- bowl and sponges/mitts
- cotton wool
- tissues
- two test tubes or similar, and orangewood sticks (for sensitivity test)
- headband
- client consultation record.

Preparation of self

Before carrying out a treatment you must prepare yourself physically, paying due consideration to high standards of professionalism and hygiene. Cleanliness is essential to protect both you and the client from cross-infection. You must also prepare psychologically and give due thought to the type of treatment required.

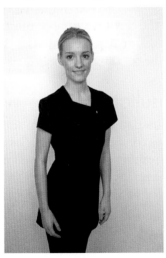

△ **Figure 3.6** Therapist dressed appropriately

Personal hygiene

A daily bath or shower should be taken to maintain cleanliness of the skin, hair and nails and to remove stale sweat odours.

- An antiperspirant should be used to prevent excessive sweating and the odour of stale sweat.
- Hair should be clean and neat; it should be kept short or tied back from the face. Hair must never fall forward around your face and shoulders or touch the client.
- Nails must be well manicured and kept short; nails should not protrude above the fleshy part of the fingertip, as long nails may harbour dirt and micro-organisms. Nail polish should not be worn as some clients may be sensitive to the product and an allergic reaction may result. Polish would also hide dirt under the nails.
- Hands must be well cared for; they must be smooth and warm. You should protect your hands with rubber gloves when doing chores. A good-quality hand lotion should be used night and morning. Gloves should be worn in cold weather. You should not carry out treatments with cuts or abrasions on your hands. Small areas may be covered with a waterproof plaster.
- Jewellery should be removed or kept to a minimum of wedding ring and small ear studs. Rings, bracelets and watches can harbour micro-organisms or can injure the client if dragged on the skin. Long earrings and necklaces may jangle, producing a noise that is disturbing to the client.
- Uniform should be crisp, well laundered and changed frequently (at least every other day). The style should allow free unrestricted movement of the arms during massage.
- Well-fitting, low-heeled or flat shoes without holes or peep-toes will protect the feet and avoid pressure points. Support tights will help prevent tired legs and varicose veins.
- If you are suffering from colds or infections it is preferable that you do not treat clients. The wearing of a surgical mask will, however, greatly reduce the risk of cross-infection.
- You must wash your hands frequently, particularly before touching a client, at the end of every treatment and if necessary during treatment should you have to blow your nose or pick up an item that dropped on the floor, etc.
- Teeth must be cleaned regularly and breath must be kept free from odours.

Best practice   **B**

Ideally, working uniform should not be worn out of the workplace, to prevent micro-organisms being brought into the workplace. It is best to change at work.

Psychological preparation

Preparing the mind enhances concentration and co-ordination and contributes to expertise and effectiveness of the treatment.

○ Develop a calm, tranquil but positive attitude. It is important to feel secure, confident and relaxed your-self as this is transmitted to the client both by your attitude and through your hands.

○ Develop coordination between mind and body. The hands and body must move as a whole. Think of your foot position, posture, arm and hand positions.

○ Develop sensory awareness, i.e. the ability to sense and visualise structures through the hands. Through the sensory receptors in the hands you learn to identify bony points, degrees of tone or tension in muscles, and variations found on different tissues and different clients. This ability only comes through practice and the experience of treating a variety of different types of client, e.g. young, old, thin, obese, well toned, poorly toned, tense or relaxed.

○ Learn to synchronise speed and rhythm so that these remain consistent throughout the treatment. These will vary depending on the effects required. Maximum effectiveness of the treatment will occur only if these factors are co-ordinated.

Getting to know the client

○ When you take on a new client it is important that you get to know each other and establish a good rapport and mutual trust. Meet the client in a friendly, welcoming manner, smile and introduce yourself. Find out how they would like to be addressed, by their first name or surname.

○ Take the initiative, put them at ease and make them feel comfortable. Be flexible and adaptable in your approach, try and assess the type of person you are dealing with.

○ Find out as much as you can about the client; discuss their needs and what they expect from the treatments.

○ Speak clearly and listen to their responses; make sure that you understand them and that they understand you; be sensitive and supportive to their needs.

○ Watch and be aware of their body language. Their posture, gestures, expressions can tell you a lot about the client. Are they assertive and calm (indicating confidence) or are they timid and appear nervous (indicating shyness or lack of confidence)? Are they familiar with treatments, or is this their first experience? Be prepared to adapt your attitude and approach accordingly.

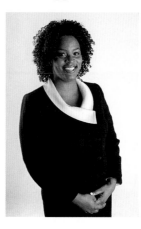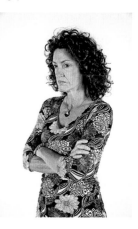

△ **Figure 3.7** Positive and negative body language

○ Explain the consultation procedure clearly to a new client. Consider the client's modesty and privacy at all times.

○ Ensure that the client is sitting comfortably. Sit with them, making sure that you have everything that you require for the consultation.

Client consultation

This involves questioning, observation and analysis to assess the client's condition and identify any contra-indications to treatment. The assessment must be thorough and accurate and all the facts should be carefully recorded on the client's consultation record.

This information will enable you to set the objectives/ goals (what the client wants to achieve as a result of the treatment) and then plan the most beneficial treatment for the client. Remember that this data is the starting point from which future improvements can be measured.

Initial consultation

The consultation is a very important part of the treatment: sufficient time must be allowed so that it is not rushed. This is the time to gather and exchange information.

The initial consultation will be the longest and provide detailed information, which must be accurately noted on a consultation record. This must be filed in a safe and accessible place and used each time the client attends for treatment.

The client should be seated comfortably for the consultation. Position yourself alongside or opposite. The environment should feel warm and private.

Detailed consultation is important. Its purpose is to:

○ introduce yourself and get to know the client
○ establish a rapport with the client and put her/him at ease
○ develop mutual trust and gain the client's confidence
○ gain information on the client's past and present state of mental and physical health

○ gain insight into the client's lifestyle, responsibilities, work environment, leisure activities, etc.
○ identify the client's needs and expectations of the treatment
○ identify any contra-indications
○ establish the most appropriate form of treatment and to discuss and agree this with the client
○ explain the treatment fully to the client, including the procedure, expected effects, timing and frequency
○ agree a treatment plan, the timing and cost with the client so that they fully understand the financial commitment, and obtain a signature to confirm
○ answer queries and questions related to the treatment and allay doubts and fears.

The information gathered will help you to formulate the best treatment plan to meet the needs of the client. The short- and long-term objectives should be discussed and agreed.

Treatment objectives include:

○ to improve skin condition
○ to improve facial and body contours and muscle condition.

Essential information

The following personal, medical and lifestyle factors should be recorded on the consultation record, together with skin and figure analysis. The information gathered will provide a baseline from which the appropriate treatment is planned, the effectiveness of the treatment can be judged and any necessary changes or adjustments made.

Sample consultation record

Personal details

Name: (include title, Mr, Mrs, Miss, Ms or other) _____

→ Some clients may want to be addressed more formally than others. Also, when contacting clients by post or email you will know how to address them.

Address: (include postcode) _____

→ To ensure correspondence arrives promptly.

Date of birth: _____

Under 20☐   21–30 ☐   31–40 ☐   41–50 ☐   51-60 ☐

61–70 ☐   71+ ☐

→ Some clients do not want to acknowledge their age but will feel comfortable ticking a category.

Telephone: day: _____   evening _____

Fax _____

Email _____

→ These are quick and efficient methods of contacting the client especially if you have to cancel or rearrange an appointment at short notice.

Client Objectives _____

→ Important to find out short and long term Objectives. Are they realistic and will the proposed treatment(s) meet the client's needs?

Medical details

Doctor's name   _____

Address   _____

Tel No.   _____

→ Should you need to liaise with the doctor about a contra-indication or give a progress report on treatment.

Past medical history

Surgical operations   _____

Pregnancies   _____

Serious illnesses   _____

→ These details will enable you to establish the client's state of health; the likelihood of any contra-indications as a result of past illnesses; whether particular care must be taken over certain areas; and whether medical referral is necessary. If the client suffers from a condition that is contra-indicated (see page 52), then treatment may be restricted or not permitted at all.

Present medical history

Medication   _____

General health   _____

→ These details will indicate whether facial/body electrotherapy treatments will be beneficial for the client and will also influence the type of treatment to be given. Be aware that certain medication causes thinning or inflammation of the skin, for example steroids, accutane and retinols. These may restrict or prevent treatment.

Lifestyle

Occupation

Free time

Ability to relax

Diet

Exercise

Type and number of drinks per day

Alcohol consumption

Smoker/non-smoker

→ Lifestyle, emotional and mental factors will affect the client's general appearance and will also give an insight into their health and well being. This information will also impact on the homecare advice you give the client.

Emotional and mental factors

Stress levels (on a scale of 1 – 10 with 1 = no stress,   _____

10 = very stressed) _____

Sleep pattern   _____

Energy levels   _____

Work/life balance   _____

Cautions

Contra-indications   _____

Any allergies   _____

→ Check if client has any contra-indications that may prevent or restrict treatment. It is important to find out if the client has experienced any previous reaction to products or has any known allergies which may impact on your choice of medium.

Previous experiences and outcomes

Has client received treatment in the past

How long ago

Number of sessions

Did client benefit from treatment _____

If the client has not experienced treatment before then he/she may be apprehensive. Previous experience of treatments will affect expectations and dictate preferences.

Facial assessment

Skin type _____

You cannot assess the client's skin type and condition just by looking at it through a magnifying lamp. You must gain as much information from the client about their skin, the type of products they use and the underlying causes of pustules, dilated capillaries, milia, hyper pigmentation etc that you may find. A client's skin type will change dependent on their lifestyle for example occupation, stress levels, diet etc. Be aware that a client with open pores may not necessarily have a greasy skin. They may have had greasy skin when younger but over time pores lose their elasticity and become permanently enlarged.

Skin texture and condition

Skin colour

Skin elasticity/muscle tone _____

Assess these by feeling and palpating the tissues.

Skin imperfections _____

Look for broken capillaries, especially on the cheeks and around the nose, pustules, papules, milia, comedones, open pores, fine and deep lines.

Body assessment

Height

Weight

These will help you work out the client's Body Mass Index (BMI), a measure of body fat based on weight and height. If the client is overweight you will need to discuss their current lifestyle and diet and recommend alternatives.

Body type

Endomorph, mesomorph, ectomorph or a combination.

Posture

Assess if there are any postural conditions e.g. kyphosis, lordosis and scoliosis where some muscles will be tight and shortened and others will be stretched and weakened. Very few people have perfect posture because it is influenced by both physical and psychological factors.

Areas of hard/soft fat/cellulite

General muscle tone

Note areas the client feels are a problem. The treatment plan must meet the needs of the client even though they may not be of primary concern in your professional judgement.

Fluid retention

Ensure you find out through questioning the cause of the oedema (see page 69), if in doubt advise the client to seek medical advice.

Skin condition _____

Stretch marks _____

Note dry, dehydrated, rough areas of skin and stretch marks; start thinking about retail products you could recommend for homecare. Look for conditions such as eczema, psoriasis, bruises, thread and varicose veins and how you are going to adapt the treatment.

Other factors that may affect treatment

Client's financial constraints and availability to attend on a regular basis will affect the short- and long-term objectives.

Treatment plan

From the information you have gathered you will be able to prepare a treatment plan. Your in-depth knowledge of all equipment, treatments and products at your disposal will enable you to make an informed choice of how you are going to meet the treatment objective(s) to suit the client's needs. This will detail the areas of the face/body to be included or excluded with reasons why. You will also need to consider how often the client should attend and for how long.

Aftercare and homecare advice given.

Any adverse reactions the client experienced

The type of medium chosen and why

Support used for client comfort _____

Client signature _____

This information should be recorded after each treatment to ensure good continuity of care and appropriate adaptation of future treatments. It is useful if another therapist has to take over future treatments for any reason. You must ensure the client reads and signs the consultation record as this confirms their understanding and agreement with the details recorded and also giving their consent to treatment.

Therapist signature

By signing this document you are agreeing to keep the client's information confidential.

Date

In the workplace

It would be beneficial to you and your business to find out how the client heard about you for future marketing opportunities.

Data Protection Act 1998

A business that stores details about their staff and clients whether manually or on a computer should register with the Data Protection Register.

The Act protects people's personal details from being freely available to others. The Data Protection Register issues businesses with a code of practice. The main points are:

○ Keep staff and clients' records safe and secure.

○ Record personal information that is relevant.

○ Release information to third parties only after seeking consent from the individual.

○ Provide the individual access to their information if requested to do so.

Remember

Clients can ask to look at their records at any time so ensure all your notes are strictly professional.

Be aware !

You must not disclose or discuss your client's details with a third party without the client's permission.

Learning point L

Open and closed questions: To gain as much information as possible from your client use open questions, for example, 'How would you describe your sleep pattern?' Closed questions are useful for 'yes' and 'no' answers, for example, 'Does your skin react to products?'

Activity A

Read through the questions in Table 3.2 and identify which are open questions and which are closed questions. The first pair have been completed for you, as an example.

▽ **Table 3.2** Sample questions to establish past and present medical history

Question	Open Q	Closed Q
	√	√
Have you been ill recently?		√
When were you last ill?	√	
Have you visited the doctor recently?		
Are you on any medication?		
If so, what medication are you taking?		
Have you suffered any serious illness in the past?		
If so, what was the problem?		
Have you had any operations in the past or are you awaiting one in the near future?		
Do you recall any close relative who has suffered from a stroke or heart attack?		
Have you any other medical problems?		

Sample questions to establish life style and stress levels

The following questions are designed to help you lead the client into a general conversation. Introduce the questions as you talk to the client.

○ Do you have children or older relatives to care for?

○ How many children do you have, and how old are they?

○ Are they very demanding and require a lot of attention or are they fairly independent?

○ Do you go to work?

○ What is your occupation?

○ What is your daily routine? Are you busy and active all day or are you sitting at a desk for long periods?

○ Do you do the cooking, cleaning and all the housework?

○ Do you ever feel stressed?

○ Do you sleep well every night?

○ Do you make time just for yourself each day, to unwind and enjoy yourself?

○ What are the ways in which you relax?

○ Do you take any form of regular exercise? What activity do you enjoy the most?

○ Do you regularly walk at least three times a week for thirty minutes?

○ What is your eating pattern?

○ Do you eat regularly?

○ Have you ever had an eating problem?

○ Are you or have you ever been on a diet?

○ Do you eat a healthy balanced diet? Do you eat at least five portions of fruit and vegetables every day with moderate carbohydrate and little fat?

○ Do you drink plenty of water or diluted fruit juice: between 1½ and 3 litres a day?

Be aware

Water makes up approximately 60 per cent of body weight. Your organs and tissues need water to function. When your body is dehydrated you may experience headaches, tiredness and lack of concentration.

○ Do you drink a lot of coffee? How many cups per day?

Be aware

Caffeine is a drug found in coffee, tea and soft drinks. It stimulates the central nervous system, increases alertness and improves concentration levels. The effect on the body depends on the amount you consume and how your body copes with it. Too much and you may experience 'highs' and 'lows'.

○ Do you drink alcohol on a regular basis? How many units a week do you drink?

Be aware

Government guidelines on sensible drinking change, so make sure you keep up to date.

○ Are you a smoker? How many do you smoke a day? Have you ever tried to give up smoking?

○ Do you know that smoking has a detrimental effect on your health and skin?

Be aware

Smoking causes carbon monoxide levels in the blood to increase. This reduces the amount of oxygen to the skin and also encourages the formation of free radicals. These are responsible for tissue damage and premature ageing of the skin. Smoking causes the skin to appear sallow and dry with prominent lines, particularly around the eyes and mouth. Research suggests that smoking causes more deaths and disabilities than any other factor.

○ What treatments have you had before? Were they beneficial?

Learning point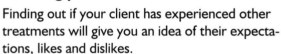

Finding out if your client has experienced other treatments will give you an idea of their expectations, likes and dislikes.

○ Which treatment did you enjoy the most?

○ Which was the most beneficial?

○ How much time can you devote each week to treatments?

These are a few examples of the questions you can ask to establish a client's lifestyle. You will require further specific questions for facial work and others for body work. Having talked to the client at length and recorded your findings, you can now proceed to the looking, palpating and testing.

Learning point

The definition of 'palpating' is to assess the tissues by the sense of touch and pressure.

Activity

Try writing a list of questions you would ask for facial work and another list for body work.

These initial questions will give you vital information about the client's suitability for treatment. It is your responsibility to be aware of conditions that are contra-indicated to treatment. Through questioning, observation and analysis you must assess each client carefully.

Contra-indications

Electrical treatments are given to improve specific conditions of the face or body. The treatment must be beneficial and help the client to achieve their desired results. If there is any risk of harming the client or making any condition worse, treatments must not be carried out, even if the client requests them.

Contra-indications specific to particular treatments are listed in the relevant chapters of this book. The contra-indications in Table 3.3 are those from the National Occupational Standards for Beauty Therapy. You must be aware of these.

You have a legal responsibility under the Health, Safety and Welfare legislation to protect yourself and your clients from harm. Remember that if clients are harmed in any way they may make a claim against you. You must therefore ensure that you have not been negligent in any way, that you have selected the appropriate treatment and that you have a written record of the consultation, the treatment given and the aftercare advice.

During the consultation you must decide whether the selected treatment is safe and suitable for the client. If the client is suffering from any condition that could be aggravated or made worse by the treatment, it obviously *must not* be carried out. These conditions are known as 'contra-indications' to treatment. Knowledge of the potentially harmful effects of inappropriate treatment is extremely important and so is the ability to recognise contra-indications.

The effects of the treatment may be harmful in certain circumstances. The following explanations will help you to understand why some treatments *may not be carried out* or *may be restricted* if certain conditions are present.

It is important to gain as much information about the condition during the consultation. You will need to take into account the treatment(s) that will meet the needs and expectations of the client without compromising their health and safety.

▽ **Table 3.3** Contra-indications and the reasons for them

Contra-indication	Reason
Acute infectious disease and fever	The client will feel hot, feverish and generally unwell. The body's immune system is already fighting the infection. As electrotherapy treatments increase blood and lymphatic circulation, this will exacerbate the condition and make the client feel worse.
Anxious, tense clients	Clients may find some treatments uncomfortable due to the noise of the machine or the sensations experienced. Prepare a treatment plan that will meet their needs and expectations without increasing feelings of anxiety.
Broken capillaries	Treatment may cause further damage. Avoid the area or suggest an alternative treatment.
Bruising	May cause further damage resulting in increased bleeding. Bruises must be allowed to heal before giving treatment, unless they are small and it is possible to work around them.
Cancer	Any client with cancer or a history of cancer must not be treated as there may be a risk of cancer cells being carried to other parts of the body via the circulating blood or the lymphatic system. Seek GP's consent. Be particularly aware if a client complains of intractable pain on rest, unexplained loss of weight, feeling generally tired or unwell.
Chemotherapy, radiotherapy	The client will be under medical supervision. In line with acceptable work ethics and professional code of practice you must seek medical consent before carrying out any treatment.

(Continued)

(Continued)

Contra-indication	Reason
Cuts and abrasions	The broken skin may have a higher moisture content, which will increase the intensity of the current with some machines where the client forms part of the electrical circuit. This will cause discomfort to the client. There is also a risk of cross-infection. Small cuts may be insulated with petroleum jelly, or covered with a waterproof plaster or avoid the area.
Defective sensation	Thermal and/or tactile sensitivity test(s) must be carried out in the area to be treated to ensure the client can distinguish between hot and cold sensations and feel the difference between sharp and soft objects. The client must be able to report any discomfort. This will ensure the treatment will not cause injury or harm to your client, potentially resulting in a claim against you.
Diabetes	Clients with diabetes may have impaired sensitivity and poor circulation therefore will not be able to give accurate feedback on the intensity of the current. Healing may also be slow. Great care must be taken to avoid damage to the skin or any other injury. If in doubt seek GP's consent.
Drink or drugs	Treatment must not be given to clients under the influence of drink or drugs, as the client may not be in control of their faculties.
Dysfunction or disorders of the nervous system: such as multiple sclerosis, strokes, Parkinson's disease, etc.	When the conductivity of nerve impulses may be abnormal; where muscles may exhibit increased tone (spasticity) which may be made worse by the treatment; where skin sensation may be impaired. These clients must only be treated with GP's consent.
Epilepsy	Find out as much as possible about the client's condition. If it is controlled, the treatment may be safe to carry out but if in any doubt seek GP's consent. Do not leave anyone who suffers from epilepsy unattended in a room or on the couch.
Facial and body piercing adornments	Treatment may be uncomfortable for the client as the applicator may pull or catch on the piercing. If the adornment is made of material that conducts an electrical current the client may experience a shock, especially with machines where the client forms part of the circuit, for example galvanic, electro-muscle stimulator, high frequency and micro-current. Avoid the area or cover the adornment.
Fragile, loose skin	There is a danger of overstretching loose skin and of breaking down fragile, thin skin, causing open wounds. Particular care must be taken with diabetics and anyone on steroid treatments as the skin may be fragile and healing may be slow. Superficial treatments with light pressure only must be used.
Heart conditions	The increase in the blood circulation may put too much pressure and stress on the heart. Seek GP's consent.
High blood pressure	Blood pressure varies with age, weight and fitness, but some people have consistently high blood pressure. Treatments can frequently help, especially if the client is worried about a particular area of their body. Medical advice should be sought if the client is not currently on medication.

(Continued)

(Continued)

Contra-indication	Reason
Injectable treatment (recent)	The skin may be red, tender and painful with bruising and swelling. The skin needs time to settle down and heal before having further treatment. Injectables include Botox, which blocks signals to muscles, stopping them contracting, therefore the client will not want treatments that will have an adverse effect on these areas. Fillers plump out lines and wrinkles, adding fullness to the face: do not treat as some electrotherapy machines may dislodge the filler.
Low blood pressure	The client may feel dizzy or faint if they sit up or get off the couch too quickly following treatment. Always supervise and give assistance if necessary.
Medication	Treatment may cause an adverse reaction. If unsure seek medical advice.
Medication causing thinning or inflammation of the skin (for example steroids, accutane, retinol)	The skin will be sensitive so avoid stimulating treatments, as these will exacerbate the condition. The products used for treatments may cause an allergic reaction in some clients.
Metal pins, plates, excessive dental fillings or bridgework	Metal is a good conductor, therefore the intensity of the current will increase in the area and may cause the client discomfort. Avoid the area or suggest an alternative treatment.
Micro-pigmentation (recent)	There is a risk of cross-infection due to possibility of open wounds as the skin has been pierced. The skin will be sensitive and needs time to heal before treatments can be carried out safely.
Muscle injury or spasm	Will aggravate the condition and cause more damage to the muscle.
Pacemaker	The current may interfere with the electrical impulses to the heart. Seek GP's consent.
Phlebitis and thrombosis	Phlebitis is a painful condition where the lining of the vein becomes inflamed and may result in a clot forming on the vein wall, known as thrombosis. Any pressure applied to the vein or increase in the force of the circulation may dislodge the clot. The clot will then be carried in the blood stream with potentially fatal consequences. **Do not treat.** Treatment of the legs is a definite contra-indication and it is safer not to treat the body as there will always be a slight risk. Facial treatments may be carried out with care. Seek medical advice.
Pregnancy	In the late stages of pregnancy or if the client is experiencing any problems with her pregnancy, seek medical advice. Do not give treatments that involve the current penetrating the tissues, for example galvanic, electro-muscle stimulator (EMS) and micro-current as there may be a risk to the foetus.
Dermabrasion/chemical peels /IPL/laser/ epilation (recent)	May aggravate the tissues as the skin will be sensitive after treatment and needs time to heal.
Scar tissue (recent)	Scar tissue is composed of thick, fibrous connective tissue that has limited blood circulation and defective sensation. The scar tissue must be allowed to heal completely before treatment is given to the area. If treatment is given before healing is complete, there is a danger of further damage to the tissues, delaying the healing process.

(Continued)

(Continued)

Contra-indication	Reason
Scleroderma (a connective tissue disease that affects the skin, muscles and blood vessels)	Treatment may aggravate the condition and cause discomfort to the client. Seek medical advice.
Skin diseases	There is a risk of cross-infection.
Skin disorders, for example eczema and psoriasis	The skin for both conditions is red with flaky dry patches. Treatment will cause more sensitivity in the area and exacerbate these conditions. Avoid the area or suggest an alternative treatment.
Undergoing medical treatment	In line with acceptable work ethics and professional code of practice, seek medical consent before carrying out treatment.
Undiagnosed lumps, swelling and inflammation	Recommend the client seeks medical advice as there may be an underlying problem that prevents treatment.
Varicose veins	Should be avoided as the tissues around the vein may be fragile and easily damaged. There is a tendency for the stagnating blood to form clots, which may be dislodged by the treatment. (See also phlebitis and thrombosis.)

Observation and analysis

Prepare the client for a face or body analysis, considering their comfort and modesty at all times. Explain each step fully, encouraging the client to ask questions, and answer clearly. It is most important that they know and understand what you are doing and why it is necessary.

Facial treatments

Having gathered the essential information from the client, you need to complete the consultation record to decide on the most appropriate treatment for their facial skin.

You need to consider the following aspects of the skin and record the information under these headings:

○ Skin type
○ Skin conditions
○ Texture
○ Colour
○ Elasticity and muscle tone
○ Imperfections.

Skin types

Remember

Involve your client when assessing their skin. You cannot decide on their skin type by just looking and feeling, you have to talk to them and listen to their responses. Ask about their skincare routine and their preferred product types. Make sure your knowledge of your retail line(s) is up to date and that you explain the benefits clearly, selecting the correct products for the skin type. The client will be more likely to buy products that are based on your professional recommendation.

Learning point

The combination of sebum and sweat forms the acid mantle on the surface of the skin. This helps to keep the moisture within the skin and also protects it from the invasion of bacteria. Using harsh products can temporarily destroy the acid mantle, which may cause irritation, dehydration and infection.

▽ **Table 3.4** Skin types

Skin type	Explanation	Pores	Texture	Oil	Moisture	Additional notes
Normal (Balanced)	A normal skin type is referred to as a balanced skin, as there is sufficient oil and moisture produced to keep the skin soft and supple.	Small	Fine	Balanced	Balanced	This is the ideal skin type.
Dry	A dry skin lacks oil and moisture. The sebaceous glands do not secrete sufficient sebum to lubricate and form a protective layer over the skin to prevent the loss of moisture from the upper layers. There may be signs of premature ageing, with fine and deep lines around the eyes, mouth and neck, as dry skin tends to age more quickly than other skin types. Causes of dry skin include: hormone imbalance, central heating, sunbathing, crash diets, smoking and medication.	Small to large	Fine to coarse	Insufficient	Insufficient	Large pores and a coarse texture could be present on a dry skin, as the client may have had a greasy skin when younger, resulting in the pores losing their elasticity.
Oily	An oily skin produces too much sebum in the ducts and hair follicles, which causes enlarged pores that are prone to comedones (blackheads) and blemishes. As the sebum builds up on the surface of the skin it affects the natural shedding of skin cells, causing the skin to look thick, dull and sallow. The overproduction of sebum is due to hormone imbalance.	Large	Coarse	Over-production of sebum	Usually good as sebum helps to keep moisture within the skin	This skin type may become dehydrated if unsuitable products are used that strip the skin's protective acid mantle.
Combination	This can be a combination of two different skin types. The most common being an oily T-zone on the forehead, nose, inner cheeks and chin, while the outer region is drier.	Medium to large	Coarse on the T-zone, finer on the outer region	Over-production of sebum in the T-zone	Good in the T-zone if the correct skin care routine is followed	There are many more sebaceous glands located in the T-zone area. This is where the majority of comedones are found.

Skin conditions

The following are referred to as skin conditions. They can accompany any of the above skin types.

Sensitive skin

A sensitive skin flushes very easily and reacts quickly to temperature change. It is also prone to allergic reactions. Common substances can cause irritation, leaving the skin red and blotchy. Dilated capillaries may be present on the cheeks and around the nose.

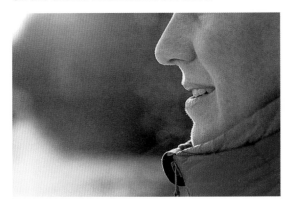

△ **Figure 3.8** Sensitive skin

> **Learning point**
> Advise clients to use hypoallergenic products for sensitive skin.

Dehydrated skin

This is characterised by a lack of moisture in the skin. It can be due to incorrect skin care routine such as using too harsh a product; over-exposure to the sun and central heating; or insufficient fluid intake. The skin may feel taut and itchy, with superficial flaking of the skin and a loss of plumpness.

Mature skin

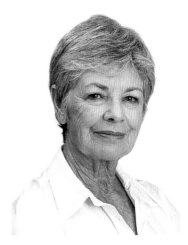

△ **Figure 3.9** Mature skin

The natural ageing process occurs over a period of time and is predetermined by genetic make-up. Changes take place for the following reasons:

○ Muscles lose their tone and those that are attached directly to the skin will cause the overlying skin to stretch, producing lines.

○ The loss of underlying fat will result in hollowed cheeks and eye sockets.

○ The protein fibres in the dermis, collagen and elastin will degenerate, causing the skin to loose its plumpness and elasticity.

○ Cellular activity decreases, causing skin tags and uneven pigmentation, for example liver spots.

○ Desquamation slows down, leaving the skin looking dull.

Congested skin

Usually associated with a greasy or combination skin. The sebaceous glands secrete excess sebum, which can harden and become blocked in the pores. As the sebum builds up on the surface of the skin it affects the natural shedding of skin cells, causing the skin to look thick and coarse, dull and sallow. Sweat glands continue to function but the sweat cannot be excreted as the pores are blocked, which adds to the problem. Pustules and papules may be present if the pores become infected.

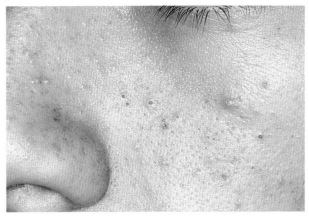

△ **Figure 3.10** Congested skin

Moist skin

This is skin that feels slightly wet or damp to the touch. It is usually an indication that the body is perspiring too much.

Oedematous skin

This is an accumulation of fluid in the tissues, which is a sign of an underlying problem that may need to be referred to a health professional.

Skin colour

In treatment terms this refers to the quality of the skin's colour or its tone. For example, whether or not the skin is pale or flushed, dull or bright, sallow or glowing. The colour can be improved by the increase in circulation created by treatment.

Learning point
The genetically determined skin colour is dependent on the amount of the pigment melanin in the skin. Melanin is produced by melanocytes, which are found in the basal layer of the epidermis. The function of melanin is to protect the skin from sun damage and ultraviolet radiation. The degree of melanin in different genetic groups varies. All groups have the same amount of melanocytes but more melanin is produced in darker skin tones. This helps to protect the skin from sun damage and delays the ageing process.

Skin elasticity

Collagen and elastin are two proteins found in the dermis. Collagen gives skin its firmness and strength, elastin gives skin its elasticity. A young skin will look firm and supple but as the skin ages, collagen and elastin fibres start to weaken and character lines begin to appear.

To test skin elasticity, pinch the skin gently between your thumb and index finger on the cheek area and release. Assess how well the skin springs back and record the result: good, average or poor. Repeat above the jaw-line and on the neck.

Muscle tone

Muscles of the face are attached to bone, to adjoining muscles or to the skin. During the ageing process muscles lose their tone and elasticity and character lines begin to form around the muscles of facial expression.

Facial contours

A client with good muscle tone will have well-defined facial contours. As the skin ages, muscles lose their tone and facial contours become slack and heavy, particularly around the jaw line, giving a jowl effect.

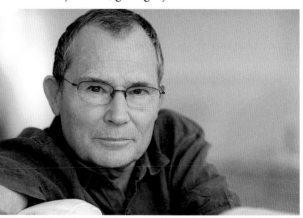

△ **Figure 3.11** Dropped contours

Skin imperfections

Dilated capillaries

Loss of elasticity of the capillary wall causes capillaries to permanently dilate. They are usually found on the cheeks and around the nose. The condition can be caused by over-exposure to the sun or other extremes of temperature (for example water that is too hot or too cold) and skin injury. They are more often found on dry and sensitive skins.

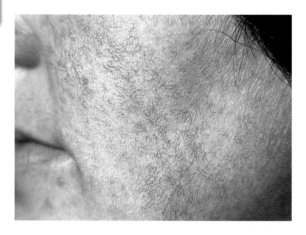

△ **Figure 3.12** Dilated capillaries

Pustule

A pustule is a vesicle (an elevation of skin), containing pus. Pustules often develop when hair follicles are infected by bacteria. They are usually found on greasy skin or where there is acne. Avoid the area to prevent the risk of cross-infection.

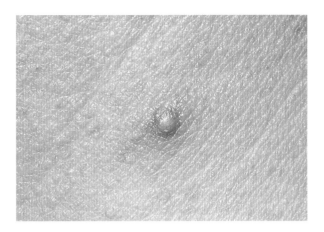

△ **Figure 3.13** A pustule

Papule

A papule is a solid raised area of skin that is red in colour and can be painful. It does not contain fluid but may develop into a pustule.

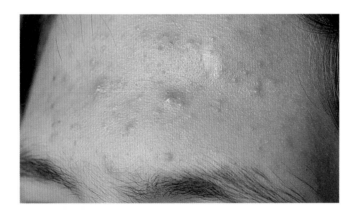

△ **Figure 3.14** A papule

Milia

This is an accumulation of sebum trapped under a fine cuticle of skin covering the mouth of the hair follicle. These small, white, pearly nodules are found around the eyes and upper cheek area, usually on clients with dry skin. Milia can be extracted by using a sterile micro-lance to pierce the fine cuticle of skin after a steam, or by disincrustation treatment when the skin has been pre-warmed.

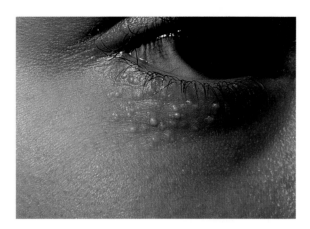

△ **Figure 3.15** Milia

Comedone

This is a build-up of excess sebum in the hair follicle, which becomes a hardened plug as the sebum mixes with the keratinised cells at the surface of the skin. The brown/black appearance of a comedone is due to the fatty substance in sebum oxidising when exposed to air.

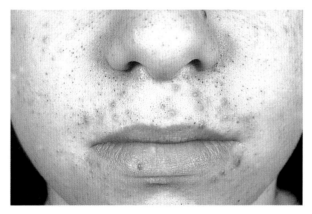

△ **Figure 3.16** Comedones

Open pores

These are caused by the build-up of excess sebum at the opening of hair follicles.

The pores become stretched and over time lose their elasticity and remain enlarged.

Remember

A client's skin type can change due to their lifestyle, stress levels and health, so do not assume the client has a greasy skin because they have open pores.

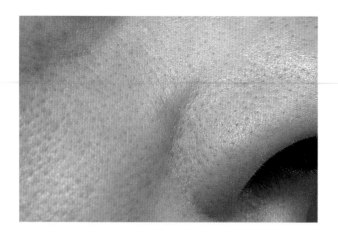

△ **Figure 3.17** Open pores

Body treatments

When you have gathered the essential information from the client you need to complete the consultation record to decide on the most appropriate treatment to meet their body treatment needs.

Information should be recorded under the following headings:

○ Height
○ Weight
○ Body type
○ Posture
○ Measurements
○ Types of fat
○ Muscle tone
○ Fluid retention
○ Skin condition
○ Stretch marks.

Height

To accurately measure height, the client should be barefoot and the measuring scale should be fixed to the wall. The client should stand with the heels together and the back as straight as possible. The head should be level, with eyes looking straight ahead and shoulders should touch the wall.

Weight

Weight measurement is needed to calculate the client's body mass index (BMI), a measurement of the proportion of body fat. If a client wishes to lose weight, and if this is appropriate, their weight can be monitored at each visit as an aid to motivation. In this case the client should be weighed at the same time of day, where

possible, and in the same amount of clothing (ideally, underwear only). If the client prefers to remain dressed, you can allow about 1 kg (2 lbs) for outer clothing. Note the weight on the consultation record. It can then be measured against the healthy weight range or BMI tables for the client's height.

> **Be aware** !
>
> People generally weigh more towards the end of the day. Pre-menstrual water retention can also increase weight temporarily.

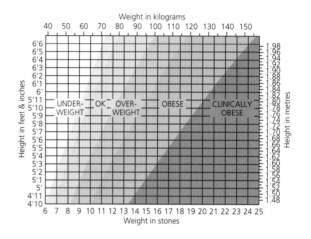

△ **Figure 3.18** BMI chart

Body type

Endomorph

These are short, stocky, curvaceous and plump, often pear-shaped with small hands and feet. For this group, weight and fat gain is easy and weight loss is difficult.

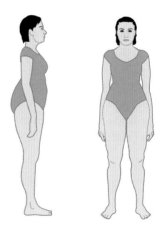

△ **Figure 3.19** Endomorph

Mesomorph

These are muscular and stocky, with well-developed shoulders and slim boyish hips, giving an inverted triangle shape. They gain weight and fat slowly but increase muscle strength easily.

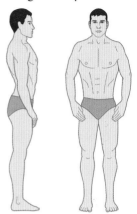

△ **Figure 3.20** Mesomorph

Ectomorph

These are long-limbed, slim and slightly muscular. They do not easily gain weight.

Individuals are predominantly of one type but may have aspects of another.

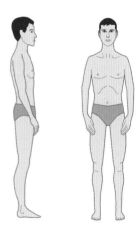

△ **Figure 3.21** Ectomorph

Posture

Posture is used to describe the alignment of the body, in other words how the body is held. Very few people have perfect posture because it is influenced by both physical and psychological factors throughout life.

When you first meet a client, observe how they walk, stand and hold themselves: this alone will give some information regarding posture. Are the movements evenly balanced or is there tilting, stooping or unevenness in the way they move?

When the client has undressed, a more accurate assessment can be made.

Clients with poor posture will also benefit from exercises to correct posture; these can be given after treatment or as part of homecare advice.

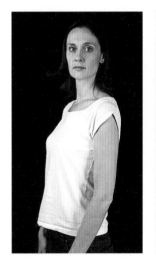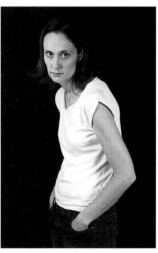

△ **Figure 3.22** Good and poor posture

Postural assessment

Ask the client to adopt a normal stance and assess the posture from the front, side and back. A plumb line may be used to check body alignment from the side. It should pass through the lobe of the ear, the point of the shoulder, the greater trochanter at the hip joint, behind the patella and in front of the ankle joint.

From the front

Head position:

○ Are the ear lobes level? If they are not there is a muscle imbalance. The sterno-cleido-mastoid and the upper fibres of the trapezius are tight on the lower side, while those on the other side will be stretched.

Shoulders:

○ Are they level, or is one higher than the other, indicating muscle imbalance? The upper fibres of the trapezius and levator scapulae are tight on the raised side.

○ A difference in level may also indicate scoliosis, so check for that also. This is a lateral curvature of the spine, which may be a long C curve or an S curve. The muscles that will require strengthening will be those on the outside of the curve. The muscles that require stretching will be those on the inside of the curve. (A slight difference is considered normal.)

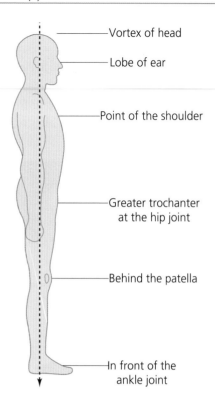

Vortex of head

Lobe of ear

Point of the shoulder

Greater trochanter at the hip joint

Behind the patella

In front of the ankle joint

△ **Figure 3.23** Checking posture using a plumb line

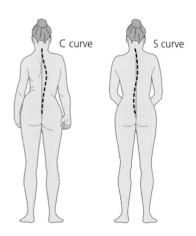

C curve   S curve

△ **Figure 3.24** Scoliosis

○ Are both shoulders held high? This indicates tension in the muscles on both sides. The right and left upper fibres of the trapezius and the levator scapulae are tight.

○ Are the shoulders drawn forward, rounded? This indicates muscle imbalance. The pectoral muscles are tight, but the middle fibres of the trapezius and rhomboids are stretched.

○ Are there hollows above the clavicles? This indicates muscle tension, which may be due to respiratory problems such as asthma.

Breasts:

○ Are the breasts held high or sagging? If there is breast sag and round shoulders, correction of the posture may help to lift the breasts.

Waist:

○ Are the waist angles on the right and left level? If one is lower than the other, there may be spinal deformity or a difference in leg length.

Anterior superior iliac spines:

○ Are they level? If not, there may be spinal deformity or a difference in leg length.

○ Are they dropped forward? This indicates a lordosis. This is an exaggerated curve of the lumbar spine where the pelvis is tilted forwards.

The weak stretched muscles that require strengthening are:

○ the abdominals – rectus abdominus, internal oblique and external oblique

○ the hip extensors – gluteus maximus and the hamstrings.

The tight muscles that require stretching are:

○ the trunk extensors – erector spinae and quadratus lumborum

○ the hip flexors – ilio-psoas.

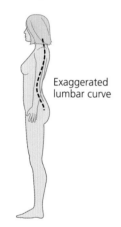

Exaggerated lumbar curve

△ **Figure 3.25** Lordosis

○ Are they dropped backwards? This indicates a flat back (or sway back). This is a condition where there is little or no lumbar curve and the pelvis is tilted backwards. It may be accompanied by kyphosis of the thoracic spine. The weak, stretched muscles that require strengthening are the back extensors – erector spinae (in some cases the abdominals and gluteus maximus are weak).

The tight muscles that require stretching are the hamstrings on the posterior thigh.

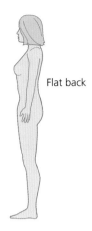

△ **Figure 3.26** Flat back

Patellae:

○ Do they point forwards? If not, there may be knock knees (genu valgum) or bow legs (genu varum).

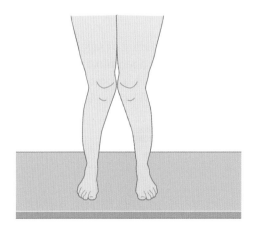

△ **Figure 3.27** Knock knees

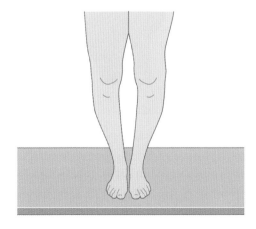

△ **Figure 3.28** Bow legs

Toes:

○ Do they point forwards? If they point outwards there may be flattening of the medial arch and flat feet.

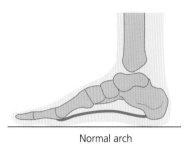

△ **Figure 3.29** Flat feet

○ If they point inwards or outwards, the weight distribution over the foot will be wrong, causing foot problems.
○ Look for bunions, where the big toe deviates towards and sometimes lies across the other toes and there is swelling at the metatarso-phalangeal joint.

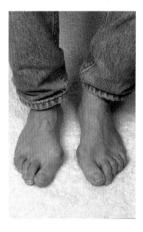

△ **Figure 3.30** Bunion

○ Look for hammer toes, where the inter-phalangeal joints are deformed.

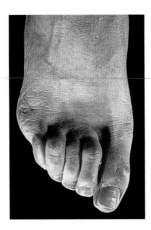

△ **Figure 3.31** Hammer toes

From the side

Use a plumb line.

> **Remember**
>
> This should fall through the lobe of the ear, the point of the shoulder and the hip joint, behind the patella and just in front of the lateral malleolus.

Head position:

○ Is the neck or cervical curve exaggerated and the chin forward? This means that the neck extensors, the upper fibres of the trapezius at the back of the neck, are tight and the neck flexors are weak.

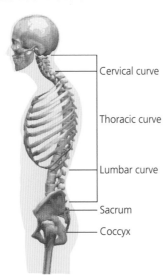

△ **Figure 3.32** Cervical curve exaggerated and chin forward

Thoracic curve:

○ Is there kyphosis? This is an exaggerated curve of the thoracic region. The weak, stretched muscles that require

strengthening are the middle fibres of trapezius, the rhomboids and the middle part of erector spinae.

The tight muscles that require stretching are the pectoralis major and the neck extensors.

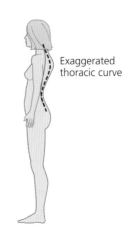

△ **Figure 3.33** Kyphosis

Abdomen:

○ Is the abdomen protruding or sagging forwards, indicating weakness of the abdominal muscles? The pelvis may be tilted forward. This is known as visceroptosis, as the weak abdominals allow the viscera to sag forward.

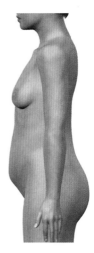

△ **Figure 3.34** Visceroptosis

Lumbar curve (see page 62):

○ Is there lordosis, i.e. an exaggerated lumbar curve with the spine curved inwards. (See front aspect.)

○ If the lumbar region is flat, which is much less common, the erector spinae and quadratus lumborum will be weak.

Buttocks:

○ Are the buttocks well toned with strong muscles, or are the gluteal muscles weak and sagging?

Knees:

○ Are the knees hyper-extended?

From the back

Head:

○ Are the ear lobes level or is the head tilted, indicating muscle imbalance? (See front aspect.)

Shoulders:

○ Are they level? (See front aspect.)

○ Are there winged scapulae, i.e. the inferior angle and medial border of the scapulae lift away from the chest wall? This indicates a weakness of the serratus anterior and the lower fibres of the trapezius.

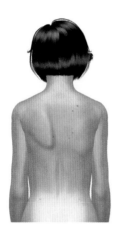

△ **Figure 3.35** Winged scapula

Spine (see page 62):

○ Is there scoliosis, i.e. a lateral deviation of the spine? This may be an **S** or **C** curve to the right or left. If you are unsure, pull a finger down the spinous process: the red line should be straight, and will show up any deviation. A scoliosis may be structural (present from birth), or it may be postural, and will straighten out when the body is flexed forward.

Buttocks:

○ Are the buttock folds level? If they are not, scoliosis, lateral pelvic tilt or different leg length may be present.

Heels:

○ Are these square and firmly planted on the ground? If not, the weight distribution will be uneven.

Correction of the posture

Where required, the correction of the posture should be discussed with the client, and the following process

should be explained. This exercise should then form part of the homecare advice given to the client, perhaps suggesting they practise in front of a mirror.

Correction of the posture should begin at the feet. Each position should be maintained as the subsequent one is practised.

Feet

Stand with the feet 10 to 15 centimetres apart, with the toes pointing forward. The weight should be evenly distributed between the balls of the feet and the heels.

Practise the following:

○ Raise the toes off the ground, feel the weight evenly distributed between the balls of the feet and the heels. Then lower the toes.

○ Sway the body forward, feeling more weight on the balls of the feet.

○ Sway the body backwards, feeling more weight on the heels.

○ Position the body so that the weight is evenly distributed between the balls of the feet and the heels. Lift the medial arch slightly, but do not curl the toes.

Knees

○ Press the knees backwards hard, ease the knees by bending them slightly, then find the mid-point and pull the kneecaps upwards by tightening the quadriceps muscle.

○ If the knees are hyper-extended, ease them slightly and pull the kneecaps upwards as just shown.

○ If the knees are bowed or knock-kneed, tighten the kneecaps, rotate the thighs outwards and tighten the buttocks to bring the kneecaps to point forward. Check the feet again after performing these movements.

Pelvis

○ Tilt the pelvis forwards and then backwards; pull it forwards again tightly, tucking the tail under, and hold this balance. Pull the abdomen in and breathe out as the pelvis is pulled forward, then hold this position while breathing normally.

Thorax

○ Pull the thorax upward from the waist as you breathe in, drawing the shoulders backwards and downwards. Hold this position while breathing normally. Do not thrust the chest forwards.

Neck and head

○ Elongate the neck and pull the chin backwards. Feel as though someone is pulling the hair upwards at the crown.

Check the feet, knees, pelvis and thorax again, hold this position and then relax. Practise this correction several times a day and during various activities; correct the posture during inhalation and hold the balance during exhalation.

If the new posture is maintained while walking around, it will eventually become habitual.

Taking measurements

Where a treatment is part of a client's weight loss goal, body measurements can be a useful guide to progress. Sometimes when weight has not changed, body shape may still have improved with the toning of muscle, so measurements will reflect this and help motivate the client. Some clients will not be interested in individual body measurements, but for those who are, it is important that the measurements are accurate. Do not pull the tape measure too tight, but ensure it fits snugly over the area. Again, wearing minimal clothing is preferable. All measurements must be taken from a fixed point so that records are accurate, (for example, a fixed measurement above or below the navel, or above a point at the top of the patella when measuring thighs).

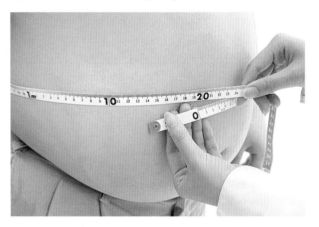

△ **Figure 3.36** Taking client's measurements

Distribution of fat

There are different types of body fat or adipose tissue: hard and soft adipose tissue and cellulite. The type and location on the body should be noted.

Hard adipose tissue

This type of fatty tissue is quite solid and well established. It can be difficult to distinguish from muscle, as it is similarly hard to pick up and it can be found over well-toned muscle. Care should be taken to correctly identify hard adipose tissue, as hard fat is more difficult to shift than soft fat.

Soft adipose tissue

This type of fatty tissue is easier to pick up and feels quite separate from the muscle layer beneath. Soft adipose tissue is relatively easy to shift by following a suitable diet and exercise regime.

Trapped adipose tissue

Deposits of fat are sometimes found trapped between bundles of muscle fibres. This is more common in people who have a history of regular training, but who no longer do so, such as former athletes or dancers. Trapped fat is slow to respond to diet or exercise.

Cellulite

Cellulite is more common in women than men and can be present on slim figures as well as those who are overweight. It is easily recognised and often described as having an 'orange peel' appearance, where the skin appears lumpy and dimpled. This rippling of the tissue is caused by water retention and the stagnation of toxins and waste products in adipose cells. Because these cells have poor blood circulation, toxins are not efficiently removed from the area, causing the orange peel effect.

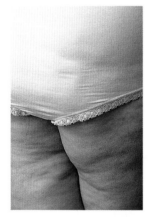

△ **Figure 3.37** Cellulite

If the skin ripples and looks like orange peel when the tissue is pressed between the palms of both hands, it is cellulite. The dimpling is sometimes noticeable without applying any pressure in more advanced stages.

Areas subject to cellulite:

○ inner, upper and backs of the thighs

○ buttocks

○ hips

○ stomach

○ lower back

○ inside and back of upper arms

○ inside the knees

○ ankles.

Some factors that contribute to the formation of cellulite include:

○ insufficient water intake

○ lack of proper exercise

○ poor circulation

○ sluggish digestion

○ poor eating habits

○ poor breathing

○ sedentary living

○ tension

○ fatigue

○ constipation.

Muscle tone

It is possible to obtain some indication of muscle strength by applying manual resistance to muscle action and feeling the degree of tone within the muscle. This will only provide a rough guide, as it is not possible to quantify the strength but only to categorise it as poor, moderate, good, very good or excellent. Muscles that are easily tested this way are the biceps and triceps, the abdominals, gluteus maximus and the hip abductors and adductors.

The following tests can be performed on the couch to give an initial guide to the client's strength and general mobility. Assess and record the outcome as poor, moderate, good, very good or excellent.

Biceps

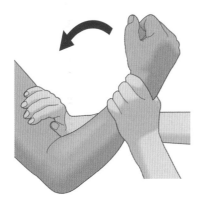

△ **Figure 3.38** Assessing muscle tone of biceps

Ask the client to bend the elbow to the mid point of the range. Place one hand over the biceps on the anterior aspect of the upper arm. Grasp the wrist with the other. Instruct the client to bend the elbow while you stop the movement. Feel the increased tone with the hand placed over the muscle.

Triceps

With one hand cover the triceps on the posterior aspect of the upper arm. Keep the other hand around the wrist. Instruct the client to straighten the elbow against resistance. Feel the increased tone with the hand placed over the muscle.

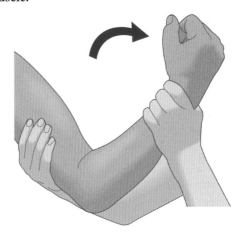

△ **Figure 3.39** Assessing muscle tone of triceps

Abdominals (particularly rectus abdominus)

With the client lying supine (face up) on the couch, the strength of the abdominal muscles can be determined by the following sequence. This test can be split into three phases: only clients with good muscle tone will be able to progress to Phase 3.

Place your hand on the abdominal area to feel the strength of the muscle. Ask the client to breathe in and on the out breath to lift the *head*, with chin towards chest to look at their toes. For some clients this test may be all they can manage due to poor muscle tone.

Place your hand on the abdomen with the other hand ready to support the client's back if needed. Ask the client to breathe in and on the out breath to lift the *head and shoulders*, with chin towards chest to look at their toes.

Ask the client to bend their knees, feet flat on the couch. Place your hand on the abdomen with the other ready to support their back. Ask the client to breathe in and on the out breath to lift *head, shoulders and vertebrae* gently off the couch to perform a curl up.

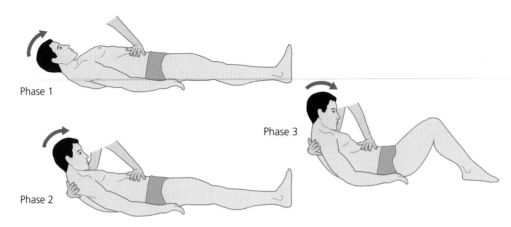

Phase 1

Phase 3

Phase 2

△ **Figure 3.40** Assessing the muscle tone of the abdomen

Gluteus maximus

With the client lying prone (face down), place one hand over the gluteus maximus on the left and the other on the back of the left leg (gastrocnemius). Instruct the client to raise the leg while you apply resistance. Feel the increased tone in the buttock. Repeat for the right side.

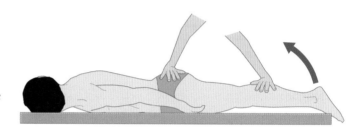

△ **Figure 3.41** Assessing muscle tone of gluteus maximus

Abductors

With the client lying supine (face up), legs straight, place one hand over the abductors on the outer aspect of the thigh above the greater trochanter and the other hand under the ankle to cup it. Instruct the client to 'push out' towards you. Resist the movement, using the hand at the ankle to push inwards. Feel the increased tone in the abductors. Repeat for the other side.

pull the leg inwards towards the other leg. Resist the movement, using the hand at the ankle to pull outwards. Feel the increased tone in the adductors. Repeat for other side.

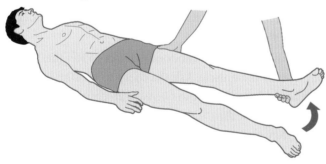

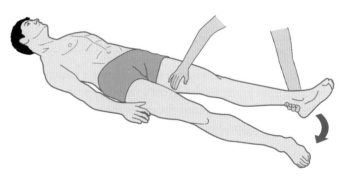

△ **Figure 3.42** Assessing muscle tone of abductors

Adductors

With the client lying supine (face up), legs straight and with one leg pushed outwards, place one hand over the adductors on the inner aspect of the thigh (upper third) and the other hand under the ankle. Instruct the client to

△ **Figure 3.43** Assessing muscle tone of adductors

Fluid retention

A client with puffy or swollen ankles, and sometimes hands, may be suffering from fluid retention. This puffiness is referred to as oedema. There are a number of possible causes:

○ not drinking enough water

○ eating too much salt

○ eating lots of processed foods.

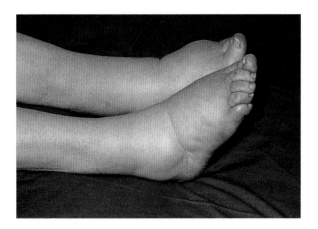

△ **Figure 3.44** Fluid retention

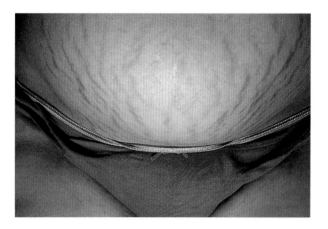

△ **Figure 3.45** Stretch marks

Also, people who stand for long periods of time, such as those working in shops, can suffer from gravitational oedema. Fluid retention is also common before menstruation, when it can affect the abdomen and breasts.

To test for fluid retention, press the client's skin in the oedematous area. If it remains indented and does not immediately spring back, this is a sign of fluid retention. Massage will help the lymphatic system to drain away the excess fluid.

Skin conditions

Bodies show age just as quickly as faces. Care of the body as with care of the face is based on a regular routine. Note areas of skin that are dry and dehydrated, particularly the lower legs, thighs, back and chest. Advise the client on retail products that will rehydrate, soften and nourish the skin.

Stretch marks

Stretch marks are caused by stretching of the skin due to rapid weight gain, pregnancy and weight training. The reticular layer in the dermis is the main support layer of the skin. It contains collagen and elastic fibres that give skin its firmness and elasticity. When these fibres are continuously over-stretched they break down, causing scarring in the dermis. They appear on the surface of the skin as purplish-reddish coloured lines that fade over time. The main areas affected are the breasts, hips, thighs and abdomen.

Research suggests that stretch marks are caused by the hormone glucocorticoid, secreted by the adrenal cortex. Levels of this hormone increase during weight gain, pregnancy and weight training. It prevents the fibroblasts in the dermis from synthesising collagen and elastic fibres that provide the support for the skin.

Selecting the treatment

When you have completed a detailed analysis you will have identified the problem areas. Discuss your findings tactfully with the client and ask if they agree with your assessment. You must then agree the goals and possible outcomes and select the treatment.

It is vitally important that you accurately identify the client's condition and select the most suitable and effective treatment, as the result you achieve will depend on this. You will require an in-depth knowledge of all the equipment, treatments and products at your disposal so that you can make an informed choice.

Activity

As a student, remembering all the treatments may be quite difficult while you are just starting. It is therefore a good idea to list on separate cards the different facial conditions and skin types, the different body conditions and suitable treatments. You can then practise matching the treatments to the conditions as a revision activity.

Once you have decided on the best treatment possible you must discuss it fully with the client, giving reasons why you consider it to be the most suitable and beneficial treatment for them.

You must then discuss:

○ the *timing* of each session
○ the *number* of sessions recommended per week
○ the *length* of the course
○ and most important of all, the *cost* per treatment/ course, including cost of any recommended products.

Most businesses offer an incentive for a course of treatment – this may include free products or the offer of free sessions at the end of the course.

Make sure that the client understands their commitment. Encourage them to ask questions and answer them fully. You must agree everything with the client. When they are satisfied, make sure that they sign an agreement/consent form.

Contra-actions

During the consultation the client should be made aware of the reactions or responses that may be experienced either during or after treatment. A client's reaction to treatment will differ depending on their physical and emotional state.

Contra-actions during treatment

The expected outcomes of the treatment are usually positive responses and include a feeling of relaxation and a sense of well-being. Occasionally, however, adverse effects may occur during treatment. Always be alert to any abnormal changes happening to the client and be prepared to deal with them.

The following contra-actions may occur during treatment.

An allergic reaction to the medium

Action: Stop the treatment. Cleanse the skin with a hypo-allergenic product and apply a cool compress to soothe the area. Record details on the consultation record for future reference.

> **Learning point**
>
> If the reaction occurs during body treatments when you already have a lot of the medium on the body, recommend a shower, where feasible, to remove it. If there is no shower then cleanse the area and apply cool damp towel(s).

> **Be aware** !
>
> If a client usually reacts to products, carry out a skin test 24–48 hours prior to treatment. Apply a small amount of product by the elbow crease or behind the ear. A positive response includes tingling, erythema, inflammation and swelling. If any of these occur, instruct the client to cleanse the area thoroughly. A negative response will be no reaction at all to the product. Record details on the consultation record for future reference.

Heightened emotional state

This can occur due to the release of suppressed feelings and emotions.

Action: liaise with the client to find out if they would like you to:

○ carry on with the treatment
○ fetch a glass of water
○ sit and chat
○ give them a tissue and continue with treatment
○ stop the treatment and have some personal space.

Profuse sweating

Action: place the client in a semi-reclining position; offer a glass of water to help hydrate the body; remove excess sweat from the area; check that the room temperature is suitable and allow client to rest for a few minutes. Ask the client how they feel about continuing with the treatment.

Nausea

Action: place the client in a semi-reclining position; offer water to sip slowly; allow them to rest and discuss options on whether to continue, cut down or stop the treatment.

Headache

Action: place a cool compress on client's forehead; offer a glass of water and discuss options to continue, cut down or stop the treatment.

Area becoming very hot and red

Action: remove the medium and place a cool compress over the area and discuss options to continue, cut down or stop the treatment.

Restlessness and irritability

Action: stop the treatment while you talk to the client about how they feel and what they want to do.

Feeling faint

Action: place client in supine or recovery position; apply a cool compress to the forehead; make sure there is sufficient fresh air in the room; offer a glass of water and allow client to rest for 5–10 minutes. Discuss what they want to do in terms of treatment.

See Chapters 5–12 for information on contra-actions that may occur *after* treatments.

Preparation for the treatment

For both facial and body treatments you must:

○ maintain client privacy at all times

○ ask the client to remove all jewellery and place it in their bag for safe-keeping

○ provide a robe or towel if the client needs to undress.

For facial treatments, depending on the type of treatment, ask the client to remove their jumper, shirt/blouse, shoes, belt (if it has a metal buckle), jewellery and hair accessories that contain metal.

> **Be aware**
>
> During indirect high frequency and galvanic treatments the client has to hold an electrode so they become part of the electrical circuit. If the electrode comes into contact with metal for example a belt buckle or similar the current will intensify and could cause an electric shock.

If it is the first body treatment and therefore entails an assessment, ask the client to remove clothing down to their underwear. Provide a robe or large towel to maintain modesty. Place a couch roll paper on the floor for the client to stand on as they undress in case they have athlete's foot or verrucae. This will help prevent cross-infection.

> **Best practice** ⓑ
>
> When offering body treatments it is advisable to give clients disposable footwear, especially those who have contagious foot conditions.

Positioning the client

The position of the client will depend on the treatment. Position the client correctly on the couch, making sure that they are well supported and relaxed. Cover the client and make sure they are warm and comfortable. Always help the client on and off the couch, to ensure that they cannot fall and injure themselves. (See Table 3.5.)

Sensitivity tests

A sensitivity test is carried out before electrotherapy treatments to ensure sensory nerves in the skin are not damaged and the client can give accurate feedback on sensations felt during treatment. There are two types of test. The type given depends on the machine to be used:

○ *thermal test* – to test sensitivity to hot and cold. Use two test tubes: one containing hot water and one containing cold water. Tell the client to close their eyes. Touch randomly over the face (or body), in the area to be treated, with the hot and cold test tubes, asking the client to identify which one is touching them.

○ *tactile test* – to test sensitivity to sharp and soft. Using an orangewood stick and cotton wool, proceed as for hot and cold test asking client to identify the sharp and soft objects.

If the client is able to identify hot and cold and sharp and soft, their sensation is intact and the treatment may proceed. If they are repeatedly unable to identify one or the other, their sensation is defective and treatment should not be carried out. Failure to perform these tests could invalidate your insurance should harm come to your client during treatment.

> **Learning point**
>
> In the event of injury to themselves, your client may take legal action against you. This is the purpose of public liability insurance.

Carrying out the treatment

Any treatment must be carried out skilfully and with care. Always practise the highest standards of hygiene and safety.

Do your very best for every client, explaining each procedure as you go along and checking that the client is happy and comfortable throughout. Ask them to tell you if at any point they feel uncomfortable. Be on the alert for any contra-actions that may arise during treatment.

Time the treatment carefully, giving each area equal attention and aim to complete the treatment in the allocated time span.

Table 3.5 Positioning the client for treatment

Position		Suggestions for comfort
Prone lying (face down).		In the prone position it is more comfortable for the client if the feet project over the edge of the bed. This prevents stretching of the ligaments at the front of the ankle. The head may be turned to one side. A pillow under the abdomen may be more comfortable and will round out a hollow back.
Supine lying (face up) or half-lying (back raised at an angle).		In the supine or half-lying position, a pillow to support the head will improve comfort. A pillow under the knees and thighs will also improve comfort and aid relaxation.
Recovery position on the side, lying with under arm and leg behind and upper arm and leg bent to support the body.		In the recovery position, a pillow under the head and a pillow supporting the upper leg improves comfort.

Be aware ❗

Running over specified treatment times could result in loss of business from unhappy clients and loss of earnings.

Be aware ❗

It is vital that you follow the manufacturer's instructions regarding timing and procedure of the treatment as well as cleaning and maintenance of equipment. If you do not, you risk causing injury to the client and invalidating your insurance should a problem with the treatment arise.

The underpinning information and the details of preparation, procedure and technique for each treatment can be found in Chapters 5–12.

Recording details

Develop the habit of accurately and neatly recording all the details as you progress through each stage. Do not leave it until the end as important information may be forgotten.

All the information you have gathered and stored is confidential. It is important that this confidentiality is maintained in accordance with the Data Protection Act (1998).

If you exceed the time allocated, analyse why and make adjustments next time.

Learning point

Important points to add to the consultation record are:

○ treatment performed

○ length of treatment

○ products used

○ equipment used and settings

○ outcome of sensitivity test if applicable

○ your initials (if you work with others).

Evaluation of treatment

After each treatment it is important to assess how effective the treatment has been. You must decide whether the treatment has produced the effects that you were expecting, and whether the goals you set at the beginning have been met.

In order to evaluate the treatment you will need to obtain feedback: this means gathering all the information you can that will indicate the effectiveness of the treatment. An analysis of the results of the treatment will enable you to make changes or modifications next time, if you feel that you have not achieved your goal.

You will obtain information through:

○ touch, sensing through your hands whether the tissues feel more toned

○ looking at the area to see what changes have been produced

○ asking the client how they feel and whether the treatment met their needs.

As a result of the information you obtain from this feedback you will be able to decide if changes need to be made and to formulate a strategy for the next treatment. You will be able to make a judgement as to whether your selected treatment has been as effective as you hoped.

Through palpating the tissues (feeling and pressing them with your hands) you will sense whether the tissues feel more relaxed: see page 74.

Discuss any changes that you intend making next time, explaining the reasons why they are needed. Ask if there is anything the client would like to change. Record the results of the feedback and the strategy for following treatments on the consultation record. Always refer to these each time the client attends. Give aftercare and homecare advice as appropriate.

Learning point

Evaluating the treatment and your own performance forms the basis of good reflective practice. It should become second nature as you become familiar with routines and develop your skills.

Aftercare and homecare advice

The client must be given advice and guidance on the routine to follow immediately after treatment and in the interval between treatments. Recommend retail products to reinforce the effectiveness of the treatment to maintain optimum results. The advice given will obviously vary depending on the treatment given.

Allow the client time to relax and sit up slowly, helping them into a semi-reclining position. Offer a glass of water to help rehydrate the body. This is an ideal time to discuss homecare advice with the client.

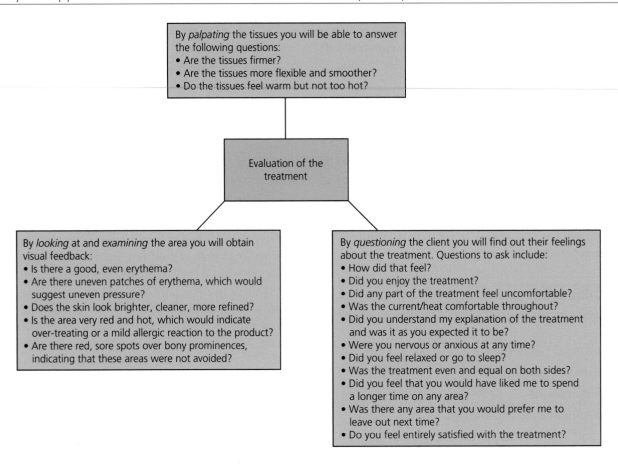

By *palpating* the tissues you will be able to answer the following questions:
- Are the tissues firmer?
- Are the tissues more flexible and smoother?
- Do the tissues feel warm but not too hot?

Evaluation of the treatment

By *looking* at and *examining* the area you will obtain visual feedback:
- Is there a good, even erythema?
- Are there uneven patches of erythema, which would suggest uneven pressure?
- Does the skin look brighter, cleaner, more refined?
- Is the area very red and hot, which would indicate over-treating or a mild allergic reaction to the product?
- Are there red, sore spots over bony prominences, indicating that these areas were not avoided?

By *questioning* the client you will find out their feelings about the treatment. Questions to ask include:
- How did that feel?
- Did you enjoy the treatment?
- Did any part of the treatment feel uncomfortable?
- Was the current/heat comfortable throughout?
- Did you understand my explanation of the treatment and was it as you expected it to be?
- Were you nervous or anxious at any time?
- Did you feel relaxed or go to sleep?
- Was the treatment even and equal on both sides?
- Did you feel that you would have liked me to spend a longer time on any area?
- Was there any area that you would prefer me to leave out next time?
- Do you feel entirely satisfied with the treatment?

△ **Figure 3.46** Evaluation of the teratment

In the workplace

Remember that time is money and your place of work may not allow any extra time between appointments for feedback and preparation of the room for the next client. Use your common sense and allocate time within the treatment.

Homecare advice

Homecare advice is very beneficial for the client, as it involves them in the treatment and encourages them to take control of their condition. It also provides a link between one treatment and the next. The advice given will obviously depend on the client's need and condition, for example:

○ After a facial, reinforce to the client the importance of following a regular skin care routine using suitable products.

○ The overweight client or a client with cellulite will need dietary advice.

○ For the tense, overworked client you may suggest that they try to reduce their workload, set aside time to rest and practise breathing and relaxation.

Each place of work will carry its own line of retail products available for the client to purchase. It is important that you familiarise yourself with the features and benefits of the range, which may include attending relevant training courses, so that you are able to advise your clients appropriately.

In the workplace

It is likely that you will earn commission from retail sales and thus increase your earning potential. It is important, however, to balance this with meeting the needs of your clients. Always act with integrity.

Retail products for the face include:

○ **Cleanser and toner**

Recommend the client uses a cleanser twice daily, morning and night. Cleanser is essential for removing daily grime, excess oil and make-up without upsetting the natural pH of the skin. Use a toner after cleansing to remove any residue, refine the pores and refresh the skin.

○ **Moisturisers**

These soften and lubricate the skin. They prevent the loss of moisture from the skin; they do *not* add moisture to the skin. The ingredients form a film over the surface of the skin preventing moisture from evaporating. Use a minimum SPF15 product.

○ **Exfoliants**

Exfoliators slough off dead skin cells from the surface of the skin to prevent the skin looking dull and lifeless. Using this product on a regular basis helps to rejuvenate the condition of the skin.

○ **Face masks**

Identify skin concerns and recommend a mask that will specifically tackle them. The mask ingredients will draw out impurities from the superficial layers of the skin, exfoliate dead skin cells and help remove congestion.

○ **Eye creams and eye masks** to moisturise, hydrate and decongest to reduce puffiness and dark circles. Know

your products: some eye creams should only be applied on the lower eye socket.

○ **Night creams** usually have high levels of active ingredients to help boost skin repair, rejuvenate and replenish the skin.

Retail products for the body include:

○ body exfoliant/scrub to help to remove dead skin cells and keep skin soft and smooth

○ body moisturising lotion to nourish and improve texture of the skin

○ body brushing/abrasive glove/loofah to increase blood circulation to the area and remove dead skin cells (particularly good for cellulite).

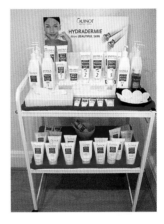

△ **Figure 3.47** Range of retail products for face and body

Homecare advice after a facial treatment

Clients should be told to avoid the following for 24 hours:

○ applying foundation or powder to the face, to allow the skin time to settle

○ self-tanning treatments, as the product may cause the skin to react

○ touching the skin after treatment unless hands are clean

○ sunbathing and sunbeds, as the skin will be more sensitive

○ heat treatments, as the skin has already been stimulated and needs time to settle

○ swimming, as the chlorine in the water may irritate the skin.

Refer to the consultation record and discuss any lifestyle changes that would help to improve the effectiveness of the treatment. Recommend a course of treatment to meet the client's short- and long-term goals.

Homecare advice after a body treatment

Clients should be told to avoid the following for 24 hours:

○ self-tanning treatments, as the product may cause the skin to react

○ sunbathing and sunbeds, as the skin will be more sensitive

○ heat treatments, as the skin has already been stimulated and needs time to settle

○ swimming, as the chlorine in the water may irritate the skin.

Also advise clients that in general, wearing tight clothing, such as tight jeans, belts or underwear, applies pressure and restricts the circulation.

Clients should use a sunblock (SPF30+) after treatments on face and on body if sunbathing.

Refer to the consultation record and discuss any lifestyle changes that would help to improve the effectiveness of the treatment. Recommend a course of treatment to meet the client's short- and long-term goals.

General homecare advice after facial and body treatments

○ Drink 6–8 glasses of water (or suitable alternatives) a day to help prevent dehydration.

○ Take time to relax before continuing with daily tasks.

○ Avoid tea and coffee for the rest of the day, as they contain caffeine.

○ Follow a light diet for the rest of the day.

○ Avoid smoking as it produces toxins in the body.

○ Avoid drinking alcohol, as it will dehydrate the body.

○ Take plenty of exercise and keep mobile during the day. If in a sedentary occupation, it is advisable to walk around, swing the legs and stretch at regular intervals.

○ Advise client of options available if you feel they need specific help from a healthcare practitioner. (This may include doctor, chiropractor, physiotherapist, osteopath.)

Relaxation

Relaxation means being free from tension and anxiety, which are normally caused by the stresses of life and upset the body balance. It is impossible to remove all the stressors in life and a certain amount of stress is desirable as it can produce feelings of excitement and aids motivation. The ability to relax is extremely important as it combats stress and reduces its harmful effects, which include fatigue, lethargy, illness and psychological problems. Clients who lead very busy lives or are coping with worries or dealing with unhappy situations may find it very difficult to relax. Advising them and showing them ways of reducing stress and promoting relaxation can form an important part of treatment. Once they have recognised the difference between the tense state and the relaxed state they can continue to practise at home.

Preparation for relaxation

The first consideration is to create the right environment to promote the relaxation response. For example; a warm, well-ventilated area; away from distracting noise; low lighting; a comfortable place to sit or lie down; relaxing music if desired.

Relaxation techniques

There are many techniques that may be used to encourage the client to relax. They may be combined for maximum effect.

The relaxation response involves the client's response to a quiet soothing environment: total concentration on a particular object while trying to let go of all tension. This is sometimes sufficient to promote the relaxed state and can be practised anywhere.

Visualisation or imagining involves visualising pleasantly soothing situations conducive to relaxation, e.g. lying on a beach, looking at a tranquil scene.

Progressive relaxation aims to develop awareness of the difference between feelings of tension and relaxation. Contraction followed by relaxation of all the muscle groups is performed, working around the body. This is a very effective method of promoting relaxation.

Progressive relaxation technique

The client should lie down somewhere comfortable. Suggest they take a few minutes to settle by closing the eyes and concentrating on the sensation of tension and relaxation. Practise breathing in deeply and letting go of tension on the out breath.

> **(L)**
> **Learning point**
> Suggest the client has a warm bath to help them relax before practising this technique.

The technique is to contract each muscle group and then to relax it, feeling the tension in the muscles float away. The relaxation (the letting go) should happen on the outward breath.

Beginning with the feet, repeat each movement three times:

○ Pull the feet up hard (dorsi-flexion), and let go.
○ Push the feet down hard (plantar flexion), and let go.
○ Push the knees down hard against the surface on which you are lying, and let go.
○ Push the leg down hard, and let go.
○ Tighten the buttock muscles hard, and let go.
○ Pull the abdominal muscles in hard, and let go.
○ Raise the shoulders, and let go.
○ Press the shoulders into the surface on which you are lying, and let go.
○ Press the arms into the surface, and let go.
○ Curl the fingers to make a fist, and let go.
○ Press the head into the surface, and let go.
○ Screw up and tighten the face, and let go.
○ Tighten all the groups together, and let go.

Best practice — B
It is a good idea to have cards showing this sequence available for the client to take away with them.

Breathing exercises

Breathing exercises are given to maintain and improve the expansion of the chest. This increases the amount of oxygen taken into the lungs and increases the amount of carbon dioxide out of the lungs. Breathing in is known as *inspiration*, and breathing out is known as *expiration*. The muscles of respiration are the external intercostal muscles and the internal intercostal muscles (which lie between the ribs) and the diaphragm, which lies horizontally, separating the thoracic cavity from the abdominal cavity. The contraction of these muscles will increase the capacity of the thorax from side to side, from front to back and longitudinally from top to bottom.

Effects of breathing exercises

Breathing exercises are very beneficial. They can:

○ improve the mobility of the thorax
○ increase the intake of the oxygen, which will improve metabolism

○ increase the output of carbon dioxide thus eliminating this waste product more quickly
○ improve the condition of the lungs
○ loosen lung secretions
○ aid venous flow: the changing pressure created in the thorax aids the flow of blood in the veins and the flow of lymph in the lymphatic vessels
○ improve posture through the increased mobility of the thorax.

Breathing technique

Position: sitting on a chair or lying supine (face up). Remove any tight restricting clothing.

Deep breathing concentrates on three areas of expansion, namely, apical, costal and diaphragmatic.

Apical breathing: place the hands on the upper chest below the clavicle, breathe in deeply through the nose and expand the chest under the hands. The chest will move up and forward as you breathe in. Then breathe out through the mouth and the chest will move back as you breathe out. Try not to allow movement in the other parts of the chest. Repeat three times.

Costal breathing: place the hands on the side of the ribs, above the waist. Breathe in deeply through the nose and feel the ribs moving out sideways. Breathe out through the mouth and the ribs will move back as you breathe out. Repeat three times.

Diaphragmatic breathing: place the hands in front, above the waist. Breathe in deeply through the nose and feel the lower chest and abdomen moving forward as you breathe in. Breathe out through the mouth and pull the abdomen back in as you breathe out. Repeat three times.

Then breathe deeply using all areas of the chest as follows: breathe in deeply through the nose, hold to count of five, then breathe out for as long as possible through the mouth. Repeat three times.

Learning point — L

Practise yourself before discussing with clients to ensure that you fully understand the movements.

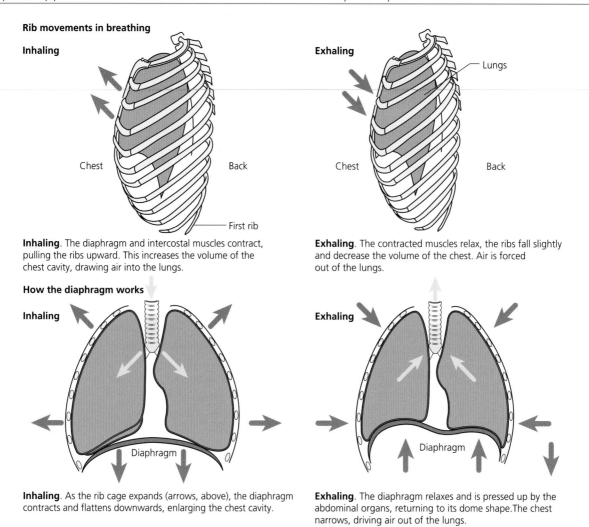

Rib movements in breathing

Inhaling

Chest   Back

First rib

Inhaling. The diaphragm and intercostal muscles contract, pulling the ribs upward. This increases the volume of the chest cavity, drawing air into the lungs.

Exhaling

Lungs

Chest   Back

Exhaling. The contracted muscles relax, the ribs fall slightly and decrease the volume of the chest. Air is forced out of the lungs.

How the diaphragm works

Inhaling

Diaphragm

Inhaling. As the rib cage expands (arrows, above), the diaphragm contracts and flattens downwards, enlarging the chest cavity.

Exhaling

Diaphragm

Exhaling. The diaphragm relaxes and is pressed up by the abdominal organs, returning to its dome shape. The chest narrows, driving air out of the lungs.

△ **Figure 3.48** The mechanism of respiration

Be aware

Deep breathing can make one feel dizzy and faint because the amount of oxygen and carbon dioxide in the body is changing and the balance between these chemicals is disturbed. If this occurs then it is important to rest for a few minutes until the feeling passes and the balance is restored. This must be explained to clients before they are encouraged to practise at home.

Home practice of posture correction

You must ensure that the client is always aware of the difference between good and poor posture. Poor posture may be the result of long-term habits. These habits must be changed through constant practice of correct positions.

Explain this to the client and give simple pointers, which they must practise as often as possible. Good posture will become automatic through constant practice.

○ Look straight ahead with the eyes level.

○ Pull the chin in, then relax into a neutral position (neither pulled in nor craned forward).

○ Feel that the crown of the head is being pulled up towards the ceiling.

○ Keep the neck straight but not tense.

○ Pull the shoulders back and down; do not hold the chest forward.

○ Hold the tummy in and tuck the tail under.

○ Balance your weight evenly through the buttocks if sitting, or through the feet when standing.

Common postural problems and corrective exercises

Kyphosis

This is an exaggerated curve of the thoracic region.

The weak, stretched muscles that require strengthening are the middle fibres of trapezius, the rhomboids and the middle part of erector spinae.

The tight muscles that require stretching are pectoralis major and the neck extensors.

Corrective exercises for kyphosis

Sitting or stride standing – gently drop the head forward pulling chin in, press the head back making a long neck and raise.

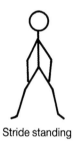

Stride standing

△ **Figure 3.49** Stride standing

Lax stoop sitting – raise the trunk gradually from the base of spine upwards.

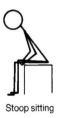

Stoop sitting

△ **Figure 3.50** Stoop sitting

Lying, arms at right angles with elbows bent – retract the shoulders pressing back of hand into the floor.

Prone lying, hands clasped behind back – keep chin in, pull shoulders back and lift head and shoulders off the floor.

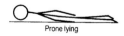

Prone lying

△ **Figure 3.51** Prone lying

Lordosis

This is an exaggerated curve of the lumbar spine, where the pelvis is tilted forwards.

The weak stretched muscles that require strengthening are:

○ the abdominals – rectus abdominus, internal oblique and external oblique
○ the hip extensors – gluteus maximus and the hamstrings.

The tight muscles that require stretching are:

○ the trunk extensors – erector spinae and quadratus lumborum
○ the hip flexors – ilio-psoas.

Corrective exercises for lordosis

Crook lying – press small of back into the floor and pull tummy in, tilting the pelvis.

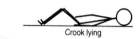

Crook lying

△ **Figure 3.52** Crook lying

Crook lying – keep chin in and raise head and shoulders to look at the knees; progress to curl up.

Prone kneeling – arch the back to stretch the lumbar spine and return to horizontal.

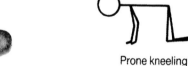

Prone kneeling

△ **Figure 3.53** Prone kneeling

Prone kneeling – keep the back straight, raise alternate legs out and up; keep knee bent.

Scoliosis

This is a lateral curvature of the spine, which may be a long **C** curve or an **S** curve.

The muscles that will require strengthening will be those on the outside of the curve. The muscles that require stretching will be those on the inside of the curve.

Corrective exercises for scoliosis

Stride standing – reach up into the air with the arm on the concave side of the curve; reach towards the floor with the other hand. Stretch, hold, relax.

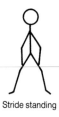

Stride standing

△ **Figure 3.54** Stride standing

Stride standing – side flex the trunk towards the convex side, where the muscles are stretched. Slide the hand down the side and return.

Prone lying – stretch the arm on the concave side up above the head along the floor; stretch the other down towards the feet. Hold and relax.

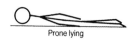

Prone lying

△ **Figure 3.55** Prone lying

Prone lying – stretch the arm on the concave side up above the head and the opposite leg down along the floor. Hold and relax.

Flat back

This is a condition where there is little or no lumbar curve and the pelvis is tilted backwards. It may be accompanied by kyphosis of the thoracic spine.

The weak stretched muscles that require strengthening are the back extensors, namely erector spinae (in some cases the abdominals and gluteus maximus are weak).

The tight muscles that require stretching are the hamstrings on the posterior thigh.

Corrective exercises for flat back

Sitting – lean forward, taking the pressure from the buttocks on to the thigh, then extend the back to create a lumbar lordosis. Hold for a count of ten, then release.

Prone lying – raise alternate legs.

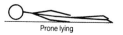

Prone lying

△ **Figure 3.56** Prone lying

Prone lying – raise both legs (this exercise is allowed for this condition).

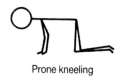

Prone kneeling

△ **Figure 3.57** Prone kneeling

Prone kneeling – arch and hollow the back.

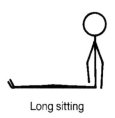

Long sitting

△ **Figure 3.58** Long sitting

Long sitting – rotate the pelvis forward, then lean backwards to arch lower back.

Evaluation of own performance

To judge how you have performed, ask yourself the following questions:

○ Did I make sure that everything was in place prior to the client's arrival? i.e. the room (to ensure a suitable, quiet environment), the couch (clean linen, towels and pillows), the trolley (neatly laid out with all commodities to hand).

○ Did I abide by the salon's health, safety and hygiene policies?

○ Did I adopt a friendly, relaxed, professional, competent manner?

○ Did I respect the client's privacy and dignity?

○ Did I observe the client's body language?

○ Did I adapt my approach to suit the type of client?

○ Did I make the client feel at ease?

○ Did I communicate well with the client; was I polite, sensitive and supportive?

○ Did I carry out a detailed client consultation and record the information and get it signed by the client?

○ Did I note all contra-indications and take the required action?

○ Did I allow the client the opportunity and time to express their needs and expectations?

○ Did I listen closely to what they were saying?

○ Did I select the most suitable treatment and set long-term goals?

○ Did I explain everything clearly to the client and did they understand my explanation?

○ Did I agree the treatment plan, cost and timing with the client and obtain their written consent?

○ Did I maintain eye contact with the client?

○ Was I aware of my own body language?

○ Did I make the client feel secure, comfortable and cared for?

○ Did I select the best possible treatment to suit the client?

○ Did I select the most suitable lubricant and make sure I did not waste any?

○ Did I wash my hands before touching the client and after treatment?

○ Did I adopt the correct posture and position to avoid strain, injury and fatigue?

○ Did I check the safety of the electrical equipment: plugs, cable, leads, terminals?

○ Did I check the current and ensure that the intensity was at zero?

○ Did I check the well-being of the client during the treatment?

○ Did I evaluate the treatment outcomes?

○ Did I offer homecare advice?

○ Did I discuss retail products to suit the client's needs?

○ Did I review the treatment plan with the client?

○ Did I keep within the time constraints for a viable cost-effective treatment?

○ Did I dispose of all waste into a lined bin with a lid?

○ Did I clean the treatment area and leave it tidy?

EVALUATION OF OWN PERFORMANCE

Name:

Date:

Think about each question carefully and assess how well you think you did and then score each one as follows:

RED   Needs improving

AMBER   Average/OK

GREEN   Good

Questions	RED	AMBER	GREEN	Comments

This exercise will also help you to prepare for your assessments, as it demonstrates pointers to successful performance.

Learning point (L)

Although this may seem to be a very long list of questions, they should become second nature to you during training, so that this thorough self-evaluation is automatic.

Activity (A)

Carry out facial and body treatments on clients. Complete an evaluation of your performance using the questions above and the traffic light system.

QUESTIONS

Multiple-choice questions

1. Public Liability Insurance covers you if:
   a one of your employees is injured on your premises
   b an employee fails to notify you of a health and safety hazard
   c a client has an accident on your premises
   d a client becomes ill on your premises.

2. Too much carbon dioxide in the atmosphere can cause the client to feel:
   a lethargic
   b relaxed
   c alert
   d energised.

3. The most suitable lighting in the treatment room for a facial is:
   a bright and welcoming
   b soft and diffused
   c subtle and intimate
   d natural lighting only.

4. The Data Protection Act 1998 requires you to:
   a pass specific details of your business to the local authority
   b store the client's details on a computer for safety
   c protect clients' personal details from being disclosed
   d give details of your client base to a third party.

5. Which of the following is a closed question?
   a What is your daily routine?
   b Have you visited your doctor recently?
   c Why did you choose that particular treatment?
   d How do you cope with stress?

6. Smoking can cause high levels of which substance in the blood?
   a Oxygen.
   b Carbon monoxide.
   c Hydroxyl ions.
   d Carbon dioxide.

7. The acid mantle is made up of:
   a sebum and sweat
   b sweat and dead skin cells
   c bacteria and sebum
   d dead skin cells and moisture.

8. A greasy skin type is due to:
   a sunbathing
   b crash diets
   c hormone imbalance
   d smoking.

9. A protein found in the dermis is:
   a keratin
   b histamine
   c sebum
   d elastin.

10. A person described as an ectomorph will be:
    a tall and long limbed, with fat deposits around the hips
    b slim and slightly muscular
    c curvaceous with small hands and feet
    d muscular with broad shoulders and slim hips.

11. During a postural assessment you note the client has winged scapulae. This indicates a weakness of:
    a serratus anterior
    b erector spinae
    c rhomboids
    d upper fibres of the trapezius.

12. If the client has lordosis, the tight muscles that require stretching are:
    a rectus abdominus and the hamstrings
    b erector spinae and quadratus lumborum
    c gluteus maximus and the hamstrings
    d ilio psoas and rectus abdominus.

13. The adductor muscles are found on the:
    a medial aspect of the thigh
    b anterior aspect of the thigh
    c lateral aspect of the thigh
    d posterior aspect of the thigh.

14. Which of the following is the result of a contra-action to treatment?

    a High blood pressure.

    b Cuts and abrasions.

    c Burns.

    d Scabies.

15. A tactile test is to test sensitivity to:

    a hot and cold

    b a product

    c ultraviolet radiation

    d sharp and soft.

16. The purpose of a moisturiser is to:

    a prevent the loss of moisture from the skin

    b add moisture to the skin

    c remove dead cells from the skin's surface

    d help draw out impurities.

17. During the consultation you notice the client has the condition scabies. What should you do?

    a Ignore the problem and continue with the treatment, as you will be working on the facial area.

    b Highlight the problem to the client but continue with the treatment to avoid upsetting them.

    c Ask the client to leave, as the condition is contagious, and to rebook when it has cleared.

    d Advise the client tactfully to seek medical advice before you can continue with treatment.

18. Which of the following conditions is recognised by a taut and itchy skin with superficial flaking?

    a Sensitive skin.

    b Dehydrated skin.

    c Moist skin.

    d Oedematous skin.

19. To calculate the client's Body Mass Index you need to know their weight and:

    a distribution of fat

    b body type

    c type of fat

    d height.

20. It is important the client signs the consultation record to confirm they agree to:

    a the conditions under the Data Protection Act 1998

    b attend the appointments or pay the cancellation fee

    c and understand the details discussed and recorded

    d pay at the end of the treatment.

Section 3: Underpinning science

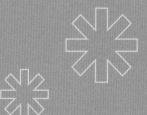

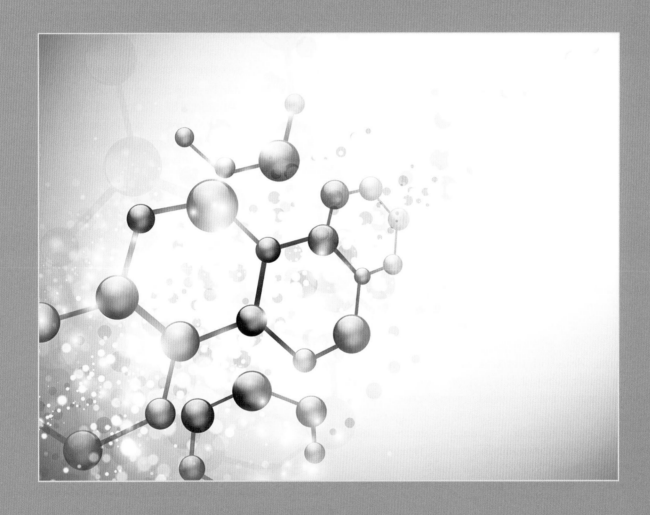

4 Basic science

Objectives

After you have studied this chapter you will be able to:

▮ list the three states of matter

▮ differentiate between an element and a compound

▮ describe the structure of an atom

▮ discuss the formation of **ions** and explain the terms **cation** and **anion**

▮ describe the flow of electrons through a conductor

▮ differentiate between conductors and non-conductors (insulators)

▮ explain the following electrical units: amps; ohms; volts; watts

▮ distinguish between closed circuit, open circuit and short circuit

▮ explain how the following devices modify current: transformer; rectifier; capacitor.

This chapter deals with the basic science that is relevant to you as a beauty therapist. It is suggested that all students study this chapter before embarking on electrical treatments as it provides background knowledge of atoms, ions, basic electricity, conductors, electrical units, Ohm's law, devices for modifying current, types of current and circuits. Where relevant, further scientific theory is to be found at the beginning of each chapter.

States of matter

Everything around us is composed of matter and all matter is made up of small particles called atoms. Matter can exist in any one of three states depending on temperature and pressure. The three states of matter are:

○ solid

○ liquid

○ gas.

In the solid state, the particles are tightly packed and regularly arranged and move or vibrate only slightly; solids are very dense. In the liquid state, the particles are more widely spaced and move more freely; liquids are usually less dense than solids. In the gaseous state, the particles are very widely spaced and move at high speed; gases have a lower density than liquids and solids.

If a solid is heated beyond its melting point it will form a liquid, and if a liquid is heated beyond its boiling point it will form a gas. The converse is also true: if a gas is cooled it will condense to form a liquid, and if a liquid is cooled it will form a solid.

Solid   Liquid   Gas

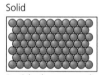 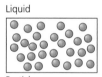 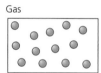

Particles have a regular pattern, are close together, they move slightly and have high density   Particles are more widely spaced, move more freely and have a medium density   Particles are widely spaced, move randomly at high speed and have a low density

△ **Figure 4.1** Particles in a solid, liquid and gas

Remember

Matter can exist as a solid, liquid or gas, depending on temperature and pressure.

Elements

Matter is made up of chemical **elements** and their various compounds. An element is a substance in its simplest form that cannot be further broken down by chemical reaction.

There are 118 known elements, and about 91 of these occur naturally. At room temperature and pressure, most elements are solid and metallic (e.g. copper, iron); some are liquid (e.g. mercury, bromine) and some are gases (e.g. hydrogen, oxygen). A compound is formed when two or more elements combine and react together.

▽ **Table 4.1** Common elements

Metal	Non-metal
Copper	Oxygen
Iron	Nitrogen
Zinc	Carbon
Sodium	Chlorine
Potassium	Sulphur
Calcium	

Compounds

Elements can combine and react together to form **compounds**. The properties of the compound will be different from the properties of the individual elements from which it is made, for example, the elements hydrogen and oxygen react to form the compound water.

Each element can be represented in shorthand by a symbol usually made up of one or two letters, for example:

Hydrogen: H   Calcium: Ca
Oxygen: O   Chlorine: Cl
Potassium: K   Sodium: Na

When two elements join together to form a compound, the symbols are combined, for example:

Sodium + chlorine gives the compound Sodium chloride. This can be represented by:

$$Na^+ + Cl^- \rightarrow NaCl$$

Atomic structure

Elements are made up of atoms. An atom is the smallest part of an element that retains its distinct chemical properties and that can take part in a chemical reaction. Atoms are made up of even smaller particles called sub-atomic particles, the main ones being protons, electrons and neutrons.

Remember

An atom is the smallest part of an element that can take part in a chemical reaction.

Two of these subatomic particles carry an electrical charge:

○ protons have a positive charge
○ electrons have a negative charge
○ neutrons have no charge, that is, they are neutral.

All the atoms of one element are identical and contain the same numbers of these particles (e.g. all atoms of helium have two electrons, two protons and two neutrons). Atoms of different elements have different numbers of particles. The arrangement of these particles in an atom follows a definite pattern.

In each atom the protons and neutrons are tightly packed together in the nucleus of the atom. The electrons orbit around the nucleus in distinct energy levels or electron shells.

Learning point

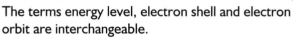

The terms energy level, electron shell and electron orbit are interchangeable.

Each orbit or energy level is capable of holding only a certain number of electrons:

○ The first level (electron shell) holds up to two electrons maximum but can hold less.
○ The second level (electron shell) holds up to eight electrons maximum but can hold less.
○ The third level (electron shell) holds up to eight electrons maximum but can hold less.
○ Further energy levels hold progressively larger numbers.

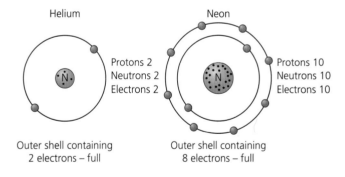

△ **Figure 4.2** Stable atoms

Learning point

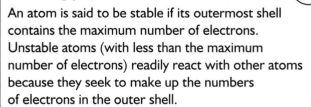

An atom is said to be stable if its outermost shell contains the maximum number of electrons. Unstable atoms (with less than the maximum number of electrons) readily react with other atoms because they seek to make up the numbers of electrons in the outer shell.

Remember

Protons have a + charge; Electrons have a – charge; Neutrons have no charge.

Because opposite charges attract each other, the negatively charged electrons are held in their electron shells by the positive charge of the protons in the nucleus. In every atom the number of positively charged protons is equal to the number of negatively charged electrons, therefore the atom has no overall charge: it is electrically neutral.

Learning point Ⓛ

The atom is always neutral because the number of protons in the nucleus is equal to the number of electrons orbiting around the nucleus.

The arrangement of particles in an atom of oxygen

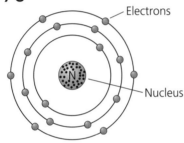

Electrons

Nucleus

The Nucleus contains 16 protons and 16 neutrons tightly packed together. The 16 electrons move rapidly around the nucleus at distinct energy levels

△ **Figure 4.3** Arrangements of particles in an atom of oxygen

○ First level has two electrons therefore is full.
○ Second level has eight electrons therefore is full.
○ Third level has six electrons therefore is not full (it could hold eight).

Atoms like this, containing fewer than the maximum number of electrons in their outer shell are said to be unstable and therefore more reactive. Atoms with the maximum number of electrons in their outer shell are said to be stable. They do not readily react with other elements, for example:

○ Helium (He) has two protons, two neutrons and two electrons.
○ Neon (Ne) has ten protons, ten neutrons and ten electrons.

Atoms of different elements combine by chemical reactions to form compounds.

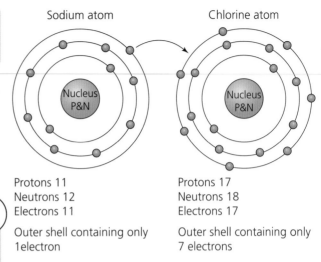

Sodium atom   Chlorine atom

Nucleus P&N   Nucleus P&N

Protons 11   Protons 17
Neutrons 12   Neutrons 18
Electrons 11   Electrons 17

Outer shell containing only 1 electron   Outer shell containing only 7 electrons

△ **Figure 4.4** Reactive atoms

Reactive atoms (see Figure 4.4) have a great 'desire' to have the maximum number of electrons in their outer shell. In order to achieve a stable electron pattern, they are able to gain or lose electrons by reacting with other elements to form compounds. The sodium atom has one electron in its outer shell; it needs to lose this to attain a stable electron pattern of eight in the outer shell. The chlorine atom has seven electrons in its outer shell; it needs to gain an electron to give the maximum eight electrons in its outer shell. Sodium and chlorine will therefore readily react together – sodium giving an electron and chlorine receiving an electron. The compound thus formed will be sodium chloride:

$$Na^+ + Cl^- \rightarrow NaCl$$

Ions

When an atom gains or loses an electron from its outer shell it becomes a charged particle called an ion.

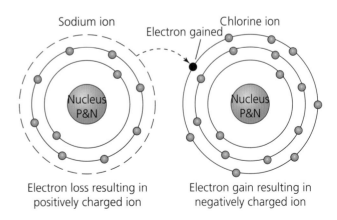

Sodium ion   Chlorine ion
Electron gained

Nucleus P&N   Nucleus P&N

Electron loss resulting in positively charged ion   Electron gain resulting in negatively charged ion

△ **Figure 4.5** Ions

When the sodium atom loses its electron (negative charge) from the outer shell, it will have one more proton (positive charge) than electrons and will therefore have a positive charge. Having lost an electron, it will be called an **ion**. A positively charged ion is called a **cation** (+).

When the chlorine atom gains an electron (negative), it will have one more electron than protons, so will have a negative charge. Having gained an electron, it will be called an ion. A negatively charged ion is called an **anion** (−).

Remember

Cations are positively charged (+). Anions are negatively charged (−).

When an atom gains or loses electrons it becomes a charged particle called an ion.

○ If an atom loses electrons it becomes a positively charged ion called a cation.

○ If an atom gains electrons it becomes a **negatively charged** ion called an **anion**.

Ions react with each other according to definite laws:

○ Ions with the same charge repel (move away from each other).

○ Ions with the opposite charge will attract (move towards each other).

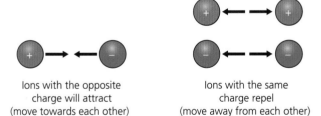

Ions with the opposite charge will attract (move towards each other)

Ions with the same charge repel (move away from each other)

△ **Figure 4.6** Ions react with each other according to definite laws

Learning point (L)

Remember this as it is the fundamental principle on which some galvanic treatments work.

Electricity

Electricity is the movement of electrons from one atom to another. It may be static or dynamic. Electricity can be produced in three ways:

○ Static electricity produced by friction.

○ Current or dynamic electricity produced by chemical reactions.

○ Current or dynamic electricity produced by magnetic fields (electro-magnetic induction).

Static electricity

Certain substances when rubbed together produce electrical charges, or static electricity. The electrons from one material can be transferred to the other material. The material losing electrons becomes positively charged, while the one gaining electrons becomes negatively charged.

Remember

These charges obey certain laws of physics: like charges repel each other, while opposite charges attract each other.

This can be demonstrated when brushing hair. The friction of brushing removes electrons from the atoms of the hair. These electrons collect on the brush, giving it a negative charge. Loss of electrons leave the hair with a positive charge. Since like charges repel and opposite charges attract, the hairs will fly apart, but will be attracted to the brush. Small crackling noises will be heard and sparks seen in the dark as energy is released.

Current electricity

An electric current is a flow of free electrons through a material called a **conductor**, such as a wire. It flows from an area of excess of electrons to an area of deficiency. In order to achieve current flow an electric force must exist between the two ends of the conductor. This is known as potential difference (PD) and is measured in volts.

Some materials, such as metals, are good conductors of electrical charge. This is because the electrons in their outer shell are weakly held to their atoms and can easily be made to flow through the material.

Remember

Electric current flows from an area of excess of electrons to an area of deficiency.

In other materials, the electrons are firmly held to their atoms, are reluctant to be detached and cannot be made to flow through the material. These are known as non-conductors or insulators. All materials offer some resistance or impedance to the flow of current.

▽ **Table 4.2** Examples of conductors and insulators

Conductors	Insulators
Copper	Rubber
Zinc	Plastic
Carbon	Glass
Brass	Dry wood
Good conductors are materials whose electrons are weakly held to their atoms and can easily be made to flow through the material.	
Insulators have electrons that are firmly held to their atoms and cannot flow through the material.	

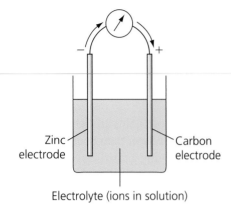

△ **Figure 4.7** A simple cell

As previously stated, the flow of electrons through the conductor requires a potential difference (PD) to exist between the ends of the wire. The greater the PD, the greater the intensity of the current. This current can be generated by chemical reactions, such as in batteries or cells; or by using magnetic fields in generators (mains electricity).

Production of electricity by chemical reaction

A simple cell or battery is a means of converting chemical energy into electrical energy. It produces *direct current*. When two different elements (usually metals) called electrodes, which are connected by a wire, are immersed in a chemical called an electrolyte, an electric current is produced. The electrolyte is a chemical compound, which dissociates (splits) into ions when dissolved in water. These ions move towards or away from the electrodes, depending upon their charge.

One electrode becomes negatively charged, having an excess of electrons; the other becomes positively charged, having a deficiency of electrons. This is called polarity. Electrons will flow through the wire from the negative electrode to the positive electrode. This flow of electrons will continue until all the chemicals in the electrolyte are used up, at which time the current flow will stop.

Dry cell batteries, being easily transportable, are now widely used to power radios, torches and portable beauty therapy equipment.

The principle of how they work is the same as described above, but their construction is different. The electrolyte is a paste contained within a zinc electrode casing; the carbon rod electrode is placed down the centre. As the chemicals are used up, the battery becomes 'flat' and is disposed of.

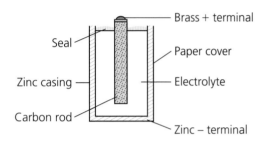

△ **Figure 4.8** Structure of a dry battery

Rechargeable batteries are available, which may be recharged by connecting them to a mains-powered battery charger. They are usually left on overnight to recharge and can then be reused when required.

The type of current produced by cells and batteries always flows in the same direction and is called direct current (DC) or constant current.

Production of electricity by electro-magnetic induction

The electricity that we obtain from the mains is produced by a dynamo or generator in large power stations. It is produced using magnetism. When a coil of wire is rotated between the north and south poles of a magnet, it cuts through the magnetic lines of force or the magnetic field and an electromagnetic force (EMF) is produced in the coil, causing electrons to flow through the wire. An EMF can also be induced by moving a magnet through a coil of wire.

Each power station will have a number of these generators for producing electricity. The long coils of wire are rotated by water power or by steam from boilers heated by coal, oil or nuclear energy. Each coil of wire is rotated at speed between the poles of a large magnet.

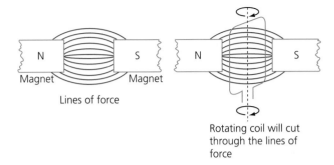

Figure 4.9 Rotating coil cutting through lines of force

As the coil rotates, it cuts through the lines of force each half revolution, and this produces what is known as an alternating current (AC). Beginning at zero, the current rises to a maximum positive value, falls to zero and then rises to a maximum negative value and returns to zero with each revolution.

One complete revolution is known as a cycle. Half the cycle will rise to maximum positive and half to maximum negative. The number of these cycles produced per second is known as the frequency of the current. Frequency is measured in **hertz** (Hz).

The frequency of the mains supply in the UK is 50 Hz (i.e. 50 cycles of current flow every second when current is switched on at the mains).The mains voltage in the UK is 240 volts. Mains voltage varies from country to country.

Units of electricity

○ The units of measurement associated with electricity are volts, amps, ohms, Hz and watts.

○ Volts are the units of measurement of the potential difference (PD). This is the pressure or force required to drive a current around a circuit. It is often referred to as the voltage and is measured by a voltmeter.

○ Amps are the units of measurement of the intensity of the current (or rate of flow). The intensity of a current is the number of electrons passing one point in one secon.d. Intensity is measured by an ammeter.

○ Ohms are the units of measurement of resistance. The intensity of the current is dependent on Potential Difference and the resistance offered to the current by the conductor.

The relationship between current flow (amps), potential difference (volts) and resistance (ohms) is expressed by Ohm's law.

Learning point

Ohm's law states that the current flowing through a circuit varies in direct proportion to the potential difference and in inverse proportion to the resistance. That is:

$$\text{current (amps)} = \frac{\text{potential difference (volts)}}{\text{resistance (ohms)}}$$

$$I = \frac{V}{R}$$

○ Hertz (Hz) are the units of measurement of frequency and apply to alternating current (AC). Frequency is the number of cycles per second (see Figures 4.10 and 4.11).

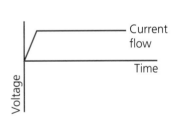

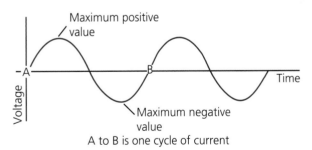

Direct current

Alternating current

Figure 4.10 Direct current and alternating current

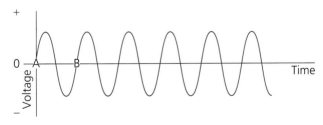

Figure 4.11 AC high frequency

○ Watts are the units of measurement of the power used when running electrical equipment and can be calculated by multiplying the intensity of current by the potential difference:

$$Watts = amps \times volts$$

Cost of electricity

The power of an appliance and the time for which it is used determines the amount of electricity used by that appliance. This quantity is measured in kilowatt-hours (kWh).

A kilowatt is 1000 watts. A kW appliance running for 1 hour uses 1 kilowatt-hour.

Electricity suppliers charge a fixed amount for each kilowatt-hour, which are known as units of electricity used. The number of units used by a house or business is registered on an electric meter that forms part of the mains circuit. Older meters consist of four dials that register thousands, hundreds, tens and units, but the more modern meters have a digital display showing the number of units used.

The cost of electricity is calculated by reading the meter and multiplying the number of units used by the cost per unit:

Cost of electricity = number of units × cost per unit (number of kilowatt hours)

Circuits

The pathway taken by an electric current is known as a circuit. In order for the current to flow, this pathway must be complete from one terminal of the electrical source to the other. If it is broken, the current flow will stop.

A **closed circuit** is an unbroken pathway between the negative and positive terminals of an electrical source. The current flows continuously in a closed circuit.

An **open circuit** is a pathway that is broken or interrupted by a switch or other device. This breaks the connection and stops the flow of current.

A short circuit occurs when the current does not pass around its designated course but takes a short cut through a path of least resistance, for example, across a break in insulation.

Components or devices used in circuits to modify (change) currents

Most beauty therapy equipment requires direct current. Batteries do not supply direct current (DC) at a high enough voltage for all treatment purposes, therefore mains current (Alternating Current – AC) is used and needs to be modified to become direct current. Machines have these components built into them.

Rectifier

A rectifier is a device for changing alternating current to direct current. This process is called rectification and is used in galvanic machines.

Transformer

A transformer is a device for altering the voltage in alternating current circuits. The voltage may be increased using a step-up transformer or the voltage may be decreased using a step-down transformer. It is used in galvanic machines.

Capacitor or condenser

A capacitor is a device that stores electrical charge and discharges it when required. It is used to smooth the impulse pattern after rectification. It is used in galvanic machines.

Rheostat or variable resistance

A rheostat is a device used to control the amount of current flowing through a circuit. It varies the resistance: the higher the resistance, the weaker the current. This is used in wax pots to control the temperature for melting the wax and in lamps to control the intensity of light.

Potentiometer

A potentiometer is a device for varying the voltage in a circuit. It is used in constant current galvanic machines to control the current during galvanic treatments.

Starter or switch

A switch or starter is a device for switching on a current; that is, starting the flow of electrons. When the client is correctly attached to the apparatus, closing the switch completes the circuit and the current will flow. When the switch is open, the circuit is broken and the current stops.

Electricity supply

Electricity is generated in large power stations at 11,000 volts. It is more efficient to transmit electricity at even higher voltages, and transformers are used to step up the voltage to 400,000 volts. This is transmitted to substations by high-voltage cables suspended on pylons, or in more urban areas, buried underground. At the substations more transformers are used to step down the voltage to suit industrial requirements (e.g. factories) and to supply private homes and businesses with a voltage of 240 volts.

▽ **Table 4.3** Devices used in circuits to modify currents

Device	Function	Effect
Transformer	Alters the voltage	Step up or step down
Rectifier	Changes AC to DC	Half wave or full wave
Capacitor	Stores electrical charge and discharges it as required	Smooths the impulse pattern
Rheostat	Controls the amount of current flowing through a circuit	Can increase or decrease the current
Potentiometer	Varies the voltage in a circuit	Current increases as voltage increases
Switch	Turns the current on or off	Makes or breaks the circuit

Mains circuit

Electricity is supplied to the home via a cable that contains two wires – one live and one neutral – which is earthed at the substation. The mains cable enters the house and passes to a sealed box where the live wire is connected to a fuse. This box can only be opened by engineers from the Electricity Board, who must investigate any faults if the fuse should 'blow'.

The mains cable then enters the meter, which registers all the units of electricity used over a period of time. It then enters the fuse box called the consumer unit. This box contains the master switch, fuses and circuit-breakers for the ring circuit, lighting circuit and others, such as for the immersion heater or cooker. If a fault develops within a circuit, the connected fuse will blow and the current flow will stop. This prevents the wire from overheating and causing fires.

Each appliance is connected to the mains circuit sockets by a flex and a plug. This plug also contains a fuse, which is designed to blow if there is electrical overload or if an appliance develops an electrical fault. When this fuse breaks the circuit, the appliance is effectively disconnected from the mains, but other appliances are not affected.

Fuses

A fuse is a safety device to stop the flow of electricity. It is the weakest point in a circuit. Fuses are found in the consumer unit (fuse box) and in the plugs that connect appliances to the mains. If a circuit is overloaded, or if the wiring or the appliance is faulty, the fuse will blow – the wire melts, breaks the circuit and the flow of electricity stops.

Cartridge fuses

These are made of short lengths of tinned copper embedded in sand and contained in a small porcelain or glass tube. The wire is attached to metal caps at each end of the tube. In the fuse box the cartridge is housed in a metal or plastic holder. They are colour coded to indicate the current rating.

Plug fuses

These are cartridge-type fuses that are fitted on to the live wire in the plug and are designed to protect the appliance. Plug cartridge fuses are all the same size but they have three different current ratings:

○ 3A rating for use with appliances up to 700 watts.
○ 5A rating for use with appliances between 700 and 1000 watts.
○ 13A rating for use with appliances between 1000 and 3000 watts.

Under the Consumer Protection Act, all new machines are supplied with a plug and correctly rated fuse. Only a person who is qualified or who has attended an appropriate course can change a plug or a fuse.

Circuit-breakers

These are modern devices designed to break the circuit if a fault is present. They may be trip switches or buttons that are designed to switch to the 'off' or 'open position' if the circuit is overloaded or faulty. The circuit-breaker can easily be reset after the fault has been found and repaired. This is done by pushing the button or moving the switch.

> **Remember**
>
> Fuses/circuit-breakers are designed to break the circuit and stop the flow of current. They are safety devices to protect the user from shock and to protect the equipment.

Sockets

In order to provide the appliance with electricity, the plug must be pushed firmly into the socket and switched on. The socket has three rectangular holes and a switch; the live and neutral holes have shutters. The earth pin on the plug is longer than the other pins – as this is pushed in the shutters move and the other pins can be pushed home. This is a safety device to prevent young children putting fingers or other articles into the live and neutral holes and receiving a shock, which could prove to be fatal.

Electrolysis

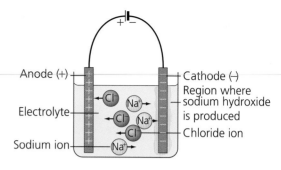

△ **Figure 4.12** Electrolysis of sodium chloride solution

Learning point

Electrolysis in this context refers to the process of passing a current through a solution, called an electrolyte, via electrodes. In beauty therapy you will also come across the term in the context of hair removal.

Electrolysis involves the passage of direct current through a solution, which results in the production of certain chemical reactions. Some chemical compounds dissolve in water to form a solution. When the compounds dissolve, they dissociate (i.e. split) into ions; either cations (+) or anions (−). These ions increase the conductivity of the solution enabling an electric current to flow easily (a solution that conducts a current is called an electrolyte).

If direct current is made to flow through such a solution, the ions will move towards the electrode with the opposite charge because like charges repel and opposite charges attract.

○ The negatively charged electrode is called the **cathode**.
○ The positively charged electrode is called the **anode**.

When the current is switched on, opposite charges will attract, therefore:

○ The cations (+) will move towards the cathode (−).
○ The anions (−) will move towards the anode (+).

The chemical reactions at these electrodes will depend upon the chemical composition of the electrolyte and the electrodes.

Remember

An electrolyte is a chemical compound that dissociates (splits) into ions and can carry an electric current.

Electrical currents used in beauty therapy
Galvanic current

A direct current is used in galvanic treatments. The direct current flows in one direction only and has polarity. When the current is flowing, one electrode will always be negatively charged (the cathode); the other will be positively charged (the anode). The treatments using direct current are:

○ facial treatments – disincrustation and iontophoresis
○ body treatments – body galvanic (iontophoresis).

High-frequency current

This is a high-frequency alternating current of around 250,000Hz used to improve the condition of the skin. There are two methods of application:

○ the direct method
○ the indirect method (or 'Viennese massage').

Muscle-stimulating currents

An interrupted direct current is usually used to produce currents of sufficient intensity and duration to stimulate motor nerves and produce contraction of muscles. The current may be modified low-frequency alternating current or more usually, modified direct current. A variety of pulses can be produced – these are arranged in 'trains' with rest periods in between. When the current flows, the muscle contracts; when the current stops, the muscle relaxes – this simulates normal movement.

Micro-currents

These are very low amperage modified direct current measured in microamps:

1 amp = 1000 milliamps
1 milliamp = 1000 microamps

These currents produce similar effects to galvanic treatment and also can be modified to produce muscle contraction.

Safety considerations when using electrical equipment

○ Always buy equipment from a reputable dealer, who can provide a good, reliable backup service.

○ Ensure that all equipment is regularly maintained and in good working order.

○ Ensure that insulation is sound, with no breaks or worn patches.

○ Ensure that all connections, such as leads, terminals and plugs, are sound and secure.

○ Have fuses replaced when necessary, by a qualified electrician. If a fuse blows repeatedly seek advice from electrician.

○ Do not overload the circuit by using multiple electrical sockets.

○ Keep electrical equipment away from water. Take particular care if pads have to be moistened with water, and do not allow water to drip over the machine.

○ Do not touch electrical equipment or leads, plugs, etc., with wet hands.

○ Make sure the equipment is stable and not in a position where it may easily be pushed or topple over.

○ Ensure that flexes do not trail over the working area.

○ Always test the current on yourself before applying it to the client.

○ Cover equipment when not in use to keep free from dust.

Remove any faulty equipment from the working area and label it clearly: FAULTY – DO NOT USE.

SUMMARY

States of matter

- The three states of matter are: **solid**, **liquid** and **gas**.
- All matter can exist in any one of these states, depending upon temperature and pressure.
- Differences between the three states of matter:
  - Solid – particles are tightly packed, move very slightly, very dense (e.g. ice).
  - Liquid – particles more widely spaced, move more freely, medium density (e.g. water).
  - Gas – particles widely spaced, move randomly at high speed, low density (e.g. steam).

Elements

- Matter is made up of chemical elements.
- An **element** is a substance in its simplest form – it cannot be further broken down by chemical reaction.
- There are 118 known elements.
- Examples include oxygen, carbon, copper, iron.

Compounds

- A **compound** is formed when elements react and combine together to form a new substance.

Atoms

- An **atom** is the smallest part of an element that retains its distinct chemical properties and which can take part in a chemical reaction.
- An atom has a nucleus containing protons with a positive charge, and neutrons with no charge. Electrons with a negative charge orbit around the nucleus at different energy levels.
- The atom is neutral (it has no charge) because it has an equal number of protons (+) and electrons (–).

Definitions

- **Protons** are **positively** charged, found in the nucleus of an atom.
- **Neutrons** are **neutral** (i.e. have no charge), found in the nucleus of an atom.
- **Electrons** are **negatively** charged, found orbiting the nucleus at different energy levels. There are up to two electrons in the first level, and up to eight in the second and third levels, etc.
- All the atoms of an element are identical, having the same number of neutrons, protons and electrons.
- Elements are different from each other because of the different numbers of protons, electrons and neutrons in their atoms.

Ions

- When atoms gain or lose electrons from their outer shell/energy level, they become ions.
- If an atom **loses** electrons, it becomes a **positively** charged ion called a **cation**.
- If an atom **gains** electrons, it becomes a **negatively** charged ion called an **anion**.

Electricity

- Electricity is the movement of electrons from one atom to another. It may be static electricity, or it may be made to move through a conductor (known as dynamic or current electricity).
- When rubbed together, substances produce static electricity, because electrons pass from one to the other.
- Dynamic electricity is produced chemically by cells and batteries, or it may be produced by magnetic fields in generators.

Current electricity

- An **electric current** is a **flow** of free electrons through a material called a **conductor**, from an area where electrons are in excess to an area deficient in electrons.
- The amount of current flowing is measured in amps.

Potential difference (PD)

- This is the force required to achieve a flow of electricity through a conductor.
- Known as **voltage**, it is measured in **volts**.

Resistance

- All conductors have a tendency to resist the flow of electrons.
- Electrical **resistance** is measured in **ohms**.
- The intensity of current flowing in a circuit depends on the voltage and the resistance to the current.
- The relationship between current flow (amps), potential difference (volts) and resistance (ohms) is expressed by Ohm's law.

Ohm's law

- This states that the current flowing through a circuit varies in direct proportion to the potential difference and in inverse proportion to the resistance.

$$I = \frac{V}{R}$$

- When the voltage increases the current increases, when the resistance increases the current decreases.

Power

- The unit of power is the watt:
  watts = amps × volts

Direct current

- Cells and batteries produce direct current (DC).
- Direct current flows in one direction only, without variation. It has polarity. One electrode will be negatively charged (the cathode) and the other will be positively charged (the anode).

Alternating current

- Generators produce alternating current (AC).
- Beginning at zero, the current rises to maximum positive value, falls to zero and then rises to maximum negative value and returns to zero. This is one cycle.
- The number of cycles per second is the frequency and is measured in hertz (Hz).
- The frequency of the UK mains is 50 Hz.
- Alternating current from the mains can be modified to provide the direct current necessary for some treatments.

Devices for modifying current

- A *transformer* changes voltage in AC circuits. It may be a step-up transformer for increasing voltage, or a step-down transformer for decreasing voltage.
- A *rectifier* changes AC to DC, it may be a half wave rectifier or full wave rectifier.
- A *capacitor* or condenser stores electrical charge and discharges it when required.
- A *rheostat* or variable resistance varies the current flowing in a circuit. It varies the resistance – the higher the resistance the weaker the current.
- A *potentiometer* varies the voltage in the circuit. It may increase the voltage thus increasing current flow or it may decrease the voltage thus reducing current flow.

Fuses

- A fuse is designed to be the weakest point in the circuit.
- It is a safety device to stop the flow of current should the circuit or appliance be faulty.

Multiple-choice questions

1. In which state are the particles that make up matter tightly packed, regularly arranged and only able to move slightly?

   a Liquid.

   b Solid.

   c Gas.

   d All of the above.

2. Which of the following statements is correct?

   a Protons are positively charged; neutrons are negatively charged.

   b Protons are negatively charged; electrons are positively charged.

   c Protons are positively charged; electrons are negatively charged.

   d Protons are positively charged; electrons have no charge.

3. The nucleus of an atom contains:

   a protons and neutrons

   b electrons and neutrons

   c protons and electrons

   d protons, electrons and neutrons.

4. Negatively charged ions called anions are formed when:

   a an atom loses an electron

   b an atom gains an electron

   c an atom loses a proton

   d an atom loses a neutron.

5. A chemical compound which dissociates (splits) into ions when dissolved in water is called:

   a an electrode

   b an anode

   c a cathode

   d an electrolyte.

6. What is the correct relationship between current, voltage and resistance?

   a Current = Voltage × Resistance.

   b Resistance = Voltage × Current.

   c Voltage = Current × Resistance.

   d Voltage = Current ÷ Resistance.

7. A device for converting an alternating current to a direct current is called a:

   a rectifier

   b transformer

   c potentiometer

   d capacitor.

8. A rheostat:

   a varies the voltage in a circuit

   b turns the current on or off

   c stores electrical charge

   d controls the amount of current flowing through a circuit.

9. What type of current is used in galvanic treatments?

   a Alternating current.

   b High frequency current.

   c Direct current.

   d Mains current.

10. Mains electricity is supplied to homes and businesses at:

    a 12v

    b 110v

    c 150v

    d 240v.

Section 4: Treatments

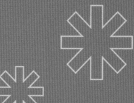

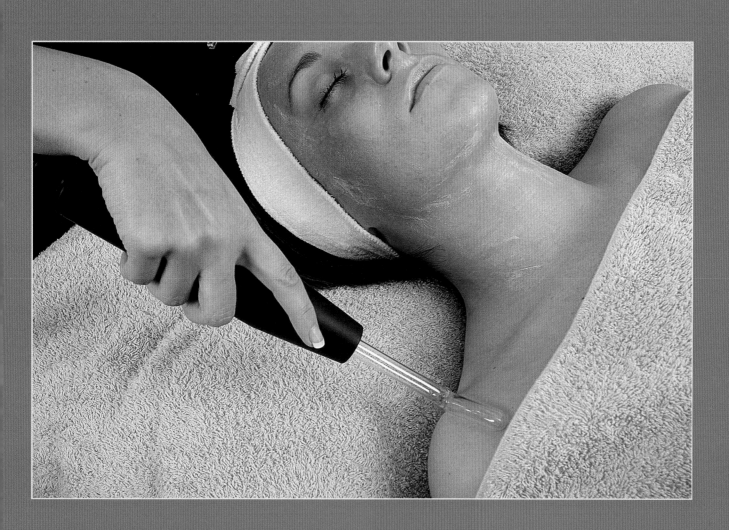

5 High frequency treatment to the face

Objectives

After you have studied this chapter you will be able to:

▮ identify the terminals on the machine

▮ describe the type of current used

▮ identify the electrodes used for each method of application

▮ describe the benefits and effects of high frequency treatments

▮ explain the contra-indications to high frequency treatments

▮ explain the dangers and precautions to high frequency treatments

▮ explain the contra-actions that may occur during and/or after treatment and the appropriate action to take

▮ carry out high frequency treatments, paying due consideration to maximum efficiency, comfort, safety and hygiene.

High frequency equipment

Figure 5.1 is a photograph of a high frequency machine and the electrodes used to deliver the current to the client. As its name implies, this machine uses a high frequency current.

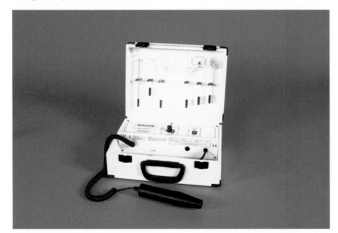

△ **Figure 5.1** High frequency machine

Remember

A current that alternates at over 100,000 cycles per second is known as high frequency.

The high frequency output of these machines is an alternating current of around 250,000 Hz at a high voltage but low current flow. This alternating current will not stimulate muscle contraction because the duration of the pulses is too short. It passes easily through the skin to produce heating effects. High frequency is used for its thermal effects.

Remember

High frequency machines contain a capacitor: this device helps to level out any unevenness in the electric current.

Machines producing high frequency currents require only two controls: an on/off switch and an intensity control. The current is delivered to the client by means of one electrode. Different electrodes are used for the following two methods of application:

○ the direct method

○ the indirect method ('Viennese massage').

These two methods have different effects on the tissues and must be selected carefully to suit the client. They are primarily used on the face but may also be used on the body – the technique and effects are similar for both.

The direct method

This method is particularly suitable for the client with greasy, seborrhoeic, acne prone skin due to its stimulating, drying effect. It may also be used on dry and mature skin.

Be aware

The treatment time for dry and mature skin must be short – around 5 minutes – otherwise the condition will be aggravated.

This method uses a glass electrode, which is moved slowly over the skin. It is sometimes known as

effluvation. The current passes from the electrode and is dispersed over the skin. The warmth generated in the tissues will produce the beneficial effects for the client. The sparking is used for its germicidal effect.

Electrodes used for the direct method

Table 5.1 shows a variety of electrodes shaped for specific purposes. They are made of glass with metal end connections. A very small amount of air, neon or mercury, is sealed inside the tube. When the electrode is pushed into its holder, the metal end makes contact with a metal plate in the holder. When the current is switched on, it flows from the machine, through the holder, to the electrode. The air or gas inside the tube ionises, the

current flows through the tube and is dispersed into the tissues under the electrode.

The electrodes glow in different colours according to what they contain:

- ○ violet if they contain air
- ○ orange if they contain neon
- ○ blue-violet if they contain mercury vapour.

Learning point

Electrodes containing mercury vapour give off ultra-violet rays. Most of these rays will not pass through the tubes as they are made of glass, which absorbs ultraviolet radiation.

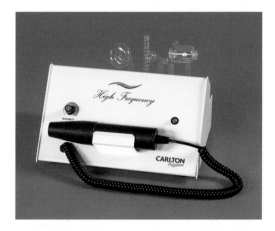

△ **Figure 5.2** High frequency machine with electrodes

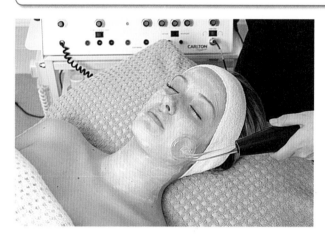

△ **Figure 5.3** Direct high frequency treatment to the face

▽ **Table 5.1** Electrodes used in treatments

Treatment	Electrode	Example	Use
Direct high frequency:	**Mushroom/facial bulb electrode (large)**		A glass electrode for the face and neck, chest and back and for sparking blemished areas, for example pustules and papules.
	Mushroom/facial bulb electrode (small)		A glass electrode suitable for use on and around the nose and chin area and for sparking blemished areas, for example pustules and papules.

(Continued)

101

(Continued)

Treatment	Electrode	Example	Use
	Horseshoe electrode		A glass electrode contoured for use on the neck.
	Roller electrode		A glass roller electrode suitable for larger areas, for example the back and chest but can also be used on the face and neck.
	Comb/rake		Glass electrodes used over the scalp and hair to stimulate the blood circulation to hair follicles, a treatment mainly carried out in hairdressing.

Learning point

The holder of some machines is made of a high insulating material that helps prevent you or your client feeling the current during treatment.

Learning point

The anti-bacterial effect can also be beneficial when treating a dry or mature skin. On this type of skin the treatment is carried out for a short time only (maximum 5 minutes) as too long a treatment will increase the dryness.

Benefits of direct high frequency

○ To dry and improve the condition of greasy skin and areas.
○ To improve the condition of blemished skin.
○ To destroy bacteria and aid healing of acne and pustular prone skin by means of sparking.

▽ **Table 5.2** Physiological effects and benefits of direct high frequency

Physiological effects	Benefits Greasy skin / greasy areas	Blemished skin / acne skin	Dry, mature / skin
Production of heat The rapidly oscillating current produces rapid motion of the molecules in the tissues which generates heat. This heating is greatest in the superficial tissues under the electrode.	√	√	√
Increased metabolic rate Metabolism is a chemical reaction capable of being accelerated by heat. An increase in metabolic rate creates a demand for oxygen and nutrients and an increase in output of waste products. This promotes healing and improves the condition of the skin.	√	√	√
Vasodilation, resulting in hyperaemia Heat causes vasodilation and an increase in the flow of blood to the area. The increase in metabolism produces an increase in metabolites which act on capillary walls producing dilation; this also increases the blood supply. In this way, oxygen and nutrients are brought more rapidly to the area and waste products are carried away. This improves the condition of the skin.	√	√	√
Germicidal effect When the electrode is held just off the skin, the current jumps across the gap forming a spark. The oxygen in the air is ionized and forms ozone, which destroys bacteria and promotes the healing of papules and pustules. As the current jumps, the spark produces ultraviolet rays, which destroy bacteria. The sparking itself may burn and destroy bacteria.	√	√	√
Drying effects The sparks stimulate nerve endings in the skin, which result in the constricting of the pores. Oxygen in the air is converted to ozone, which has a drying effect.	√	√	
Soothing effects on nerves Mild heat has a soothing effect on nerve endings, producing a feeling of relaxation.	√	√	√

❗ Be aware

Great care must be taken when sparking as too large a gap and too long a spark can destroy the tissues. Distance should be no more than 7mm or 1/4 inch away.

Contra-indications to high frequency

Be aware

Infected acne is contra-indicated, as there is a risk of cross-infection and also the current may intensify over open skin, which would cause discomfort to the client.

Learning point

Check the contra-indications listed in the manufacturer's instructions to ensure you do not invalidate your insurance policy, should the client be injured during or after treatment.

▽ **Table 5.3** Reasons for contra-indications to high frequency

Contra-indication	Reason
Asthma	Consider placing your client in a semi-reclined position with additional supports for ease of breathing during treatment. Take care if using talc as a medium, as the particles may irritate the respiratory tract. Ensure client has their inhaler within easy reach.
Bruising	May cause further damage, resulting in increased bleeding. Bruises must be allowed to heal before giving treatment, unless they are small and it is possible to work around them.
Chemotherapy, radiotherapy	The client will be under medical supervision. In line with acceptable work ethics and professional code of practice you must seek medical consent before commencing any treatment.
Cuts and abrasions	The broken skin may have a higher water content, which will increase the intensity of the current and cause the client discomfort. Insulate small cuts with petroleum jelly or cover with waterproof plaster or avoid the area.
Defective sensation	The client will be unable to give accurate feedback about the intensity of the current. Carry out a sensitivity test. If the client is unable to identify the difference between hot and cold, do not treat. Suggest an alternative treatment.
Diabetes	May have impaired sensitivity and poor circulation therefore will not be able to give accurate feedback about the intensity of the current. Some clients can be treated but be aware that the tissues are liable to bruise quite easily, and tissue healing is impaired. Carry out a sensitivity test.
Eczema	The skin is red with flaky dry patches, so the treatment will cause more sensitivity in the area and exacerbate the condition.
Epilepsy	Find out as much as possible about the client's condition. If it is controlled epilepsy, the treatment may be safe to carry out but if in any doubt seek medical advice. Do not leave a client suffering from epilepsy unattended in a room or on the couch.
Facial piercing adornments	Avoid the area or cover the adornment as it may be made of materials that conduct an electrical current and will cause a shock.
Heart conditions	The increase in blood circulation may put too much pressure and stress on the heart. Seek medical consent.
High blood pressure	This varies with age, weight and client lifestyle, but some have consistently high blood pressure. Treatments can frequently help, especially if the client is worried about their skin. Medical advice should be sought if the client is not currently on medication.

(Continued)

(Continued)

Contra-indication	Reason
Hypersensitive skin, vascular, couperose conditions	Clients with hypersensitive skin must not have stimulating treatments as these will exacerbate the condition. The products used for treatments may cause a reaction in some clients.
Injectable treatments (recent)	The skin may be red, tender and painful, with bruising and swelling. The skin needs time to heal before having treatment.
Low blood pressure	This is not usually an issue. Be aware that the client may feel dizzy or faint if they sit up or get off the couch too quickly following treatment. Always supervise and give assistance if necessary.
Metal fillings (excessive) or heavy bridge work	Metal is a good conductor, so the intensity of the current will increase in the area and may cause the client discomfort. Avoid the area or suggest an alternative treatment.
Nervous clients	The noise of the machine, the glow of colour in the glass electrode and the sparking process may make the client feel too apprehensive and pull away from the electrode, causing them a minor electric shock. Suggest an alternative treatment.
Pregnancy	There may be a risk to the foetus. Suggest an alternative treatment.
Sinus blockages	May be painful and could also aggravate the condition. Discuss options with the client.
Skin diseases	There is a risk of cross-infection.
Sunburn	The erythema following sunburn must clear completely before treatment can be given, as the tissues will be too sensitive.
Swelling in area	Treatment may make the condition worse as blood and lymph flow will increase in the area. Recommend the client seeks medical advice, as there may be an underlying problem that may prevent treatment.

Dangers of direct high frequency

The main risks of harm with high frequency current are:

○ electric shock

○ destruction of tissues: if sparking is at too great a distance, for too long a time or too frequently on the same area.

Precautions should be taken to minimise the risk of harming the client and to ensure you give an effective treatment.

▽ **Table 5.4** Precautions to take with direct high frequency

Precaution	Explanation
Examine and test the machine.	You need to check it is in good working order and ensure it will not cause harm to you or your client.
Remove jewellery, metal hair grips, belts or any other metal objects from treatment area.	Metal is a conductor of electricity and may cause a shock.
Carry out a thermal sensitivity test (see page 71).	The client must be able to give accurate feedback about the intensity of the current.

(Continued)

(Continued)

Precaution	Explanation
Warn the client of the noise from the machine.	The loud buzzing noise may make the client tense and pull away from the electrode this could result in a shock.
During treatment ensure your client does not touch any metal, for example the couch or trolley.	Metal is a conductor of electricity and may cause shock.
Rest your free hand on the pillow or hold the cable.	Do not place on the client's face as it will draw off the current or produce a mild electric shock if moved on and off.
Make sure intensity is turned down before lifting the electrode off the skin during treatment	Your client may receive a shock.
Do not spark more than 7mm/¼" away from the skin's surface.	Too large a gap, too long and too frequent a spark can destroy the tissues.
Speak to the client during treatment.	You need to ensure they are comfortable. Be alert to contra-actions.

Direct high frequency procedure

Preparation of working area

1. Place machine on a suitable stable base on the correct side of the couch.
↓
2. Check plugs and leads.
↓
3. Test the machine – Insert the mushroom electrode into the holder. Apply talc or oxygenating cream to a small area on the flexors of your forearm. Place the mushroom electrode on the flexors and use circular movements over the area. Switch on the machine and increase the intensity until you feel a tingling prickling sensation. Turn down the intensity, switch off the machine before removing the electrode.
↓
4. Clean the attachment with a disinfecting solution.
↓
5. Check intensity controls are at zero.
↓
6. Check the couch is prepared with clean linen and towels.
↓
7. Prepare trolley with:
   ○ oxygenating cream
   ○ gauze
   ○ talc
   ○ client consultation record.
↓

Preparation of self

8. Before carrying out treatment ensure you prepare yourself physically and mentally by paying due attention to high standards of professionalism. Adopt a sensitive calm, confident and understanding attitude as this approach will have a positive effect on your client.
↓

Preparation of client

9. Carry out a consultation, or if a regular client refer to the notes from their last treatment and discuss the effects and outcomes before proceeding.
↓

Best practice

Position the machine on the left side of the couch if you are right handed and the right side of the couch if you are left handed to avoid crossing over or changing hands.

Learning point (L)

As you develop your confidence with this machine, practise starting the treatment by placing a finger on the electrode, switch on the machine and place the electrode on the client's skin before removing your finger. Continue to turn up the intensity to client's tolerance.

10. Check for contra-indications.

↓

11. Check contact lenses and all jewellery have been removed.

↓

12. Place the client in a well-supported and comfortable position.

↓

13. Protect hair and clothing as appropriate.

↓

14. Explain the treatment to the client. They will experience:
    - ○ a tingling, warming sensation
    - ○ noise produced by the machine
    - ○ the smell of ozone.

Explain what to expect if sparking is to be included in the treatment. Reassure as necessary.

↓

WASH YOUR HANDS

15. Carry out a sensitivity test.

↓

16. Cleanse and tone the skin.

↓

17. Carry out a skin analysis.

Treatment technique for direct high frequency

18. Select appropriate electrodes depending on client's needs. Use the large or small mushroom electrode first to introduce the treatment.

↓

19. Apply suitable medium to the area to facilitate movement of the electrode.

↓

20. Place the mushroom electrode on the skin. Switch on the machine and increase the intensity to client's tolerance. This may have to be decreased over bony areas.

↓

21. With your free hand hold the cable away from the client. Work over the area using circular movements.
    Mushroom electrode – use circular movements. This electrode can also be used to spark papules and pustules.
    Horseshoe electrode – use in a continuous up-and-down movement from one side of the neck to the other, covering base to under jawline.
    Roller electrode – use on the décolleté and back in sweeping movements.

↓

22. Lower the intensity to zero and switch off the machine before removing the electrode from the client's skin. Change the electrode as necessary.

↓

23. Keep in verbal contact with the client to monitor progress of the treatment and be alert to contra-actions.

↓

24. Remove the medium and tone the skin.

↓

25. Continue with the facial routine depending on client's needs.

↓

26. Update the consultation record with salient points about the treatment for future reference. This will include the outcome of the sensitivity test.

Learning point

Gauze can be used with the oxygenating cream to help prevent too much or too little slip when working over the face. It also provides a uniform layer leaving a miniscule gap between the ozone and the skin, making the current more effective. Cut out holes for the nose to enable the client to breathe easily.

Learning point

Oxygenating cream or talc can be used as the medium. The cream encourages the production of oxygen, which is beneficial for the tissues. Talc is sometimes used as it has a drying effect on the tissues. It also aids the movement of the electrode over the tissues.

Remember

Ensure the client cannot touch any metal during treatment, for example the couch or trolley.

Remember

Keep the electrode in contact with the skin to prevent the client receiving a shock.

Learning point

The more superficial the movement, the greater the stimulation.

Learning point (L)

Although manufacturers give treatment times for different skin conditions, these are for guidance only. You must always observe the client's skin reaction during the application and respond appropriately.

Be aware (!)

Ensure the client knows what to expect if you need to spark papules and pustules.

Be aware (!)

Take care when applying talc as the particles may irritate the respiratory tract of some clients, particularly those who are asthmatic.

Be aware (!)

Method for sparking: 3 sparks per area at low intensity.

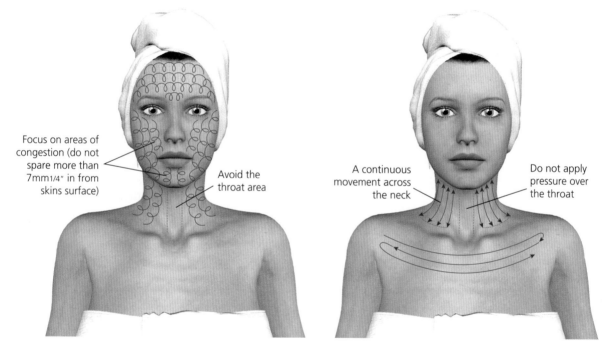

Focus on areas of congestion (do not spare more than 7mm1/4" in from skins surface)

Avoid the throat area

A continuous movement across the neck

Do not apply pressure over the throat

△ **Figure 5.4** Treatment technique for direct high frequency

Timing of treatment

○ Greasy skin conditions: 4–7 minutes, depending on sensitivity.

○ Dry, mature skin: 2–5 minutes.

Refer to manufacturer's instructions for specific guidance.

Contra-actions to direct high frequency

○ Excessive erythema: caused by intensity being too high and/or prolonged treatment. Place a cool compress on the skin and apply a suitable product or mask that will help to calm and soothe the tissues.

○ Destruction of tissues caused by sparking at too great a distance from the skin; for too long or too frequently. Advise the client to regularly apply a soothing healing cream and if possible to avoid applying make-up to the area until the skin heals.

Recommendations for direct high frequency

Direct high frequency treatment is especially beneficial to help improve conditions associated with greasy, seborrhoeic and acne skins. This includes open pores, comedones, pustules and papules. The treatment refines pores and the ozone has a drying, healing and anti-bacterial effect. To complement this treatment, advise the client to have a steam treatment to warm and soften the tissues followed by disincrustation, as this deep cleanses the skin by opening the pores and removing excess sebum. Complete the treatment with direct high frequency, using oxygenating cream to nourish the tissues and help refine the pores followed by a mask. This could be recommended as a course of treatment once per week for six weeks. Reinforce with suitable retail products to maintain the result achieved between treatments and then review.

> **Remember**
> Always seek feedback from your client and give appropriate aftercare advice (see pages 73–4).

Cleaning

To clean the attachments, wipe over with a disinfecting solution and when dry, place in a sanitiser. Take particular care not to wet the metal contact at the base of each attachment. Always refer to manufacturer's instructions for guidance.

> **Learning point** (L)
> If you experience a lot of electric shocks from the high frequency machine it may be because the electrode holder has become contaminated with the media used during treatments and has not been cleaned thoroughly. Creams conduct the high frequency current so ensure you always wipe over the holder and the area where the electrodes are inserted into the holder.

The indirect method ('Viennese massage')

This method is primarily used for dry, dehydrated and mature skin although it would also be beneficial for clients who feel tense and stressed. This method uses a saturator, which is held firmly in the client's hand. The holder is held in the other hand. When the current is switched on, it passes through the holder into the saturator and 'charges' the client. As you massage the client, your fingers on the client's skin make you part of the circuit. Current discharges from the skin to your fingers. This is a warming and relaxing treatment.

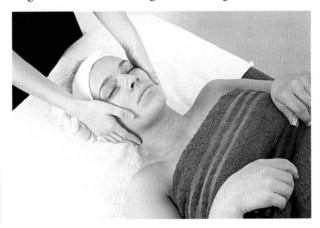

△ **Figure 5.5** Indirect high frequency treatment to the face

The electrode used for the indirect method

The electrode used is known as a saturator. It may be made of metal or glass and again fits into a holder. The client holds the holder in one hand and the saturator is held firmly in the other hand.

The current passes through the holder into the saturator and 'charges' the client. As you massage the client, your fingers on the client's skin make you part of the circuit. Current is 'drawn off' through your fingers.

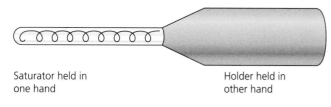

Saturator held in one hand
Holder held in other hand

△ **Figure 5.6** Electrode used for indirect high frequency treatment

▽ **Table 5.5** Electrodes used

Machine	Electrode	Use
Indirect high frequency	**Saturator**	This may be made of metal or glass. The glass electrode contains a metal spiral inside the glass that produces a gentle effect on the tissues.

Benefits of indirect high frequency

○ To improve dry and dehydrated skin conditions.
○ To improve sluggish circulation.
○ To improve the condition of mature and tired skin with fine lines.
○ To promote relaxation for stressed and tense clients.

▽ **Table 5.6** Physiological effects and benefits of indirect high frequency

Physiological effects	Dry/dehydrated skin	Sluggish circulation	Mature and tired skin with fine lines	General stress and tension
Warmth is produced in the superficial tissues.	√	√	√	√
Vasodilation of surface capillaries producing hyperaemia and erythema.	√	√	√	√
The increase in blood flow to the area will bring nutrients and oxygen to nourish the tissues and will remove waste products. This will improve the condition of tissues.	√	√	√	√
The increase in metabolic rate due to heating will also improve the condition of the skin.	√	√	√	√
The mild warmth and slow massage has a sedative effect on the sensory nerve endings and produces relaxation of the tissues.				√
The friction produced by the massage movements aids desquamation (loss of dead skin).	√	√	√	
Stimulates sebaceous glands.	√	√	√	

Contra-indications

See page 104.

Dangers of indirect high frequency

Again, the main danger with high frequency current is electric shock. Precautions should be taken to minimise the risk of harming the client and to ensure you give an effective treatment.

▽ **Table 5.7** Precautions to take with indirect high frequency

Precaution	Explanation
Examine and test the machine.	You need to check it is in good working order and ensure it will not cause harm to you or your client.
Remove jewellery, any metal hair grips, belts etc.	Metal is a conductor of electricity so may cause a small shock.
Carry out a sensitivity test for hot and cold (see page 71).	The client must be able to give accurate feedback about the intensity of the current.
Apply talc to the client's hand holding the saturator.	Water is a conductor of electricity; talc will absorb any moisture on the hand and prevent a shock.
The client must be told to hold the saturator firmly – one hand holding the holder and the other holding the saturator firmly.	Sparks will occur if the saturator is loosely held. If the client loses contact with the saturator they have broken the electrical circuit and will experience a shock.
Explain the treatment to the client using terminology that they will understand.	This is to ensure the client knows what to expect and therefore can relax and enjoy the treatment.
Warn the client about the noise the machine will make.	The loud buzzing noise may make the client tense and pull away from your hands, or release the saturator, which could result in a shock.
During treatment ensure you and your client do not touch any metal, for example the couch, trolley and stool.	Metal is a conductor of electricity and may cause shock.
Always keep one hand in contact with the client when turning the machine on and off.	Remember that removing one hand from the face intensifies the current through the other hand, avoid creating discomfort, especially over bony areas such as the forehead.
Speak to the client during treatment.	You need to ensure they are comfortable. Be alert to contra-actions.

Indirect high frequency procedure

Preparation of working area

1. Place machine on a suitable stable base on the correct side of the couch.

   ↓

2. Check plugs and leads.

   ↓

3. Test the machine – Insert the saturator electrode into the holder. Apply oil or cream to a small area on the flexors of your own forearm and hold the saturator with this hand. Leave your index finger and thumb free to switch on the machine and turn up the intensity. Place the fingers of your other hand on your flexors and use circular movements over the area. Switch on the machine and turn up the intensity until you feel warmth. Turn down the intensity and turn off the machine before releasing the saturator.

   ↓

4. Clean the attachment with a disinfecting solution.

   ↓

5. Check intensity control is at zero.

   ↓

6. Check the couch is prepared with clean linen and towels.

   ↓

7. Prepare trolley with
   - suitable massage oil/cream
   - client consultation record.

   ↓

Preparation of self

8. Before carrying out treatment ensure you prepare yourself physically and mentally paying due attention to high standards of professionalism. Adopt a sensitive calm, confident and understanding attitude as this approach will have a positive effect on your client.

   ↓

Preparation of client

9. Carry out a consultation, or if a regular client refer to the notes from their last treatment and discuss the effects and outcomes before proceeding.

   ↓

10. Check for contra-indications.

    ↓

11. Check contact lenses and all jewellery have been removed.

    ↓

12. Place the client in a well-supported and comfortable position.

    ↓

13. Protect hair and clothing.

    ↓

14. Explain the treatment to the client. They will feel warmth as you massage over the area. Warn them of the noise produced by the machine and not to break contact with the saturator. Reassure as necessary.

    ↓

WASH YOUR HANDS

15. Carry out a skin sensitivity test.

    ↓

16. Cleanse and tone the skin using suitable products.

    ↓

17. Carry out a skin analysis.

    ↓

Best practice B

Position the machine on the left side of the couch if you are right-handed and the right side of the couch if you are left-handed to avoid crossing over or changing hands.

Be aware !

Rings or other metal jewellery must not be worn on the hand that holds the saturator.

Be aware !

If the client cannot remove their wedding ring ask them to hold the electrode holder with that hand and hold the saturator in the hand free of rings.

Treatment technique for indirect high frequency

18. Apply a suitable medium to the face, neck and chest depending on client needs.

↓

19. Ask the client to hold the saturator firmly, and if necessary, talc the hand to absorb any perspiration as moisture will intensify the current.

↓

20. Place one hand on the client's face and, using small circular movements, begin to massage the area.

↓

21. Switch on and turn the machine up slowly within the client's tolerance.

↓

22. Place the other hand on the opposite side of the face and massage slowly with both hands covering the face, neck and shoulders similar to your manual facial massage movements. Warmth should be felt in your hands.

↓

23. Keep in verbal contact with the client to monitor progress of the treatment and be alert to contra-actions.

↓

24. Maintain contact with **at least one** hand as loss of contact of both hands could result in a shock to you and the client.

↓

25. At the end of the treatment, remove one hand from the client's skin, reduce the current intensity slowly to zero and switch off the machine.

↓

26. Remove the medium.

↓

27. Continue with the facial routine depending on client's needs.

↓

28. Update the consultation record with salient points about the treatment for future reference. This will include the outcome of the sensitivity test.

Be aware

It is advisable to ask the client to hold the saturator on top of the towel/cover so you can ensure they do not lose contact at any time, for example to scratch, to fiddle with clothes etc.

Learning point

Assess how tolerant the client is to the current by starting the treatment on the face as there is less padding so it is usually more sensitive than the neck and chest.

Be aware

Clients will feel the intensity of the current more on areas with little supporting tissue. Be alert and ready to turn down the intensity over these areas but always keep one hand in contact with the skin.

Be aware

Avoid tapotement and percussion movements as your hands will break contact with the skin, breaking the circuit and thereby causing discomfort to you and your client.

Be aware

If you need to remove one hand to adjust controls, for example, the client will experience increased intensity under the remaining hand. This will be most intense (and uncomfortable) if you only leave your fingertips in contact with the client's skin.

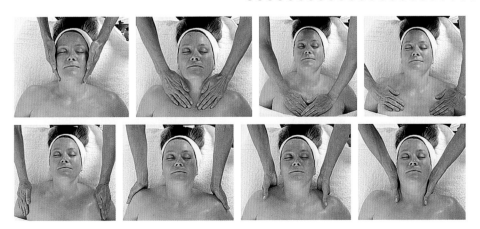

△ **Figure 5.7** Indirect high frequency movements over the décolleté, neck and face: use your manual massage movements

Timing of treatment

Apply for 10–15 minutes, depending on client's skin type, skin reaction and client tolerance. Refer to manufacturer's instructions for specific guidance.

Contra-actions to indirect high frequency

○ An allergic reaction to the medium. Cleanse the skin with a hypo-allergenic product and apply a cool compress to soothe the area. Record details on the consultation record for future reference.

○ Excessive erythema: caused by intensity being too high and/or prolonged treatment. Place a cold compress on the skin and apply a suitable product or mask that will help to calm and soothe the tissues.

Recommendations for indirect high frequency

Indirect high frequency is a very relaxing treatment that has deeper effects than a manual massage. To complement this treatment, follow with a vacuum suction treatment to increase lymphatic drainage, cleanse the pores by loosening blockages and comedones and aid desquamation. Complete the treatment with a face mask to suit the client's needs.

Remember

Always seek feedback from your client and give appropriate aftercare advice (see pages 73–4).

Cleaning

To clean the attachments wipe over with a disinfecting solution and when dry place in a sanitiser. Take particular care not to wet the metal contact. See manufacturer's instructions for specific guidance.

SUMMARY

High frequency

- A high frequency current is a rapidly oscillating current of over 100,000Hz (cycles per second).
- The frequency produced by beauty therapy equipment is around 250,000Hz.
- It passes easily through the skin to produce heating effects.

- It will *not* stimulate muscles to contract as the frequency is too high and, therefore, the pulse duration is too short.
- High frequency current may be applied to the body in two ways: the direct method and the indirect method ('Viennese massage').

The direct method

- With the direct method, the current is applied to the skin by means of a glass electrode. It is used for its warming and stimulating effects. Sparking is used for its germicidal effect. Sparking must be carried out with care, it must be done quickly and the gap between the electrode and the skin should be less than 7mm or 1/4 inch. If sparking is done slowly and with too big a gap, the tissues may be destroyed.
- Skin types that benefit from direct high frequency treatment are: greasy skin, acne and blemished skin with comedones, pustules and papules.
- The treatment time for greasy skin is 4–7 minutes, depending on sensitivity.

The indirect method

- With the indirect method, the current is carried to the client via a saturator electrode, which is held in the client's hand. The current is then 'drawn off' through your fingers as you massage the skin. You form part of the circuit for the indirect method.
- It is used for its warming and relaxing effect.
- Skin types and conditions that benefit from indirect high frequency are: dry skin, dehydrated skin; sluggish circulation; mature and tired skin with fine lines.
- The treatment time is 10–15 minutes, depending upon the skin type and client tolerance.

QUESTIONS

Oral questions

Direct high frequency

1. Name the type of current used in direct high frequency treatments.
2. Why is this treatment suitable for a client with greasy skin?
3. What is meant by the term 'germicidal effect'?
4. How does direct high frequency produce its germicidal effect?
5. Why would you instruct the client to remove jewellery?
6. Why is direct high frequency a suitable treatment for mature skin?
7. If a client experiences excessive erythema, what should you do?
8. What is a safe distance for sparking?
9. How can sparking destroy tissues?
10. During treatment, where should your free hand be placed and why?
11. How do you gain feedback from the client after treatment?
12. How would you clean the electrodes after treatment?

Indirect high frequency

1. What does high frequency current mean?
2. Why is this treatment called indirect high frequency?
3. Why is this treatment suitable for clients with dry, dehydrated and mature skin?
4. What do you understand by metabolic rate of the cells?
5. What would happen if you removed both hands from the client's skin before turning the current off?
6. Why should you apply cream to the face before starting the treatment?
7. What type of massage movements should you avoid? Give reasons for your answer.

8. What are the approximate timings of this treatment?
9. When may you need to stop the treatment?
10. Why is it important to ensure that the client places their hands on top of the cover during treatment?

Multiple-choice questions

1. The high frequency current is used to:
   a open the pores of the skin
   b heat the superficial tissues
   c increase muscle tone
   d introduce substances into the skin.

2. If the mushroom electrode glows violet it contains:
   a neon
   b ultraviolet rays
   c mercury vapour
   d air.

3. Which of the following electrodes is usually used to spark pustules and papules?
   a Mushroom.
   b Rake.
   c Horseshoe.
   d Roller.

4. Why should you avoid moving your hand on and off the client's skin during a direct high frequency treatment? It will:
   a minimise the risk of cross-infection
   b increase the intensity of the current
   c produce a mild electric shock
   d irritate the client.

5. When sparking pustules and papules, the maximum distance between the electrode and the skin's surface is:
   a 3 mm
   b 7 mm
   c 10 mm
   d 12 mm.

6. Gauze can be used with oxygenating cream to:
   a increase the intensity of the current
   b protect the tissues from becoming too warm
   c improve the effectiveness of the current
   d encourage the production of more oxygen.

7. Which of the following treatments would complement a direct high frequency treatment for a client with a greasy skin?
   a Desincrustation.
   b Electro-muscle stimulation.
   c Warm oil mask.
   d Indirect high frequency.

8. What effect does ozone have on the skin?
   a Soothing.
   b Stimulating.
   c Heating.
   d Drying.

9. Why is it advisable to apply talc to the client's hand that holds the saturator?
   a To ensure the client does not lose contact.
   b To help reduce the noise of the machine.
   c To absorb any moisture on the skin.
   d To enable the client to grip the electrode.

10. Which of the following massage movements should you avoid during an indirect high frequency treatment?
    a Tapping.
    b Kneading.
    c Effleurage.
    d Vibrations.

11. Why should you advise the client to remove jewellery before a high frequency treatment?
    a To ensure it does not get damaged.
    b To adhere to salon policy and regulations.
    c To prevent an electric shock occurring.
    d To avoid causing an allergic reaction.

12. Why is it important to keep one hand in contact with the skin during an indirect high frequency treatment?
    a To reassure the client.
    b To 'draw off' more current from the client.
    c To ensure there is a continuous flow of current.
    d To prevent the client experiencing an electric shock.

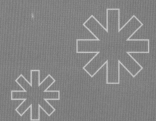

6 Mechanical massage: gyratory and audio-sonic

Objectives

After you have studied this chapter you will be able to:

▮ distinguish between the different types of mechanical massage equipment

▮ describe the benefits and effects of mechanical massage

▮ explain the contra-indications to mechanical massage

▮ explain the dangers and precautions of mechanical massage

▮ explain the contra-actions that may occur during and/or after treatment and the appropriate action to take

▮ select the appropriate massage equipment to suit the needs of the client

▮ carry out treatment paying due consideration to maximum efficiency, comfort, safety and hygiene.

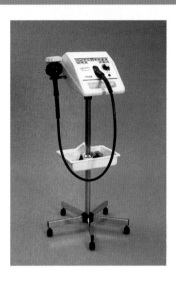

△ **Figure 6.1** A gyratory massager

Figure 6.1 is a photograph of just one type of equipment used for mechanical massage. Mechanical massage is the manipulation of body tissues using machines. Generally, mechanical massage is used in conjunction with other treatments to relieve muscle tension and muscle pain, to improve the circulation and to improve certain skin conditions. Providing the client is on a reducing diet, the heavier vibrations may help to disperse fatty deposits from specific areas of the body.

Many different types of appliances are manufactured to produce effects similar to those of a manual massage. They vary from the small, hand-held equipment designed to treat small, localised areas, to the large, heavy gyratory massagers used for deeper effects on large areas of the body. Although the effects are similar to those of manual massage, the sensation felt by the client is very different. The treatment is rather impersonal and the use of a machine rather than the touch of hands may not be as pleasing to some clients.

In practice, most mechanical massage treatments should be combined with some manual massage, thus gaining the more personal aspects of manual massage combined with the depth and power of vibratory equipment. Using mechanical massage equipment is certainly less tiring for you than performing a long, vigorous manual massage. The effects produced are similar for all types of massage equipment, but are deeper and greater with the heavier machines. The treatment is very popular with clients as they feel invigorated and consider that the desired results will be achieved.

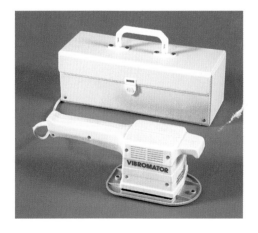

△ **Figure 6.2** A hand-held massager

Gyratory massager – body

Gyratory massagers enable you to perform a deep and thorough massage. The floor-standing gyratory massager, shown in Figure 6.1, provides a deep body massage.

Portable hand-held body massagers are available (as shown in Figure 6.2). Some of these may be heavy to use as all the electrical components are held in the hand. They do not achieve the same depth, but are a useful machine for mobile therapists. The principles of treatment are the same for all models.

The floor-standing gyratory massager includes vibration and percussion. It provides a deep, vigorous massage, which is a very effective and popular treatment.

It has all the working electrical components housed in a box supported on a stand; only the moving head is held in the hand. A rotary electric motor turns a crank attached to the head. The head is driven to turn in a gyratory motion, moving round and round, up and down and side to side with pressure, providing a deep massage. A variety of attachments that screw on to the head are available. They are designed to simulate the movements of manual massage.

▽ **Table 6.1** Examples of different heads for the gyratory massager

Applicator	Example	Use
Curved sponge

Curved sponge | **Effleurage:** arms and legs |
| Round sponge |

Round sponge | **Effleurage:** back, hips and buttocks, abdomen |
| Hard rubber multiple prong |

Hard rubber multiple prong | **Petrissage:** hips, buttocks and upper thighs for a deeper effect |
| Four half-ball (eggbox) |

Four half-ball | **Petrissage:** hips, buttocks and upper thighs for a deeper effect |

(Continued)

(Continued)

Applicator	Example	Use
Single ball (lighthouse)	Single ball	**Petrissage:** use on the back to help breakdown nodules and either side of the spine to help relieve tension
Single half ball		**Petrissage:** use in a circular or stroking movement on the colon to increase peristalsis
Double ball (two half ball)	Two half-ball	**Petrissage:** use either side of the spine to help relieve tension
Fine spiky	Fine spiky	**Percussion effect:** use to stimulate nerve endings and increase the blood flow to the area. Helps to improve the texture of the skin by increasing desquamation
Directional stroking adaptor		**Percussion effect:** pushes up and down on the skin similar to a pummelling effect which also helps to increase lymphatic drainage in the area. Attach the adaptor to the head first and add a suitable applicator depending on the effect required and the area being treated

Benefits of gyratory massager for body

○ For spot reduction of fatty deposits in conjunction with other treatments and reduced food intake.

○ To relieve muscular tension.

○ To reduce muscular aches and pains.

○ To improve poor circulation.

○ To improve skin colour and the texture of dry, flaky, rough skin.

▽ **Table 6.2** Physiological effects and benefits of gyratory massager

Physiological effects	Spot reduction of fatty deposits	Relieve muscular tension	Reduce muscular aches and pains	Improve poor circulation	Improve skin colour and the texture of dry, flaky, rough skin
As with manual massage, the main effect is stimulation of the circulation. The movements speed up the flow of blood in the veins, removing deoxygenated blood and waste products more rapidly. This affects the arterial circulation bringing oxygenated blood and nutrients to the area. Lymph drainage via the lymphatic vessels is also increased.	√	√	√	√	√
Increased blood supply will increase the metabolic rate in the tissues. This will improve the condition of the tissues.	√	√	√	√	√
Increased blood supply and friction of the heads will raise the temperature of the area, so will aid muscle relaxation and relieve pain.		√	√	√	
Pain in muscles may also be relieved due to rapid removal of waste products, such as lactic acid.		√	√		
Surface capillaries dilate giving an erythema. This improves skin colour.				√	√
The desquamating effect of the heads may improve the texture of the skin.	√				√
The continuous heavy pressure on adipose tissue and increased circulation to the area may aid the dispersion of fatty deposits, if the client is on a reducing diet.	√				

Contra-indications to gyratory massager (body)

> **Learning point** ⓛ
> Check the contra-indications listed in the manufacturer's instructions to ensure you do not invalidate your insurance policy should the client be injured during or after treatment.

▽ **Table 6.3** Reasons for contra-indications to gyratory massager (body)

Contra-indication	Reason
Acute back and spinal problems (e.g. disc trouble)	May aggravate the condition and cause further problems. Recommend the client seeks medical advice.
Bony areas	Because of the lack of depth of tissue, the client may experience the vibrations more intensely on these areas. Also, bruising and dilated capillaries may result. Avoid these areas.
Bruising	May cause further damage resulting in increased bleeding. Bruises must be allowed to heal before giving treatment, unless they are small and it is possible to work around them.
Chemotherapy, radiotherapy	The client will be under medical supervision. In line with acceptable work ethics and professional code of practice, you must seek medical consent before commencing any treatment.
Cuts and abrasions	There is a risk of cross-infection. May also cause discomfort. Cover small cuts with plaster and/or work around these areas.
Diabetes	A client with diabetes may have impaired sensitivity and poor circulation. Treatment may cause bruising, dilated capillaries and discomfort. Find out more about their condition and if in doubt seek GP's consent.
Dilated capillaries	May cause further damage if the pressure is too deep. Proceed with treatment if the area can be avoided.
Elderly clients with thin, crêpey skin and lack of subcutaneous fat	There is a danger of overstretching loose skin and of breaking down fragile, thin skin, causing open wounds. Suggest an alternative treatment.
Epilepsy	Find out as much as possible about the client's condition. If it is controlled epilepsy, the treatment may be safe to carry out but if in any doubt seek medical advice. Do not leave anyone suffering from epilepsy unattended in a room or on the couch.
Hairy areas (very)	Select applicators that will not catch and pull the hairs to prevent client discomfort.
Lymphangitis (a bacterial infection of the lymphatic vessels)	There is a risk of cross-infection and also the disease can spread via the bloodstream with fatal consequences. **Do not treat.**
Menstruation (first 2–3 days)	Omit the abdomen during the first 2–3 days of a period as it may cause a heavier blood flow. Also blood loss contributes to feelings of faintness.
Pacemaker	The mechanical vibrations may interfere with the rhythm of the pacemaker. Seek GP's consent.
Pregnancy	The heavier vibrations will be too deep and uncomfortable for the client and may be a risk to the foetus. Suggest an alternative treatment.
Scar tissue and operations (recent)	The scar tissue must be allowed to heal. If treatment is given before healing is complete, there is a danger of further damage to the tissues, delaying the healing process. Avoid the area.
Skin diseases	There is a risk of cross-infection.

(Continued)

(Continued)

Contra-indication	Reason
Skin tags, warts or pigmented moles	Applicator may pull on them causing abrasions and discomfort. Avoid the area.
Thrombosis or phlebitis	Avoid treatment if a client suffers from either or both of these conditions (known as thrombophlebitis). Dislodging or fragmenting a blood clot is the greatest danger of treatment to the legs. Death could result if medical treatment is not administered quickly.
Varicose veins	Should be avoided, as the tissues around the vein may be fragile and easily damaged. There is a tendency for the stagnating blood to form clots, which may be dislodged by the treatment.

Dangers of gyratory massager (body)

There is a risk of damage to internal organs. Do not treat an abdomen with poor muscle tone.

Precautions should be taken to minimise the risk of harming the client and to ensure you give an effective treatment.

Be aware

Particular care should be taken when selecting heads for treating the abdominal wall. Abdominal organs have no bony framework for protection – their only protection is provided by the muscles and tissues of the abdominal wall. Overstretched muscles with poor tone offer less protection. This must be considered when treating the abdomen. The heavier petrissage heads should only be used on well-toned abdominal muscles with a covering of adipose tissue (e.g. the younger, overweight client).

▽ **Table 6.4** Precautions to take with gyratory massager for body

Precaution	Explanation
Test the machine.	You need to check it is in good working order and ensure it will not cause harm to you or your client.
Carry out a tactile sensitivity test (see page 71).	If the client cannot tell the difference between sharp and soft, they have defective sensation and the treatment should not be carried out.
Cover the applicators with disposable/washable covers.	This will reduce the risk of cross-infection and prevent the disintegration of sponge and rubber applicators resulting from continual washing.
Hold the head away from the client when switching on the machine.	This is in case the applicator is insecure and becomes detached.
Heavy and prolonged treatments.	This can cause bruising and dilated capillaries. To prevent this happening keep the applicator moving and ensure the surface of the applicator is parallel to the surface of the body. If one side lifts off the body there is a danger of damaging the tissues with the hard edge of the applicator.
Avoid heavy petrissage or percussion over bony areas.	This will prevent resonance, bruising and dilated capillaries.
There are units that offer variable speeds from 20 to 60 cycles per second. Select the correct speed to meet the needs of the client.	Using an inappropriate speed could cause bruising and discomfort.

Gyratory massager procedure

Preparation of working area

1. Place machine on the correct side of the couch.
   ↓
2. Check plugs and leads.
   ↓
3. Test the machine: secure an applicator to the head, point it down towards the floor, switch on the machine, turn up the intensity, then turn down and switch off the machine.
   ↓
4. Ensure the applicators are clean. Use disposable covers whenever possible.
   ↓
5. Check intensity control is at zero.
   ↓
6. Check the couch is prepared with clean linen and towels.
   ↓
7. Prepare trolley with:
   ○ unperfumed talc
   ○ disposable/washable covers
   ○ client consultation record.
   ↓

Preparation of self

8. Before carrying out treatment ensure you prepare yourself physically and mentally, paying due attention to high standards of professionalism. Adopt a sensitive calm, confident and understanding attitude, as this approach will have a positive effect on your client.
   ↓

Preparation of client

9. Carry out a consultation, or if a regular client, refer to the notes from their last treatment and discuss the effects and outcomes before proceeding.
   ↓
10. Check for contra-indications.
    ↓
11. Check jewellery has been removed from the area.
    ↓
12. Place the client in a well-supported and comfortable position.
    ↓
13. Protect hair and clothing if appropriate.
    ↓
14. Explain the treatment to the client. They will feel the pressure of the applicator on the part and a sensation of warmth. The pressure should be to their tolerance.
    ↓
15. Carry out a tactile sensitivity test.
    ↓
16. Cleanse the area using an appropriate product.
    ↓

Best practice **B**

Position the machine on the left side of the couch if you are right-handed and the right side of the couch if you are left-handed to ensure you are in control of the dials.

Best practice **B**

Recommend the client has a preheat treatment or use hot towels to warm and soften the tissues to increase the effectiveness of the treatment.

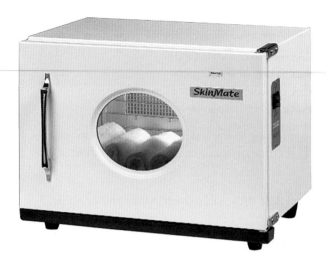

△ **Figure 6.3** Hot towel cabinet

Technique for gyratory massager

17. Select the appropriate applicators to suit the needs of the client.

↓

WASH YOUR HANDS

18. Apply an appropriate medium to the area using manual effleurage strokes.

↓

19. Use the curved sponge on limbs and the round sponge on other areas, to introduce the gyratory massager and to continue to warm the tissues.

↓

20. Apply in long sweeping strokes following the direction of venous return and natural contours of the body. The stroke should be smooth and of a pressure suited to the tissues being worked on.

↓

21. At the end of the stroke break contact or return with superficial strokes.

↓

22. Re-apply medium if necessary using manual massage.

↓

23. Change the applicator to one that simulates petrissage movements. Use a circular kneading motion applying upward pressure and work with venous return.

↓

24. Use the other hand to support the tissues and lift them towards the applicator.

↓

25. Intersperse use of the applicators with manual massage movements.

26. Continue with the body routine depending on client's needs.

↓

27. Update the consultation record with salient points about the treatment for future reference. This will include the outcome of the tactile sensitivity test.

Learning point ⓛ
Do not change the heads too often as this breaks the continuity of the treatment.

Be aware !
If using talc, apply sparingly and with care. Airborne particles can cause respiratory problems.

Remember
Switch the machine on, holding the head below the level of the couch to prevent injury should the applicator become detached.

Remember
Keep the surface attachment parallel to the surface of the body at all times. If one side lifts off the body there is a danger of damaging the tissues with the hard edge of the head.

Learning point ⓛ
The short prong (spiky) applicator is ideal for a desquamating effect and for increasing the circulation, producing erythema.

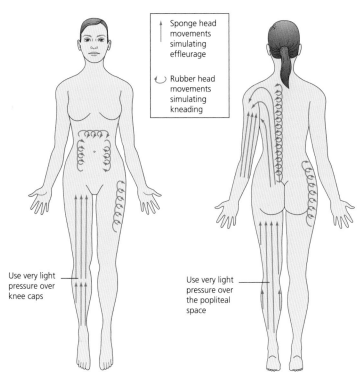

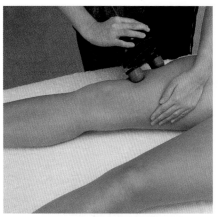

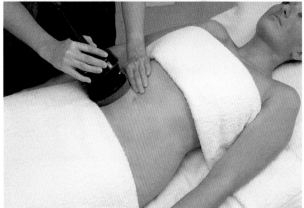

△ **Figure 6.4** Direction of strokes for gyratory massager

Timing of treatment

The degree of erythema and client tolerance dictates the length of the treatment.

Refer to manufacturer's instructions for specific guidance.

△ **Figure 6.5** Treatment technique

Contra-actions to gyratory massager

○ Bruising and dilated capillaries: caused by too much pressure, prolonged treatment over an area or failure to keep the applicator surface parallel to the surface of the body. Advise the client to apply a soothing, healing product over the area and to avoid wearing tight clothing.

○ Excessive erythema: caused by a sponge applicator that is worn, prolonged treatment over an area especially with the fine spiky applicator, insufficient medium to help with slippage. Place a cool compress over the area and apply a soothing product.

○ Irritation and itching: caused by a sponge applicator that is worn or prolonged treatment with the fine spiky applicator. Ensure all medium is removed, place a cool compress over the area and apply a soothing product.

Recommendations for gyratory massager

This is a popular treatment for clients with localised adipose deposits and muscular aches and pains. Treatment time ranges from 30 to 45 minutes depending on client's needs. It is recommended clients book a course of 6–10 treatments and have 2 or 3 treatments per week. A preheat treatment will help to soften and warm the tissues. Vacuum suction would be a beneficial treatment to follow gyratory massager as it will increase lymphatic drainage in the area. Body galvanic (iontophoresis) to follow would help to soften areas of fat/cellulite and aid its absorption.

Cleaning of applicators

Remove and dispose of protective covers. Clean the washable covers and applicators with hot water and detergent, rinse and allow them to dry, store in a sanitiser.

Refer to manufacturer's instructions for specific guidance.

Remember

Always seek feedback from your client and give appropriate aftercare advice. See pages 73–4.

Gyratory massager – face

As the name suggests, this mechanical massager is for use on the face, neck and décolleté and should be used in conjunction with manual massage. Again, a variety of different applicators are used for different functions, such as cleansing, exfoliation, massage and treating fine lines.

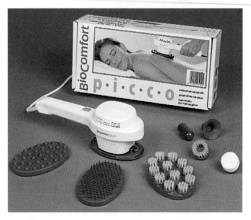

△ **Figure 6.6** Light-weight massager

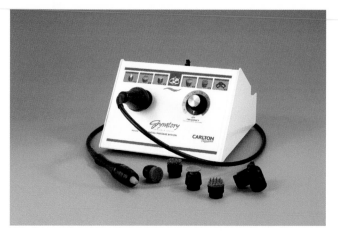

△ **Figure 6.7** A gyratory facial massager

▽ **Table 6.5** Applicators used in gyratory facial massagers

Applicator (*names of applicators may vary for different manufacturers)	Example	Use
Sponge		Cleansing
Coarse sponge		Exfoliation
*Rubber (for deeper petrissage type movements)		Massage and lymphatic drainage
Multiple prong		Aiding the penetration of medium
*Rubber tip		Treatment of fine lines and to increase circulation to the area

Benefits of gyratory facial massager

○ To stimulate dry, dehydrated or mature skin.

○ To improve a sluggish, dull looking skin.

○ To aid deep cleansing of the tissues using appropriate applicators and products.

○ To promote relaxation of muscle fibres.

▽ **Table 6.6** Physiological effects and benefits of gyratory facial massager

Physiological effects	Dry, dehydrated and mature skin	Sluggish, dull looking skin	Deep cleansing effect	Relax muscle fibres
An increase in circulation to the treated area, bringing nutrients and oxygen to the area and removing waste products increases metabolic rate. This improves the condition of the tissues.	√	√	√	√
It produces vasodilation, giving hyperaemia and erythema, improving the colour of the skin.	√	√	√	
The increase in circulation and the friction of the heads raises the temperature of the area. This promotes relaxation, relieves pain and may stimulate the activity of sebaceous glands.	√	√	√	√
The friction of the heads aids desquamation; this removes the surface layer of cells, improving the condition of the skin.	√	√	√	

Contra-indications to gyratory facial massage

▽ **Table 6.7** Reasons for contra-indications to gyratory facial massager

Contra-indication	Reason
Bony features or mature skin with poor elasticity	There is a danger of overstretching loose skin and of breaking down fragile, thin skin causing open wounds. Treatment over bony areas may be uncomfortable for the client. Suggest an alternative treatment.
Bruising	May cause further damage resulting in increased bleeding. Bruises must be allowed to heal before giving treatment unless they are small and it is possible to work around them.
Chemotherapy, radio-therapy	The client will be under medical supervision. In line with acceptable work ethics and professional code of practice you must seek medical consent before commencing any treatment.
Headaches or migraines	Client will feel tense and unable to relax and enjoy the treatment. The increase in blood circulation to the area may cause more discomfort and exacerbate the condition. Do not treat.
Inflammation	The skin will be red, swollen and sensitive; the inflammatory process may also stimulate the nerves causing pain. The treatment will cause further discomfort as the skin needs time to heal.
Sinus problems	May be painful and could also aggravate the condition.
Skin diseases	There is a risk of cross-infection.
Vascular skin; or skin with dilated capillaries	Clients with hyper-sensitive skin must not have over-stimulating treatments as these may cause further damage. The products used for treatments may cause an allergic reaction in some clients. Suggest an alternative treatment.

Precautions to take with gyratory facial massager

There are no dangers associated with this treatment. However, precautions should be taken to minimise the risk of harming the client and to ensure you give an effective treatment.

▽ **Table 6.8** Precautions to take with gyratory facial massager

Precaution	Explanation
Test the machine.	You need to check it is in good working order and ensure it will not cause harm to you or your client.
Avoid bony areas.	Treatment on such areas will cause the client discomfort.
Avoid eye region.	The tissue around the eye area is very delicate and should be avoided to prevent bruising and discomfort to the client.
Carry out a tactile sensitivity test (see page 71).	If the client cannot tell the difference between sharp and soft, they have defective sensation and the treatment should not be carried out.
Keep the surface of the applicator parallel to the surface of the face.	If one side lifts off the area there is a danger of damaging the tissues with the hard edge of the applicator.
Do not over-treat one area.	Keep the head moving to prevent bruising and dilated capillaries.

Gyratory facial massager procedure

Preparation of working area

1. Place machine on the trolley on the correct side of the couch.
   ↓
2. Check plugs and leads.
   ↓
3. Test the machine: Insert an applicator into the head, switch on the machine and turn up the intensity, test it on the flexors of your forearm, turn down the intensity and switch off the machine.
   ↓
4. Clean the attachment with a suitable product.
   ↓
5. Check intensity controls are at zero.
   ↓
6. Check the couch is prepared with clean linen and towels.
   ↓
7. Prepare trolley with:
   ○ appropriate products
   ○ client consultation record.
   ↓

Preparation of self

8. Before carrying out treatment, ensure you prepare yourself physically and mentally paying due attention to high standards of professionalism. Adopt a sensitive, calm, confident and understanding attitude, as this approach will have a positive effect on your client.
   ↓

Best practice **B**

Position the trolley on the left side of the couch if you are right-handed and the right side of the couch if you are left-handed to avoid crossing over or changing hands.

Preparation of client

9. Carry out a consultation, or if a regular client refer to notes from their last treatment and discuss the effects and outcomes before proceeding.

↓

10. Check for contra-indications.

↓

11. Check contact lenses and all jewellery have been removed.

↓

12. Place the client in a well-supported and comfortable position.

↓

13. Protect hair and clothing.

↓

14. Explain the treatment to the client. They will feel a vibrating sensation and warmth. The depth of pressure must be comfortable for the client.

↓

WASH YOUR HANDS

15. Carry out a tactile sensitivity test.

↓

16. Cleanse and tone the skin using suitable products.

↓

17. Carry out a skin analysis.

↓

Technique for gyratory facial massager

18. Select the appropriate applicators to suit the needs of the client.

↓

19. Apply an appropriate medium to the area.

↓

20. Commence the treatment using straight lines or a circular motion depending on the applicator and the effect required; ensure coverage of all the area. Keep the applicator moving and parallel to the surface of the skin for maximum benefit. A routine might include:

   ○ cleansing
   ○ exfoliation
   ○ massage
   ○ extractions (see page 296)
   ○ application of beneficial creams.

   Refer to manufacturer's instructions for specific guidelines.

↓

21. Keep in verbal contact with the client to monitor progress of the treatment. Be alert to contra-actions.

↓

22. Remove the medium and tone the skin.

↓

23. Continue with the facial routine depending on client's needs.

↓

24. Update the consultation record with salient points about the treatment for future reference. This will include the outcome of the tactile sensitivity test.

Best practice B

In between changing the applicators, include some manual movements to spread the medium and make the treatment more relaxing and more personal.

Learning point

Although manufacturers give treatment times for different skin conditions these are for guidance only. You must always observe client's skin reaction during the application and respond appropriately.

Timing of treatment

The skin reaction indicates the length of the treatment time. When an even erythema is produced the treatment should stop. This may take 10–20 minutes, depending on client's skin type, skin reaction and client tolerance.

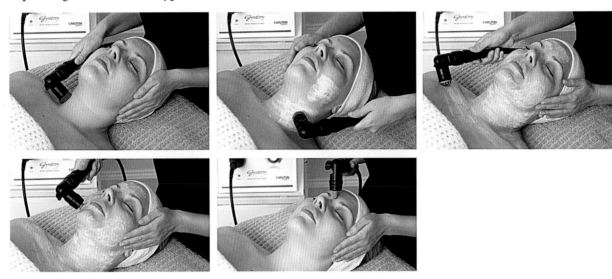

△ **Figure 6.8** Gyratory facial massager treatment technique

Contra-actions to gyratory facial massager

○ Bruising and dilated capillaries: due to prolonged treatment, applying too much pressure to certain areas and failing to monitor the client's reaction. Advise the client to apply a soothing and healing product to the area.

○ Excessive erythema: due to prolonged treatment or too much pressure. Place a cool compress on the area and apply a soothing product.

> **Remember**
> Always seek feedback from your client and give appropriate aftercare advice. See pages 73–4.

Recommendations for facial gyratory massager

Recommend a course of 4 treatments for 4 weeks. Monitor progress and review the treatment plan.

Cleaning of applicators

Wash the applicators in hot soapy water, rinse and leave to dry. Store in a sanitiser. Refer to manufacturer's instructions for specific guidance.

Audio-sonic

This is a hand-held appliance. Its name is derived from the fact that the machine produces sound waves (which can be heard as a humming sound). This vibrator generates sound waves using an electromagnet. When the current is passing one way, the coil moves forward; as the current reverses, the coil moves back. The speed of the movement is measured in Hertz and is referred to as frequency (the number of oscillations per second).

Sound waves can be divided into three groups:

○ infrasonic waves – these have a frequency of less than 16Hz (too low to be heard).

○ intrasonic waves – these have a frequency between 16Hz and 20,000Hz. This is the frequency band which the human ear can hear.

○ ultrasonic waves – these have a frequency above 20,000Hz (too high to be heard).

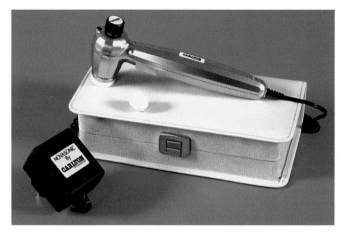

△ **Figure 6.9** Audio-sonic machine

Audio-sonic massagers use part of the intrasonic frequency band. When the applicator is placed on the area, the sound waves penetrate the tissues, causing the oscillation of molecules making up the cells. Different molecules oscillate at different inherent frequencies; when they are made to oscillate at a frequency close to their own inherent frequency they resonate more strongly, producing a beneficial effect.

Be aware !

Audio-sonic should not be confused with ultrasound therapy, which is quite different and has various medical uses.

Because the applicators do not physically move forward and backward, this appliance has a gentle action. It penetrates more deeply into the tissues (2¼"/60 mm), but is less stimulating on the surface of the skin.

There are two applicators:

○ The flat disc applicator is for general use on muscles.
○ The ball-type sound applicator is for use around joints.

Benefits of audio-sonic

○ To produce warmth and aid relaxation of muscle fibres. Particularly effective over tension nodules.
○ To relieve cramp, pain and muscle spasms.
○ To aid dispersal of aches and pain around joints.

▽ **Table 6.9** Physiological effects and benefits of audio-sonic

Physiological effects	Benefits — Aid relaxation of muscle fibres	Help relieve cramp, pain and muscle spasms	Help to relieve aches and pains around joints
It produces an increase in circulation to the treated area, bringing nutrients and oxygen and removing waste products.	√	√	√
It increases the metabolic rate, thus improving the condition of the tissues.	√	√	√
The increase in circulation raises the temperature of the area. This promotes relaxation of muscle fibres.	√	√	√
It produces vasodilation, giving hyperaemia and erythema.	√	√	√

Contra-indications to audio-sonic

> **Learning point** (L)
>
> Check the contra-indications listed in the manufacturer's instructions to ensure you do not invalidate your insurance policy should the client be injured during or after treatment.

▽ **Table 6.10** Reasons for contra-indications to audio-sonic

Contra-indication	Reason
Chemotherapy, radiotherapy	The client will be under medical supervision. In line with acceptable work ethics and professional code of practice you must seek medical consent before commencing any treatment.
Lean or bony features/areas	The sound waves resonate more intensely over bone, which could cause discomfort. Treatment can be carried out but avoid these areas.
Metal or plastic plates	Could cause discomfort or damage the implant. Do not treat the area.
Pacemaker	The frequency of the sound waves can interfere with the function of the pacemaker. Seek GP's consent.
Pregnancy	There may be a risk to the foetus. Do not treat.
Skin diseases	There is a risk of cross-infection.
Thrombosis	The increase in circulation could cause the blood clot to be transported in the blood stream to the lungs and heart, with fatal consequences. **Do not treat.**
Undiagnosed pain, especially in the legs	Recommend the client seeks medical advice as there may be an underlying problem that prevents treatment.

Dangers of audio-sonic

If a vein in the calf becomes inflamed (phlebitis), treatment may increase the inflammation. The greatest risk of harm to the client is if a clot develops in the vein (thrombosis). The treatment increases blood circulation and a clot could be dislodged and transported to the lungs and heart, with fatal consequences.

Precautions should be taken to minimise the risk of harming the client and to ensure you give an effective treatment.

▽ **Table 6.11** Precautions to take with audio-sonic

Precaution	Explanation
Test the machine	You need to check it is in good working order and ensure it will not cause harm to you or your client.
Avoid bony areas	Because of the lack of depth of tissue, treating such areas will cause the client discomfort. This can be alleviated by placing your hand on the area and applying the audio-sonic over your hand.
Avoid eye region	The tissue around the eye area is very delicate and bruises easily, which will cause the client discomfort.

Audio-sonic procedure

Preparation of working area

1. Place machine on the trolley on the correct side of the couch.

   ↓

2. Check plugs and leads.

   ↓

3. Test the machine: Insert an applicator into the head, switch on the machine and turn up the intensity, test it on the flexors of your forearm, turn down the intensity and switch off the machine.

   ↓

4. Clean the attachment with a suitable product.

   ↓

5. Check intensity controls are at zero.

   ↓

6. Check the couch is prepared with clean linen and towels.

   ↓

7. Prepare trolley with:
   - pillows or rolled towels for client comfort and additional support
   - client consultation record.

   ↓

Preparation of self

8. Before carrying out treatment, ensure you prepare yourself physically and mentally, paying due attention to high standards of professionalism. Adopt a sensitive, calm, confident and understanding attitude, as this approach will have a positive effect on your client.

   ↓

Preparation of client

9. Carry out a consultation, or if a regular client, refer to the notes from their last treatment and discuss the effects and outcomes before proceeding.

   ↓

10. Check for contra-indications.

    ↓

11. Check jewellery has been removed from the area.

    ↓

12. Place the client in a well-supported and comfortable position.

    ↓

13. Protect clothing if appropriate.

    ↓

14. Explain the treatment to the client. They will feel warmth in the area being treated. It is a very gentle treatment that penetrates deep within the tissue.

    ↓

WASH YOUR HANDS

15. Cleanse the area with a suitable product.

    ↓

16. Carry out an assessment of the area.

    ↓

> **Best practice** **B**
>
> Position the trolley on the left side of the couch if you are right-handed and the right side of the couch if you are left-handed to avoid crossing over or changing hands.

Technique for audio-sonic

17. Select the appropriate applicator to suit the needs of the client.

↓

18. Check manufacturer's guidance on the type of medium recommended.

↓

19. Select the most appropriate intensity to suit the client's needs.

↓

20. Use stroking or circular movements. Do not apply pressure with the applicator but keep it moving and parallel to the surface for maximum benefit.

↓

21. Keep in verbal contact with the client to monitor progress of the treatment and be alert to contra-actions.

↓

22. Wipe over the area with a cleansing product.

↓

23. Continue with the routine depending on client's needs.

↓

24. Update the consultation record with salient points about the treatment for future reference.

> **Be aware** !
> Some products may damage the head or the applicators of the machine.

> **Be aware** !
> If the client experiences discomfort, work on the outer perimeters of the area as the treatment will still be beneficial.

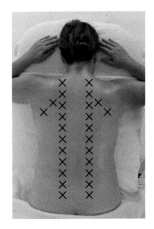

△ **Figure 6.10** Audio-sonic treatment technique

Timing of treatment

The skin reaction indicates the length of the treatment time. When an even erythema is produced the treatment should stop. This may take 5–15 minutes, depending on the tissues, skin reaction and client tolerance.

> **Be aware** !
> Do not use the machine for more than 20 minutes as it will overheat.

Contra-actions to audio-sonic

The machine produces and transmits sound waves, which have a soothing and healing effect on the tissues. If a client is experiencing pain they must consult their doctor before having this treatment. As this treatment penetrates deep into the underlying tissues, a client may find that after the first few treatments their condition has got worse. This often happens as the body deals with the accumulation of toxins and waste and starts the healing process. The reaction will vary depending on the imbalance within the body.

> **Remember**
> Always seek feedback from your client and give appropriate aftercare advice. See pages 73–4.

Recommendations for audio-sonic

This treatment is very effective for muscular problems, aches and pains around joints as it penetrates deep into the tissues. Recommend the client has a course of treatments, to include a heat treatment to warm and soften the tissues ready for a manual massage, combined with an audio-sonic treatment on the area that needs a deeper and stronger effect at cellular level.

Suggest a course of treatments. The number of treatments per week will depend on the client's condition.

Cleaning of applicators

To clean the applicators wash in warm soapy water, rinse and dry thoroughly. Store in a sanitiser.

Refer to manufacturer's instructions for specific guidance.

SUMMARY

- Mechanical massage is the manipulation of body tissues using machines.
- Types of mechanical massage equipment are: gyratory massager, hand-held massager; gyratory facial massager; audio-sonic.
- The hand-held massagers are used for small body and facial areas; the large massagers are used on large body areas.
- Mechanical massage is used to improve many conditions. It is usually combined with some manual massage. The client will then benefit from the comforting effects of touch and from the deeper effect of the mechanical massage.
- Mechanical massage will improve the circulation to the area, will relieve muscle tension and aches and pains, will aid the dispersal of fatty tissue in conjunction with diet and will improve the condition of the skin.
- There is little danger in application, except that bruising and dilated capillaries may result from heavy or prolonged treatment.
- The head moves round and round with gyratory movement. It is used on the body.
- The audio-sonic massager alternately compresses and decompresses the tissues due to the movement of an electromagnet within the head. Because the head does not physically tap on the area, it is much more gentle in action. It is used on painful tension nodules, to relieve cramp, pain and muscle spasms and aid dispersal of aches and pain around joints.

QUESTIONS

Oral questions

Gyratory massager

1. How does gyratory massager on the body differ from manual massage?
2. What are the benefits of gyratory massager on the body?
3. What advice would you give a client if they wanted gyratory massager treatment but scar tissue in the area is recent?
4. Why would you use gyratory massager on a client who was overweight?
5. Why would you use talc as the medium, not oil?
6. Why would you hold the head below the couch level to switch the gyratory massager on?
7. What gyratory massager applicators would you choose for a client with heavy hips and thighs?
8. What is happening in the tissues as you treat an area with gyratory massager?
9. How would you protect your client from cross-infection?
10. When would you use the hard, spiky, rubber applicator?

Audio-sonic

1. What are the benefits of audio-sonic?
2. How deeply do the sound waves penetrate?
3. What is happening in the tissues during the treatment?
4. What should you do if the area is bony?
5. If a client had a pacemaker how would you deal with the situation?
6. What precautions should you take before, during and after treatment?
7. What are the contra-actions to treatment?
8. What other treatments would complement audio-sonic? Give reasons.

Multiple-choice questions

1. The type of current used for a gyratory vibrator treatment is:
   a an alternating current
   b a direct current
   c a high frequency current
   d a modified direct current.

2. The single-ball applicator is mainly used on:
   a upper thighs
   b adipose tissue
   c tension nodules
   d well-toned muscles.

3. What type of test should you always carry out prior to a gyratory vibrator treatment?
   a Hot and cold test.
   b Tactile test.
   c Allergic test.
   d Skin test.

4. Which of the following is a contra-action from a gyratory vibrator treatment?
   a Broken capillaries.
   b Varicose veins.
   c Burning.
   d Feeling of relaxation.

5. What treatment would be most appropriate prior to a gyratory vibrator treatment?
   a Vacuum suction.
   b Sunbed.
   c Infrared.
   d Body galvanic.

6. Which of the following conditions would be totally contraindicated to treatment?
   a Diabetes.
   b Menstruation.
   c Epilepsy.
   d Radiotherapy.

7. The hard rubber multiple-prong applicator is similar to which manual massage movement?
   a Petrissage.
   b Tapotement.
   c Vibration.
   d Effleurage.

8. During the treatment you discover your client has tinea corporis, what should you do?
   a Make a note of it and continue with treatment.
   b Stop the treatment and recommend the client seeks medical advice.
   c Work around the areas where possible and suggest the client see their doctor.
   d Give the client the option of a manicure or pedicure treatment.

9. What type of sound waves does the audio-sonic machine produce?
   a ultrasonic.
   b infrared.
   c infrasonic.
   d intrasonic.

10. Sound waves can penetrate to a depth of:
    a 20mm.
    b 40mm.
    c 60mm.
    d 80mm.

7 Vacuum suction

Objectives

After you have studied this chapter you will be able to:

■ describe the lymphatic system and identify the main lymph nodes of the human body

■ identify the terminals on the machine

■ describe the benefits and effects of a vacuum suction treatment

■ explain the contra-indications to facial and body vacuum suction

■ explain the dangers and precautions of vacuum suction treatments

■ explain the contra-actions that may occur during and/ or after treatment and the appropriate action to take

■ carry out vacuum suction treatments, paying due consideration to maximum efficiency, comfort, safety and hygiene.

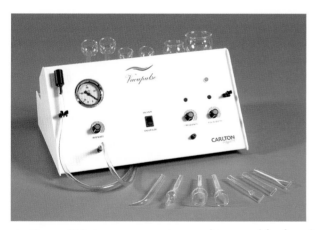

△ **Figure 7.1** A vacuum suction machine used for facial and body treatments

Figure 7.1 is a photograph of a vacuum suction machine. This particular model may be used for both facial and body work, and includes a variety of applicators. These are called ventouses for facial work and cups for body work. It is used to speed up the flow of lymph and blood and stimulate the metabolic rate. The treatment is based on the principle of creating reduced pressure within the applicator. This is moved over the area in the direction of lymphatic drainage towards the nearest

lymph nodes, into which the lymph will drain. When the pressure within the applicator is reduced to below atmospheric pressure, the tissues are lifted into it. The lymphatic and blood vessels dilate as the suction is applied, and as the applicator moves along, the rate of flow will increase. Vacuum suction treatment is effective on the face and the body.

The lymphatic system

In order to provide the most effective treatment, you must have an understanding of the lymphatic system. The lymphatic system is closely associated with the blood circulatory system. It transports a fluid, called lymph, from the tissue spaces, and returns it to the blood via the subclavian veins.

> **Learning point** L
>
> If fluid is not drained away from tissue spaces, swelling of the area will occur – this is known as oedema.

Large protein molecules and waste products are transported via the lymphatic system back to the bloodstream. Lymphatic capillaries begin as blind-end tubes and form a network throughout the tissue spaces. Their walls are very thin, allowing particles of large molecular size to pass through. Lymph capillaries join together to form larger vessels. These lymph vessels are similar to small veins in structure and have semi-lunar valves lining their walls to prevent the backward flow of lymph.

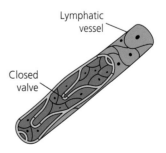

△ **Figure 7.2** A lymphatic vessel

All lymph vessels drain into lymph nodes. These are small, bean-shaped structures strategically placed in groups throughout the body. The lymph is filtered as it passes through each node: damaged cells, microbes, etc., are filtered and destroyed. In the nodes, lymphocytes multiply and antibodies are produced; these may be carried via the lymph into the circulation.

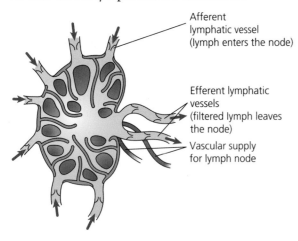

Afferent lymphatic vessel (lymph enters the node)

Efferent lymphatic vessels (filtered lymph leaves the node)

Vascular supply for lymph node

△ **Figure 7.3** A lymphatic node

After leaving the nodes, the lymphatic vessels join to form even larger lymph trunks. These empty into one of two lymphatic ducts:

○ **The thoracic duct** drains the whole of the body apart from the upper right quarter; it empties into the left subclavian vein.

○ **The right lymphatic duct** drains the right arm, right side of the head and chest; it empties into the right subclavian vein.

The speed at which lymph flows through the system depends on the:

○ contraction and relaxation of muscles.

○ negative pressure and movement of the chest during respiration.

Backward flow of lymph is prevented by valves in the vessel walls. The volume of lymph passing into the capillaries depends on the arterial pressure and pressure of the tissue fluid.

During vacuum suction treatment, it is essential to follow the course of the lymphatic vessels and end at the nearest set of lymph nodes.

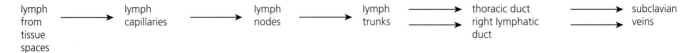

lymph from tissue spaces → lymph capillaries → lymph nodes → lymph trunks → thoracic duct / right lymphatic duct → subclavian veins

△ **Figure 7.4** Flow of lymph

Lymph nodes of the body and face

▽ **Table 7.1** Lymph nodes of the body and face

Facial nodes	Body nodes
Occipital	Supraclavicular (above clavicle)
Post auricular (mastoid)	Axillary nodes (in armpit)
Anterior auricular (parotid)	Supratrochlear nodes (at elbow)
Buccal	Inguinal nodes (in groin)
Submandibular	Popliteal nodes (behind knee)
Submental	
Superficial cervical	
Deep cervical	

See also Figure 7.9 Facial lymph nodes and Figure 7.11 Body lymph nodes.

Vacuum suction machines

Some of these are designed as facial machines and some as body machines, while others are combined machines for the treatment of the face and body (see Figure 7.1). They all consist of a machine, and a selection of ventouses for the face and cups for the body, which connect to it by plastic tubing. A suction effect is produced in the cups by sucking out air to reduce the pressure. This is done using a vacuum pump driven by an electric motor. The amount of negative pressure is registered on a gauge, and can be controlled by increasing or decreasing a regulating knob. The on/off switch controls the power from the mains. Most machines have a second outlet for blowing the air out. This air outlet can be used with an atomiser spray bottle, which can be filled with a variety of preparations, for example:

- toner: to spray the area with a fine mist that will not need blotting
- water: to remove masks and loosen setting masks
- oil: to spray an area when more slippage is required.

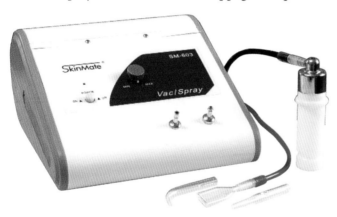

△ **Figure 7.5** SkinMate® vacuum spray

The applicators are manufactured in various sizes and shapes to suit the areas of the body to be treated: ventouses are for facial work and may vary in shape for different uses, e.g. loosening comedones; cups are for body work and vary in size to contour the area being treated. The selection of the appropriate cup to suit the body part must be carefully considered. Applicators are generally made of glass or perspex. Some have a small hole in the side to release the vacuum when required. This hole must be covered with a finger to maintain a vacuum (the finger is removed to release the vacuum).

If there is no hole, the vacuum must be released by depressing the flesh with the finger.

Be aware !

Too large an applicator will not contour the area and therefore the treatment will be ineffective. Too small an applicator may cause bruising as too much flesh may be sucked into it.

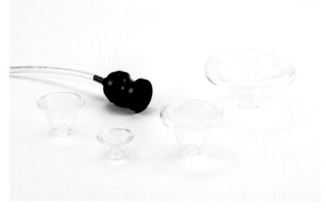

△ **Figure 7.6** Cups for vacuum suction

Facial vacuum suction

Vacuum suction may be used on the face and neck for general cleansing on normal, dry, combination and greasy skins. It can be used to loosen blocked pores and blackheads (comedones) and to improve the condition of dry, dehydrated skin.

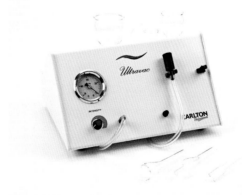

△ **Figure 7.7** A vacuum suction machine used for facial work

▽ **Table 7.2** Different ventouses used for facial vacuum suction treatments

Ventouse	Example	Use
Facial (small and large)		General cleansing and lymph drainage.
Pore blockage		Cleansing of congested areas, for example on the chin and around the nose.
Comedone		To loosen and aid the removal of comedones. This ventouse does not have a hole in the side to release the vacuum so take care not to pull it off the skin; use a finger to depress the skin to release the vacuum.
Flat head		Especially beneficial for treating lines of facial expression for example frown lines, outer eye area, labial nasal folds.

Benefits of facial vacuum suction

○ General skin cleansing on normal and combination skin. This can be carried out following steam treatment.

○ The deep cleansing of greasy skin to remove dead keratinised cells and sebum and clear follicular blockages. This is most effective following steam or disincrustation treatments to the face.

○ To stimulate dry, dehydrated, mature and sluggish skin and improve its condition.

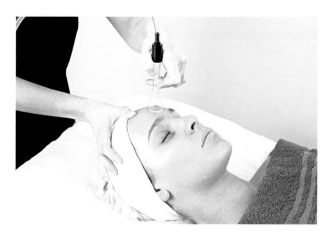

△ **Figure 7.8** Vacuum suction treatment to the face

▽ **Table 7.3** Physiological effects and benefits of facial vacuum suction

Physiological effects	Benefits	General cleansing of normal and combination skin	Deep cleansing of greasy skin	Stimulate dry, dehydrated mature and sluggish skin
It speeds up the removal of waste products via the lymphatic system.		√	√	√
It increases blood circulation to the area, bringing nutrients and oxygen, thus improving the condition of the skin.		√	√	√

(Continued)

(Continued)

Physiological effects	Benefits		
	General cleansing of normal and combination skin	**Deep cleansing of greasy skin**	**Stimulate dry, dehydrated mature and sluggish skin**
It produces vasodilation, giving an erythema and improving skin colour.	√	√	√
It stimulates cell metabolism.	√	√	√
It aids desquamation and the removal of dead keratinised cells, and improves the texture of the skin.	√	√	√
It loosens blockages and comedones, cleansing the pores.	√	√	

Contra-indications to facial vacuum suction

Learning point

Check the contra-indications listed in the manufacturer's instructions to ensure you do not invalidate your insurance policy should the client be injured during or after treatment.

▽ **Table 7.4** Reasons for contra-indications to facial vacuum suction

Contra-indication	Reason
Bruising	May cause further damage resulting in increased bleeding. Bruises must be allowed to heal before giving treatment unless they can be avoided.
Chemotherapy, radiotherapy	The client will be under medical supervision. In line with acceptable work ethics and professional code of practice you must seek medical consent before commencing any treatment.
Crêpey skin and fine texture	There is a danger of overstretching loose skin and of breaking down fragile, thin skin causing open wounds. Suggest an alternative treatment.
Cuts and abrasions	There is a risk of cross-infection from body fluids as the wounds are open. Avoid the area.
Diabetes	Clients with diabetes may have impaired sensitivity, and poor circulation. Healing may be slow. Great care must be taken to avoid damage to the skin or any other injury. If in doubt seek GP's consent.
Dilated capillaries	Suction over the area could make the condition worse. Carry out treatment if the area can be avoided.
Epilepsy	Find out as much as possible about the client's condition. If it is controlled epilepsy, the treatment may be safe to carry out as the treatment is quite soothing and gentle on the tissues but if in any doubt seek medical advice. Do not leave anyone suffering from epilepsy unattended in a room or on the couch.
Hypersensitive skin	Treatment may over stimulate the skin and there is also a risk of causing dilated capillaries and bruising. Suggest alternative treatment.
Infected acne	There is a risk of cross-infection. Do not treat.
Injectable treatment (recent)	The skin may be red, tender, painful with bruising and swelling. The skin needs time to settle down and heal before having further treatment. In particular, avoid treatment where there are fillers that plump out lines and wrinkles adding fullness to the face, as the suction effect over the area may dislodge the filler.

(Continued)

(Continued)

Contra-indication	Reason
Scar tissue (recent)	The scar tissue must be allowed to heal completely before giving treatment as there is a danger of further damage to the tissues delaying the healing process.
Skin diseases	There is a risk of cross-infection.
Sunburn	The erythema (reddening) following sunburn must clear completely before treatment can be given as the skin will be sensitive.

Dangers of facial vacuum suction

Bruising of the area may be caused by poor technique:

○ pressure too high

○ pulling ventouse off before releasing the vacuum

○ over-treating the area with too many stokes or too long a treatment

○ pushing the ventouse downwards instead of lifting and gliding.

Precautions should be taken to minimise the risk of harming the client and to ensure you give an effective treatment.

▽ **Table 7.5** Precautions to take with facial vacuum suction

Precaution	Explanation
Test the machine.	You need to check it is in good working order and ensure it will not cause harm to you or your client.
Check the rim of the ventouses for any roughness or chips.	This may cause small scratches/abrasions on the skin.
Carry out a tactile sensitivity test (see page 71).	If the client cannot tell the difference between sharp and soft, they have defective sensation and the treatment should not be carried out.
Select the correct ventouses to suit the area.	Too large a ventouse will not contour the area and therefore the treatment will be ineffective. Too small a ventouse may cause bruising and dilated capillaries as too much flesh may be sucked into the ventouse.
Check the pressure on yourself.	To ensure the machine is working correctly and the pressure can be adjusted to suit the tissues being treated.
Apply sufficient oil to the area.	To facilitate the movement of the ventouse and provide a seal.
Lift enough flesh – do not exceed 20 per cent of the ventouse.	Too much flesh sucked into the ventouse will cause dilated capillaries and bruising due to compression of the skin, which is why it is important to only lift maximum of 20 per cent.
Lift the ventouse and move it across the contours of the face and neck to the nearest set of lymph nodes. Do not work over the nodes.	This may cause swelling and sensitivity in the area.
Release the pressure before lifting the ventouse off the area.	This is to prevent dilated capillaries and bruising.
Overlap the previous stroke.	This is to ensure even coverage.
Do not overtreat the area.	This is to avoid client discomfort.
Speak to the client during the treatment.	You need to monitor progress of the treatment and be alert to contra-actions occurring.

Facial vacuum suction procedure

Preparation of working area

1. Place machine on a suitable stable base on the correct side of the couch.

   ↓

2. Check plugs, leads and tubing and ventouses.

   ↓

3. Test the machine. Switch it on and place a finger over the inlet hole (the end of the tube that will be inserted into the ventouse), turn up the intensity dial and watch the negative pressure register on the gauge, turn down the dial and switch off. *Or*: Place the ventouse on the flexors of your forearm, with a finger over the hole in the ventouse, switch on the machine and increase the intensity until the flesh is lifted into the ventouse. Remember this must then be adjusted to suit the flesh on the area being treated. Turn down the dial and switch off the machine.

   ↓

4. Wipe over the ventouse with a disinfecting solution.

   ↓

5. Check intensity controls are at zero.

   ↓

6. Check the couch is prepared with clean linen and towels.

   ↓

7. Prepare trolley with:
   - suitable medium – oil or cream
   - client consultation record.

   ↓

Preparation of self

8. Before carrying out treatment ensure you prepare yourself physically and mentally, paying due attention to high standards of professionalism. Adopt a sensitive calm, confident and understanding attitude, as this approach will have a positive effect on your client.

   ↓

Preparation of client

9. Carry out a consultation, or if a regular client refer to the notes from their last treatment and discuss the effects and outcomes before proceeding.

   ↓

10. Check for contra-indications.

    ↓

11. Check contact lenses and all jewellery have been removed.

    ↓

12. Place the client in a well-supported and comfortable position.

    ↓

13. Protect hair and clothing.

    ↓

14. Explain the treatment to the client. They will feel a gentle lifting of the tissues and warmth as you work rhythmically over their face and neck. If the lifting sensation or a feeling of pressing down on the skin becomes uncomfortable they must let you know.

    ↓

WASH YOUR HANDS

15. Carry out a tactile sensitivity test.

    ↓

16. Cleanse and tone the skin.

    ↓

17. Carry out a skin analysis.

    ↓

Best practice **B**

Position the machine on the left side of the couch if you are right-handed and the right side of the couch if you are left-handed to avoid crossing over or changing hands.

Technique for facial vacuum suction

18. Select the appropriate ventouses to suit client's needs.

↓

19. Apply a suitable medium, oil or cream to the face and neck.

↓

20. Place the ventouse on the area and adjust the suction – do not exceed 20 per cent of the ventouse.

↓

21. Lift the ventouse and glide it over the contours of the face and neck to the *nearest* set of lymph nodes.

↓

22. Break the suction before lifting the ventouse off the skin (use the release hole or depress the skin with the little finger).

↓

23. Move on to the next stroke; overlap the previous stroke until the area is covered. Repeat 5–8 times depending upon the skin reaction and whether the skin is preheated. An erythema will develop more quickly if the skin is preheated.

↓

24. Continue until the neck and face are covered.

↓

25. Use the appropriate ventouse to work over comedones and blockages or for treating lines.

↓

26. Keep in verbal contact with the client to monitor progress of the treatment and be alert to contra-actions.

↓

27. At the end of treatment switch off the machine, remove the medium and tone the skin.

↓

28. Continue with the facial routine depending on client's needs.

↓

29. Update the consultation record with salient points about the treatment for future reference. This will include the outcome of the tactile sensitivity test.

Learning point Ⓛ

The pattern of strokes in Figure 7.10 is a guide to the drainage towards the nodes named in Figure 7.9.

Learning point Ⓛ

When using a ventouse, hold it like a pencil, perpendicular to the skin.

Remember

Some ventouses have a small hole in the side to release the vacuum when required. This hole must be covered with a finger to maintain a vacuum (the finger is removed to release the vacuum). If there is no hole, the vacuum must be released by depressing the flesh with the finger.

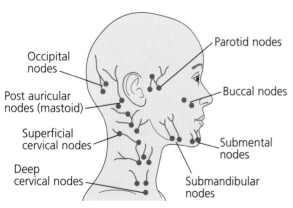

△ **Figure 7.9** Lymphatic nodes of face and neck

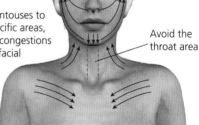

Applicator: facial ventouse for general cleansing

Overlap the previous stroke until the area is covered

Use other ventouses to focus on specific areas, for example congestions and lines of facial expression

Avoid the throat area

△ **Figure 7.10** Treatment technique for vacuum suction

Timing of treatment

Normal and combination skin: 5–7 minutes.

Deep cleansing of greasy skin: 10–12 minutes.

Dry, dehydrated, mature and sluggish skin: 7–10 minutes.

Refer to manufacturer's instructions for specific guidance.

Remember

Although manufacturers give treatment times for different skin conditions these are for guidance only. You must always observe client's skin reaction during the application and respond appropriately.

Contra-actions to facial vacuum suction

Bruising and dilated capillaries: caused by too much suction, failing to break the suction before lifting the cup off the skin, pressing the cup down instead of lifting when working towards the lymph node. Place a cool compress on the skin and apply a suitable product that will help to calm and soothe the tissues.

Remember

Always seek feedback from your client and give appropriate aftercare advice (see pages 73–4).

Recommendations for facial vacuum suction

This treatment can be used in conjunction with steam to increase the effectiveness of the treatment for most skin types and conditions. Take care, if treating sensitive skin, to avoid over-stimulating the tissues.

The facial steamer is used as a preheat treatment to warm and soften the skin and open the pores to prepare the tissues for general cleansing, aiding the removal of congestion and increasing lymphatic drainage of the area.

Disincrustation prior to vacuum suction would be beneficial for greasy and congested skin as it warms the tissues, opens the pores and has a deep cleansing effect. Vacuum suction treatment would then focus on loosening blocked pores and comedones and increasing lymphatic drainage, helping to improve the texture and tone.

A course of 6 treatments combined with steam and iontophoresis would benefit dry, dehydrated and mature skin; one every 2–3 weeks depending on the skin condition.

A greasy skin type would benefit from a treatment every week for the first three weeks to help clear congestion and comedones and improve the texture and tone of the skin, combined with steam, disincrustation and vacuum suction.

Remember

Monitor progress and review the treatment plan.

Cleaning

Wash the ventouses and tubes in hot water and detergent. Use a small brush to clean and remove oil and debris inside the ventouse and tubing. Rinse, dry and store in a sanitiser.

Refer to manufacturer's instructions for specific guidance.

Body vacuum suction

Vacuum suction on the body is always used in conjunction with other treatments.

Benefits of body vacuum suction

○ To reduce fatty deposits on the abdomen, hips, thighs, 'dowager's hump', below the neck, etc. (in conjunction with other treatments and diet).

○ To improve and reduce areas of cellulite.

○ To improve poor circulation, both lymphatic and blood.

○ To reduce non-systemic oedema and areas of fluid retention.

○ To improve the texture, tone and general condition of the skin.

▽ **Table 7.6** Physiological effects and benefits of body vacuum suction

Physiological effects	Improve and reduce fatty deposits in conjunction with diet	Improve poor circulation	Reduce non-systemic oedema and fluid retention	Improve skin condition
The flow of lymph is speeded up. The vacuum inside the cup sucks the tissues into the cup. This causes the lymph vessels to dilate and fill up with lymph; as the cup moves along it draws lymph with it. The stroke will end just before the lymph node and lymph will drain into the node. As the flow of lymph is speeded up, more waste products will be removed.	√	√	√	√
Oedema may be reduced. Because the flow of lymph in the vessels is speeded up, more lymph will be drained from the tissues thus reducing stagnation and swelling. This works well for gravitational oedema but not for oedema caused by high blood pressure, kidney problems and other systemic problems. (Seek a doctor's advice to establish the cause of the oedema.)			√	
Circulation is increased. In the same way as lymph vessels are affected, the veins will alternately expand and contract and the venous flow is speeded up. If blood flows more quickly in the veins, then the arterial side may also speed up. This increases the supply of nutrients and oxygen to the body part and speeds up the removal of waste. This will improve the condition of the tissues.	√	√	√	√
The increased circulation will produce heat and vasodilation with erythema (this improves the colour of the skin).	√	√	√	√
Cell metabolism is stimulated and this improves the condition of the skin.	√	√	√	√
The friction of the cup, the oil used on the part and the stimulation of the circulation will aid desquamation, thus also improving the condition of the skin.	√		√	√

Contra-indications to body vacuum suction

Learning point Ⓛ

Check the contra-indications listed in the manufacturer's instructions to ensure that you do not invalidate your insurance policy should the client be injured during or after treatment.

▽ **Table 7.7** Reasons for contra-indications to body vacuum suction

Contra-indication	Reason
Breast tissue	Do not treat this area as breast tissue is thinner and more fragile than the skin on the body and could easily be damaged.
Dilated capillaries (thread veins)	Suction over the area could make the condition worse. Carry out treatment if the area(s) can be avoided.
Bruising	May cause further damage resulting in increased bleeding. Bruises must be allowed to heal before giving treatment, unless they are small and it is possible to work around them.
Chemotherapy, radiotherapy	The client will be under medical supervision. In line with acceptable work ethics and professional code of practice you must seek medical consent before commencing any treatment.
Cuts and abrasions	There is a risk of cross-infection from body fluids as the wounds are open. Avoid the area.
Diabetes	Clients with diabetes may have impaired sensitivity, poor circulation and healing may be slow. Great care must be taken to avoid damage to the skin or any other injury. If in doubt seek GP's consent.
Epilepsy	Find out as much as possible about the client's condition. If it is controlled epilepsy, the treatment may be safe to carry out as the treatment is quite soothing and gentle on the tissues but if in any doubt seek medical advice. Do not leave anyone suffering from epilepsy unattended in a room or on the couch.
Hairy areas (very)	Treatment will be uncomfortable for the client because as the cup glides over the area it will pull on the hairs.
Hypersensitive skin	Treatment will cause sensitivity in the tissues and there is also a risk of thread veins. Suggest an alternative treatment.
Loose, crêpey skin and ageing thin skin	There is a danger of overstretching loose skin and of breaking down ageing thin skin causing open wounds. Suggest an alternative treatment.
Phlebitis	Phlebitis is inflammation of the vein that could result in a clot forming on the wall of the vein known as thrombosis. If pressure is applied to this area the clot could be carried by the blood circulation to the heart or lungs, with fatal consequences. Do not treat. Treatment of the legs is a definite contra-indication and it is safer not to treat the body as there will always be a slight risk.

(Continued)

(Continued)

Contra-indication	Reason
Scar tissue and stretch marks (recent)	The tissue must be allowed to heal completely before giving treatment, as there is a danger of further damage to the tissues delaying the healing process.
Skin diseases	There is a risk of cross-infection.
Sunburn	The erythema (reddening) following sunburn must clear completely before treatment can be given as the skin will be sensitive.
Thread veins	Treatment will make the condition worse. Avoid the area.
Varicose veins	If varicose veins are already present, do not use vacuum suction over the area as it will exacerbate the condition. If varicose veins are present in the calf, the thigh can be treated.

Learning point

Vacuum suction can help to prevent varicose veins as venous flow is speeded up.

Dangers of body vacuum suction

The main risk of harm with suction is bruising of the area caused by poor technique:

○ pressure too high
○ pulling cup off before releasing the vacuum
○ over-treating the area, too many stokes or too long a treatment
○ pushing the cup downwards, instead of lifting and gliding.

Precautions should be taken to minimise the risk of harming the client and to ensure you give an effective treatment.

▽ **Table 7.8** Precautions to take with body vacuum suction

Precaution	Explanation
Test the machine.	You need to check it is in good working order and ensure it will not cause harm to you or your client.
Check the rim of the cups for any roughness or chips.	This may cause small scratches/abrasions on the skin.
Carry out a tactile sensitivity test (see page 71).	If the client cannot tell the difference between sharp and soft, they have defective sensation and the treatment should not be carried out.
Select the correct cup size for the area.	Too large a cup will not contour the area and therefore the treatment will be ineffective. Too small a cup may cause bruising, as too much flesh will be sucked into the cup.
Check the pressure on yourself.	This is to ensure the machine is working correctly and the pressure can be adjusted to suit the tissues being treated.
Apply sufficient oil to the area.	This is to facilitate the movement of the cup and provide a seal.

(Continued)

(Continued)

Precaution	Explanation
Make sure appropriate pressure is used.	Too high a pressure will cause bruising and thread veins in the area.
Lift enough flesh, but do not exceed 20 per cent of the cup.	This is to prevent bruising and thread veins.
Use a lifting and gliding technique, rather than pushing the cup downwards.	This could result in bruising or thread veins.
Avoid over-treating the area with too many strokes or too long a treatment.	This could result in bruising or thread veins and cause the client discomfort.
Do not work over the nodes.	This may cause swelling and sensitivity in the area.
Release pressure before lifting the cup off the area.	This is to prevent thread veins and bruising.
Overlap the previous stroke by 1 cm (1/2 inch).	This is to ensure even coverage.
Speak to the client during the treatment.	You need to monitor progress of the treatment and be alert to contra-actions occurring.

Body vacuum suction procedure

Preparation of working area

1. Place machine on a suitable stable base on the correct side of the couch.
   ↓
2. Check plugs, leads, tubing and cups.
   ↓
3. Test the machine. Switch it on and place a finger over the inlet hole where the tube attaches to the cup, turn up the intensity dial and watch the negative pressure register on the gauge, turn down the dial and switch off. Or: Place the cup on the flexors of your forearm, switch on the machine and increase the intensity until the flesh is lifted into the cup. Remember this must then be adjusted to suit the flesh on the area being treated. Turn down the dial and switch off the machine.
   ↓
4. Wipe over the cup with a disinfecting solution.
   ↓
5. Check intensity controls are at zero.
   ↓
6. Check the couch is prepared with clean linen and towels.
   ↓
7. Prepare trolley with:
   - suitable medium – oil or cream
   - pillows or rolled towels for support
   - client consultation record.
   ↓

Preparation of self

8. Before carrying out treatment ensure you prepare yourself physically and mentally, paying due attention to high standards of professionalism. Adopt a sensitive calm, confident and understanding attitude, as this approach will have a positive effect on your client.
   ↓

Best practice B

Position the machine on the left side of the couch if you are right-handed and the right side of the couch if you are left-handed to ensure you are in control of the dials.

Preparation of client

9. Carry out a consultation, or if a regular client refer to the notes from their last treatment and discuss the effects and outcomes before proceeding.

↓

10. Check for contra-indications.

↓

11. Check jewellery has been removed from the area.

↓

12. Place the client in a well-supported and comfortable position.

↓

13. Protect clothing.

↓

14. Explain the treatment to the client. They will feel a gentle lifting of the tissues and warmth as you work rhythmically over the area. If the lifting sensation or a feeling of pressing down on the skin becomes uncomfortable they must let you know.

↓

WASH YOUR HANDS

15. Carry out a tactile sensitivity test.

↓

16. Cleanse the area using appropriate products.

↓

Technique for body vacuum suction

17. Select cups of suitable size, the largest possible to fit the area without losing suction.

↓

18. Apply oil or cream to the area to facilitate the movement of the cup and to provide a seal between the cup and the skin.

↓

19. Place the cup on the area and adjust the suction so that the skin fills 20 per cent of the cup. (Break the suction quickly if suction is too high, otherwise bruising and dilation of capillaries may occur.)

↓

20. *Lift* the cup and *glide* it in a straight line towards the nearest set of lymph nodes that drain the area.

↓

21. Break the suction by removing finger from the hole on the cup. If there is no hole, depress the flesh with the little finger under the rim of the cup or use the thumb of the other hand to depress the flesh.

↓

22. Move to the adjacent area, overlapping the last stroke by 1 cm or 1/2 inch only. Continue until all the area is covered. Return over the first stroke and cover the area between five and ten times, depending on the type of flesh and desired effect.

↓

23. Keep in verbal contact with the client to monitor progress of the treatment and be alert to contra-actions.

↓

24. At the end of the treatment, effleurage the area and remove oil from the area.

↓

Remember

Pressing the cup down instead of lifting can be painful and may cause bruising.

Remember

The pressure must be released before the cup is lifted otherwise bruising and dilated capillaries may occur.

Remember

Do not repeat the stroke over the same area without moving on – this can cause dilated capillaries.

Remember

The rhythm should be of medium even speed, not too fast or too slow. The sequence should be as follows:

○ Place the cup on the body part, filling 20 per cent of the cup.

○ Lift the cup and move it in a straight line towards the nearest lymph nodes draining that area.

○ Release the pressure.

○ The next stroke should overlap the last stroke by 1 cm or 1/2 inch if possible.

25. Continue with the body routine depending on client's needs.

↓

26. Update the consultation record with salient points about the treatment for future reference. This will include the outcome of the tactile sensitivity test.

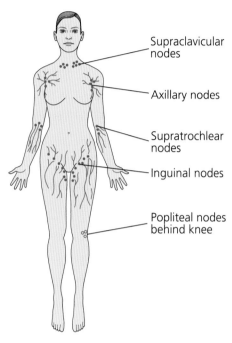

Supraclavicular nodes

Axillary nodes

Supratrochlear nodes

Inguinal nodes

Popliteal nodes behind knee

△ **Figure 7.11** Lymphatic nodes of the body

Recovery position

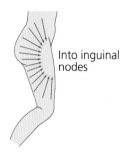

Into inguinal nodes

△ **Figure 7.13** Direction of strokes, lateral aspect

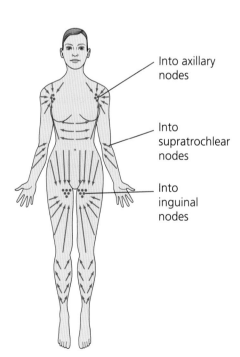

Into axillary nodes

Into supratrochlear nodes

Into inguinal nodes

△ **Figure 7.12** Direction of strokes, anterior aspect

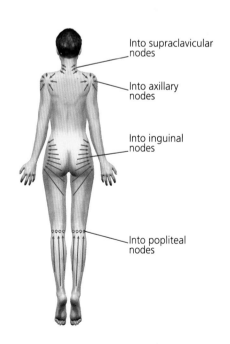

Into supraclavicular nodes

Into axillary nodes

Into inguinal nodes

Into popliteal nodes

△ **Figure 7.14** Direction of strokes, posterior aspect

Timing of treatment

The degree of erythema and client tolerance dictates the length of the treatment.

Refer to manufacturer's instructions for specific guidance.

Contra-actions to body vacuum suction

Bruising and thread veins may be caused by too much suction, failing to break the suction before lifting the cup off the skin, pressing the cup down instead of lifting when working towards the lymph node.

Place a cool compress on the skin and apply a suitable product that will help to calm and soothe the tissues. Advise the client to avoid wearing restrictive clothing in the area.

> **Remember**
> Always seek feedback from your client and give appropriate aftercare advice. See pages 73–4.

Recommendations for body vacuum suction

> **Best practice**   B
> Recommend the client has a preheat treatment or use hot towels to warm and soften the tissues to increase the effectiveness of the treatment.

Vacuum suction should form part of a treatment routine – pre-heating followed by gyratory vibrator or manual massage to warm and soften the area and increase circulation. This can be followed by electrical muscle stimulation (EMS) and then vacuum suction to increase lymph drainage.

Suggest a course of 9–12 treatments, between 2 and 4 times per week, depending on client's needs but especially if they want to lose weight. Monitor progress and review treatment plan.

If galvanic treatment has been given, do not use vacuum suction over the area of the pads as the skin may be very sensitive. Vacuum suction can be done prior to galvanic treatment to decongest the area.

Cleaning

Wash the cups and tubes in hot water and detergent, use a brush to clean and remove oil and debris from inside the cups and tubing; rinse, dry and store in a sanitiser. Check manufacturer's instructions for specific guidance.

SUMMARY

- Vacuum suction treatment speeds up the flow of lymph in the lymphatic vessels and therefore removes waste products from the area more quickly and reduces any oedema in the area. It also increases the circulation to the area, bringing oxygen and nutrients to the body part and removing waste products.

- **The lymphatic system**: small blind end tubes, called lymphatic capillaries, form a network through tissue spaces between cells; they join to form larger lymphatic vessels. These vessels drain into lymph nodes where lymph is filtered; lymph nodes also produce lymphocytes. Afferent lymph vessels enter the nodes; efferent lymph vessels leave the nodes. Lymph vessels eventually form lymph trunks, which drain into the thoracic duct or into the right lymphatic duct and then into the right and left subclavian veins.

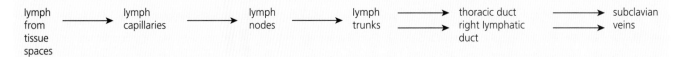

lymph from tissue spaces → lymph capillaries → lymph nodes → lymph trunks → thoracic duct / right lymphatic duct → subclavian veins

- Vacuum suction on the face is used for general and deep cleansing and to stimulate and improve the condition of dry, dehydrated skin.
- Vacuum suction is used on the body in conjunction with other treatments to improve the circulation of the blood and lymph, to aid dispersal of fatty deposits for clients on a diet, to improve areas of cellulite, and to reduce oedema.

- The treatment time will depend on the size of the area to be treated – the larger the area, the longer the time needed to cover it.
- The main danger is causing bruising of the area. Bruising may be caused:
  - if the pressure is too high
  - by pulling the cup off before releasing the vacuum
  - by over-treating the area with too many strokes
  - by pushing the cup down instead of lifting and gliding it.

QUESTIONS

Oral questions

Facial vacuum suction treatments

1. Why does the flesh rise into the ventouse?
2. How do you control the degree of suction?
3. How much flesh should be lifted into the ventouse?
4. Why would you select this treatment for the client?
5. Why would you follow a particular pattern when moving the ventouse over the skin?
6. Name the lymph nodes you would be working towards.
7. How would you release the suction at the end of the stroke?
8. Why is it important to release the suction before lifting the ventouse off the part?
9. What are the contra-actions to treatment and how would you deal with them?
10. How do you clean the ventouse and tubing after treatment?
11. How long is a vacuum suction treatment?
12. What procedure would you follow after the treatment?

Body vacuum suction treatments

1. When would you select vacuum suction as a suitable treatment?
2. What treatment could you advise prior to vacuum suction? Why would this be beneficial?
3. What precautions would you take:
   - before treatment?
   - during treatment?
4. How would you ensure good, even coverage?
5. How would you select the cup size?
6. How would you decide when to stop the treatment?
7. How would vacuum suction be combined with other treatments?
8. If the client had oedema in the area to be treated what should you do?
9. What are the contra-actions to treatment and how would you deal with them?
10. Why is it not advisable to use vacuum suction after body galvanic?
11. How long is a vacuum suction treatment?
12. What procedure would you follow after the treatment?

Multiple-choice questions

1. Which of the following is transported by the lymphatic system back to the blood stream?
   a Protein molecules.
   b Oxygen.
   c Bile.
   d Carbon dioxide.

2. Which of the following lymphatic structures produce antibodies?
   a Capillaries.
   b Trunks.
   c Nodes.
   d Ducts.

3. What affects the speed of lymph flow?
   a Liver.
   b Hormones.
   c Haemoglobin.
   d Muscles.

4. Where are the supratrochlear nodes located?
   a In front of the ear.
   b At the elbow.
   c Under the chin.
   d Above the clavicle.

5. The suction effect is produced in the cups by:
   a sucking out air to reduce the pressure
   b balancing the correct amount of air and pressure
   c forcing in air to increase the pressure
   d blowing out air to increase the pressure.

6. The flat-head ventouse is mainly used to:
   a aid the removal of comedones
   b cleanse the area
   c improve lines of facial expression
   d treat areas of pigmentation.

7. What is the maximum amount of flesh that should be lifted into the ventouse/cup?
   a 10 per cent.
   b 15 per cent.
   c 20 per cent.
   d 25 per cent.

8. Which of the following conditions is a contra-action from a vacuum suction treatment?
   a Cellulite.
   b Congested skin.
   c Scar tissue.
   d Bruising.

9. Which of the following is the correct technique when giving a vacuum suction treatment? Place the ventouse/cup on the area and:
   a glide and break suction
   b lift, glide and break suction
   c press down, glide and break suction
   d press down and break suction.

10. What condition would be totally contra-indicated to a vacuum suction treatment?
    a Phlebitis.
    b Hairy areas.
    c Cuts and abrasions.
    d Scar tissue.

11. Oil is used to:
    a protect the skin
    b prevent swelling in the area
    c improve the suction effect
    d aid the movement of the cup.

12. An excess of fluid within the tissue spaces is called:
    a osmosis
    b oedema
    c diffusion
    d inflammation.

8 Galvanic treatment

Objectives

After you have studied this chapter you will be able to:

- describe the type of current used in galvanic treatments
- list the treatments that use the galvanic current
- describe the benefits and effects of galvanic treatments
- explain the contra-indications to galvanic treatments
- explain the dangers and precautions to galvanic treatments
- explain the contra-actions that may occur during and/or after treatment and the appropriate action to take
- carry out galvanic treatments, paying due consideration to maximum efficiency, comfort, safety and hygiene.

Introduction

Galvanic treatments use a direct current. The current flows in one direction and has polarity (see page 90).

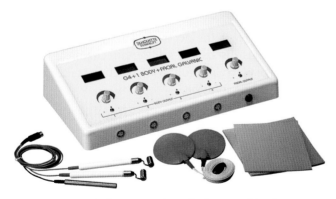

△ **Figure 8.1** Galvanic machine for face and body treatments

Figure 8.1 is a photograph of a galvanic machine. This is one of the larger models and may be used for both facial and body work. Galvanic treatments use a low-voltage direct (constant) current, sometimes called a galvanic current. This current flows in one direction only and has polarity. One electrode is negatively charged (called the cathode), while the other is positively charged (called the anode). Galvanic treatments may be used on the face or body and are given specific names, as follows.

Facial treatments:

- desincrustation – a deep-cleansing treatment. The effects at the cathode are used to remove the build-up of sebum and keratinised cells and to soften the skin of the face.
- iontophoresis (or ion repulsion) – specially manufactured products are repelled into the skin by appropriate electrodes. It is suitable for many skin types: a variety of products are available to suit different skin conditions.

Body treatments:

- body galvanic (iontophoresis) – specially manufactured anti-cellulite products are used to soften and aid the dispersal of cellulite.

Body galvanism (sodium chloride (salt) solution) is no longer used as a stand-alone treatment, but is dealt with here to explain the chemical and physical effects that are produced under the electrodes that are used in treatment. For example, the softening effect under the cathode is used to treat areas of cellulite. For the purposes of explanation (and possibly during your training), this process will be explained using a saline solution (sodium chloride) as the electrolyte. In practice, however, you would not use saline on a client.

The effects produced by these treatments are dependent on:

- the chemistry of electrolysis.

Learning point

Electrolysis in this context refers to the process of passing a current through a solution, called an electrolyte, via electrodes. In beauty therapy you will also come across the term in the context of hair removal.

155

○ the laws of physics, which state that like charges repel and opposite charges attract.

The first part of this chapter explains these principles, and it is recommended that you study and understand them before commencing treatments. This knowledge will enable you to select the most appropriate and effective treatment to suit the needs of the client. It will also enable you to fully explain the treatment to the client.

Activity (A)

Revise the sections on elements, compounds, atoms, ions and electrolysis in Chapter 4.

Electrolysis of sodium chloride solution

The purpose of this explanation is to help you to understand what happens at each electrode and between the electrodes during a galvanic treatment using a sodium chloride solution (salt solution). In the workplace you will use specially manufactured products as the electrolyte, which contain beneficial ingredients in some form of salt solution.

Learning point (L)

Electrodes are also referred to as 'poles'.

Remember

Sodium chloride is the chemical name for common salt: another term for sodium chloride solution is saline solution.

An electrolyte is a chemical compound that is capable of splitting into ions and can carry an electric current.

A solution containing common salt and water is an electrolyte. In solution the sodium chloride will dissociate (split) into ions of sodium and chloride. The water will dissociate into ions of hydrogen and hydroxyl:

Sodium chloride will ionize, giving sodium (+) ions and chloride (−) ions

$$NaCl \rightarrow Na^+ \text{ and } Cl^-$$

Water will ionize giving hydrogen (+) ions and hydroxyl (−) ions

$$H_2O \rightarrow H^+ \text{ and } OH^-$$

Negatively charged ions are called *anions* (−) and positively charged ions are called *cations* (+)

These ions move freely in the solution; when a direct current is applied to the solution by means of two electrodes, the current will flow through the electrolyte, the saline solution. The electrodes will be charged depending on their connections to the battery or machine.

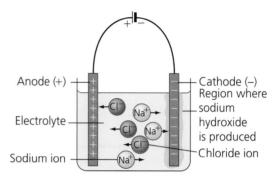

△ **Figure 8.2** Electrolysis of sodium chloride solution

One will be negatively charged, this is the cathode (−).

The other will be positively charged, this is the anode (+).

When the current is switched on, the ions will move *away from* or *towards* the electrodes. This occurs because:

○ like charges repel

○ opposite charges attract.

Therefore, the cations (+) will move towards the cathode (−) and the anions (−) will move towards the anode (+). See Figure 8.2.

The cathode (−) is the negative electrode and it attracts the positive ions; cations (+): the anode (+) is the positive electrode and it attracts the negative ions; anions (−).

When the ions reach the electrode with the opposite charge, some are discharged and certain chemical reactions take place. The following reactions take place when using saline solution:

○ At the cathode (−) the sodium ion (Na^+) reacts with the hydroxyl ion (OH^-) in the water producing the alkali sodium hydroxide (NaOH) and hydrogen (H_2) gas.

○ At the anode (+) the chloride ion (Cl^-) reacts with the hydrogen ions (H^+) in the water producing *hydrochloric acid* (HCl) and oxygen (O_2) gas.

The formation of the alkali sodium hydroxide at the cathode is used in facial desincrustation to soften the stratum corneum and to help remove hard plugs of sebum. In body galvanic it reduces and softens areas of cellulite by changes in circulation, metabolic rate and water content of the tissue through which the current passes.

At the same time, hydrochloric acid will be produced under the anode (+). This hardens the tissues and restores the acid mantle.

Galvanic machines pass direct current in one direction only. For some treatments the cathode is known as the working or active electrode, and the anode is the inactive or indifferent electrode. Other treatments may require the anode to be the working electrode and the cathode to be inactive. You must always check with manufacturer's instructions to ensure you are using the correct electrode as the working electrode. It will vary depending on the product being used. It refers to the direction of flow of the current. Machines have a polarity switch to change the direction of current flow.

The switch may be used during a treatment, for example, using the cathode as the working electrode with saline solution, the alkali sodium hydroxide formed at the cathode will be used to soften the tissues at the start of the treatment. The polarity may then be reversed for the last 2–3 minutes of the treatment so that the formation of hydrochloric acid at the anode as the working electrode can be used to tighten and refine the tissues and help to restore the natural pH balance of the skin.

> ### Learning point (L)
> A current applied to the face or body by means of two electrodes will be carried through the tissues. This happens because tissue fluid contains a high percentage of salts and is an electrolyte.

In the workplace it would not be acceptable to use a sodium chloride solution (salt), as the client would expect you to use a professional range of products for their treatment. There are many manufactured products on the market, which, in addition to some form of salt solution, contain beneficial substances to treat the skin. These products use the principles of body galvanism (sodium chloride (salt) solution) described in this chapter.

The effects of galvanic current application

Physiological effects

When galvanic current is applied to the face or body certain effects are produced at the electrodes also known as 'poles'. These effects are known as 'polar effects'. Other effects are produced in the tissues between the electrodes or poles; these are known as 'inter-polar effects'.

Polar effects

These occur immediately beneath the electrodes (poles). (See Table 8.1.)

Galvanic machines

There is a wide variety of machines on the market for facial treatments, body treatments and combined facial and body treatments. Low-voltage, direct current is produced by a battery or modified AC mains. This current is applied to the face and body using electrodes connected to the machine by leads.

- One electrode will be negative, called the cathode (−).
- The other will be positive, called the anode (+).

All machines have:

- intensity controls
- a milliammeter to indicate current flow
- polarity reversal switch to reverse the polarity should you need to do so during the treatment, from cathode (−) to anode (+) and vice versa depending on the effect required
- electrodes that are connected to the machine by leads.

> ### Be aware
> Because machines are not standardised, you may misinterpret the polarity switch and this can lead to incorrect treatment. It is vital to refer to each individual manufacturer's instruction manual to ensure understanding and correct use of the machine. Your client will be expecting positive results from the treatment.

> ### Activity (A)
> It is always vital to check the polarity output of each machine yourself. This can be done in different ways:
>
> - To check the polarity, hold both electrodes in your hand and increase the intensity: the negative electrode/pole (the cathode) will always be the more irritating. This test is the easiest to perform, but is not as definitive as the water test.
> - Hold the electrodes in a beaker of water and increase the intensity: bubbles of hydrogen will be seen at the cathode (−).

▽ **Table 8.1** Polar effects

Polar effects at the cathode (–)	Polar effects at the anode (+)	Polar effects in the tissues between the cathode (–) and anode (+)
An *alkali* is formed which is irritating to the tissues. It: ○ breaks down keratin. ○ destroys the acid mantle, reducing the skin's protective function against micro-organisms ○ saponifies sebum ○ has a drying effect on the skin.	An *acid* is formed which is irritating to the tissues. It: ○ increases the acidity of the skin ○ improves and restores the acid mantle and the skin's protective function ○ tightens and hardens the tissues.	Increased blood flow through the area. Increased lymphatic flow through the area. Improved cell metabolism.
Marked vasodilation with hyperaemia and erythema (due to heat and irritation). Heat is produced; the degree of heat depends on the intensity of the current, the time for which it flows and the skin's resistance to the current.	Less marked vasodilation, hyperaemia and erythema (due to less heat and irritation). Mild heat produced. Helps to calm the skin at the end of treatment.	Increased permeability of blood vessel walls.
Increased excitability and conductivity of nerves.	Decreased excitability and conductivity of nerves. Prolonged treatment can produce numbing of the area (analgesic effect).	
Increased tissue fluid drawn to the area – softening the tissues.	Oxygen is released improving the condition of the tissues.	Slight reduction in blood pressure.

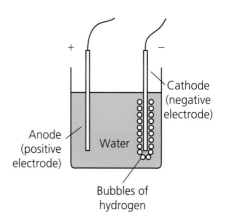

△ **Figure 8.3** Hydrogen bubbles at the cathode

Learning point

Various names are used to describe the electrode that is producing the required effect and the one merely completing the circuit. These include:

○ working and inactive
○ active and passive
○ active and indifferent
○ active and inactive
○ differential and passive.

Be aware ❗

You must always ensure that you understand all the components of the machines in order to give effective treatments.

Facial galvanic treatments

The direct or galvanic current is used in two ways on the face to improve cleanliness, tone, texture and condition of the skin. The methods are known as **desincrustation** and **iontophoresis**.

Facial desincrustation treatment

The treatment requires a source of direct current applied to the skin via two electrodes: a cathode (−), which must be the working electrode and an anode (+), which is the inactive electrode. It also requires a/specific product as an electrolyte, for example a manufactured product in the form of a gel that contains beneficial substances in a salt solution.

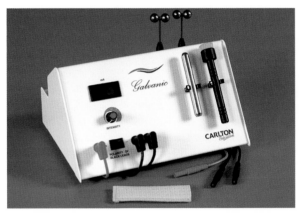

△ **Figure 8.4** A facial galvanic machine with electrodes for desincrustation and iontophoresis

> **Learning point** ⓛ
>
> A sodium chloride solution could be used as the medium, one teaspoon of salt to one pint/600mls of water. However the client would expect you to use a professional range of products for their treatment.

The alkali, formed from the product under the cathode (−), will soften the build-up of sebum, break down keratinised cells of the superficial layer of the skin, open pores and release blockages. It is therefore used as a general and deep cleansing treatment.

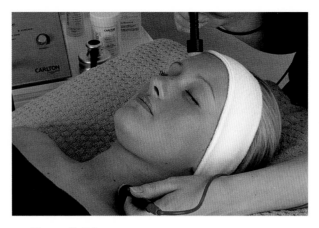

△ **Figure 8.5** Desincrustation treatment

The alkali does alter the pH of the skin, destroying the acid mantle. This is an undesirable effect and is corrected by reversing the polarity at the end of the treatment for 2–3 minutes.

Electrodes for desincrustation

The anode (+) is the inactive electrode and must be placed in a comfortable position on the client to complete the circuit.

> **Best practice** Ⓑ
>
> The bar electrode can be held in the client's hand. It must be covered with a dampened sponge cover, which must be of an even texture. You may prefer to place the bar electrode behind the client's shoulder so they can relax during the treatment.

Benefits of desincrustation

○ General cleansing of a combination, dry, dehydrated and mature skin.

○ Deep cleansing of a greasy skin.

○ Stimulation of a sluggish skin with build-up of keratinised cells and comedones.

> **Learning point** ⓛ
>
> This treatment is beneficial for acne skin as long as there is no infection present.

A careful skin analysis must be carried out before treatment to ensure that the skin type is suitable for desincrustation.

159

▽ **Table 8.2** Electrodes for desincrustation

Electrode	Example	Use
Ball or double ball		Working electrode
Tweezer electrode		Working electrode
With a disposable sponge head		Working electrode
Roller electrodes		Working electrodes for greasy skin to cover a wider area
Bar electrode		Inactive electrode(s)

▽ **Table 8.3** Physiological effects and benefits of desincrustation

Benefits Physiological effects	General cleansing of a combination, dry, dehydrated and mature skin	Deep cleansing of greasy skin	Stimulation of a sluggish skin
Effects at the cathode (−) working electrode			
The alkali formed will saponify sebum and soften the skin; the pores relax releasing the sebum. It will also break down the keratin in the superficial layers of the skin, thus softening and cleansing the area and aiding desquamation.	√	√	√

(Continued)

(Continued)

Physiological effects	Benefits	General cleansing of a combination, dry, dehydrated and mature skin	Deep cleansing of greasy skin	Stimulation of a sluggish skin
Fluid drawn towards the cathode (–) will soften the skin. This hydrating effect is only temporary.		√	√	√
It causes vasodilation with hyperaemia and erythema; the increase in circulation brings nutrients and oxygen to nourish the skin and removes waste products. This will improve the condition of the skin and improve the colour of sallow, sluggish skin.		√	√	√
Effects at the anode (+) working electrode when the polarity is reversed for the last 2–3 minutes of treatment.				
The formation of an acid restores the natural pH of the skin.		√	√	√
The acid tightens and firms the skin refining the pores.		√	√	√
The release of oxygen revitalises the skin (oxygen will be a bi-product of the reaction at the anode).		√	√	√
Inter-polar effects (effects between the two electrodes)				
Increased blood and lymph flow.		√	√	√
Increased permeability of blood vessel walls.		√	√	√
Improved cell metabolism.		√	√	√

Contra-indications to desincrustation and iontophoresis

Check the contra-indications listed in the manufacturer's instructions to ensure you do not invalidate your insurance policy should the client be injured during or after treatment.

▽ **Table 8.4** Reasons for contra-indications to desincrustation and iontophoresis

Contra-indication	Reason
Acne, pustular with inflamed areas	There is a risk of cross-infection. If it is not possible to avoid these areas, do not treat.
Asthma	Suggest an alternative treatment if the condition is severe. If treatment can be carried out place the client in a semi-inclined position with additional supports for ease of breathing during treatment. Ensure client has their inhaler within easy reach.
Bruising (extensive)	May cause further damage resulting in increased bleeding. Bruises must be allowed to heal before giving treatment, unless they can be avoided.
Chemotherapy, radiotherapy	The client will be under medical supervision. In line with acceptable work ethics and professional code of practice you must seek medical consent before commencing any treatment.
Cuts and abrasions	The broken skin may have a higher moisture content, which will increase the intensity of the current and cause the client discomfort. Small cuts may be insulated with petroleum jelly.

(Continued)

(Continued)

Contra-indication	Reason
Diabetes	Clients with diabetes may have impaired sensitivity and poor circulation therefore will not be able to give accurate feedback on the intensity of the current. Healing may also be slow. Great care must be taken to avoid damage to the skin or any other injury. If in doubt seek GP's consent.
Epilepsy	Find out as much as possible about the client's condition. If it is controlled epilepsy, the treatment may be safe to carry out but recommend the client seeks medical advice. Do not leave anyone suffering from epilepsy unattended in a room or on the couch.
Facial piercings	Avoid the area or cover the adornment as it may be made of material that conducts an electrical current that will cause a shock.
Heart conditions	The increase in the blood circulation may put too much pressure and stress on the heart. Obtain medical consent.
High blood pressure	This varies with age, weight and lifestyle of clients. Some have consistently high blood pressure. Treatments can frequently help, especially if the client is worried about their skin. Medical advice should be sought if the client is not currently on medication.
Hypersensitive skins, e.g. rosacea	Desincrustation – the cleansing process will be too harsh and will exacerbate these conditions. Iontophoresis – this is not contra-indicated, as active substances are introduced into the skin that will be beneficial for sensitive skin conditions.
Injectable treatment (recent)	The skin may be red, tender and painful, with bruising and swelling. The skin needs time to settle down and heal before having further treatment. Fillers plump out lines and wrinkles, adding fullness to the face: do not treat as the movement of the electrodes over the area may dislodge the filler.
Lack of skin sensitivity, which may be caused by damage to or pressure on nerves, neurological disorders, scarring, Bell's palsy or dental treatments, etc.	The client must be able to report any build-up of heat (hot spots) and must report if the intensity of the current is too high. Always carry out a thermal and tactile sensitivity test to check that the client can distinguish between hot and cold and sharp and soft (see page 71).
Low blood pressure	This is not usually an issue. Be aware that the client may feel dizzy or faint if they sit up or get off the couch too quickly following treatment. Always supervise and give assistance if necessary.
Metal pins or plates around the head or excessive fillings	Metal is a good conductor, therefore the intensity of the current will increase in the area and may cause the client discomfort. Keep in verbal contact with the client.
Pacemaker	The current may interfere with the electrical impulses to the heart. Do not treat.
Pregnancy	As the client forms part of the circuit there may be a risk to the foetus.
Skin diseases	There is a risk of cross-infection.
Skin disorders, eczema, psoriasis	The skin for both conditions is red with flaky dry patches, the treatment will cause more sensitivity in the area and exacerbate the condition.
Sunburn	The erythema (reddening) following sunburn must clear completely before treatment can be given as the current intensity and products could cause an adverse reaction.
Swelling	Recommend the client seeks medical advice, as there may be an underlying problem that prevents treatment.

Dangers of desincrustation

There is a danger of shock if the:

○ current is turned up or down suddenly
○ electrode(s) are lifted off the skin during treatment.

There is a slight risk of burning:

○ if the equipment is faulty
○ the intensity of the current is set too high
○ if using saline solution, the solution is too concentrated.

> **Learning point** **L**
>
> Thermal burns are the result of too much heat. Galvanic burns, or electrical burns are the result of too great an intensity of current. Chemical burns can be caused by alkalis or acids that are too highly concentrated.

Precautions should be taken to minimise the risk of harming the client and to ensure you give an effective treatment.

▽ **Table 8.5** Precautions to take with desincrustation

Precaution	Explanation
Test the machine.	You need to check it is in good working order and ensure it will not cause harm to you or your client.
Carry out a thermal and tactile test (see page 71).	This is to ensure the client can distinguish between hot and cold sensations and feel the difference between sharp and soft objects so that you know the client will be able to report any discomfort to you.
Check that all jewellery has been removed.	If the electrodes come into contact with jewellery the client may experience a shock.
Apply petroleum jelly under the eyes.	This acts as insulation to prevent 'flash' as the skin is delicate under the eyes. This is an uncomfortable sensation and may happen if the electrode moves too near the eye. Always check manufacturer's instructions as some electrodes can be used under the eye area.
Client must hold the inactive electrode firmly.	There is a danger of the client experiencing an electric shock if they lose contact with the bar electrode. To avoid this happening ask the client to place their hand on top of the covers or place the electrode behind their shoulder.
Place the working electrode on a sensitive area, such as the forehead, and turn the current up slowly.	This is to assess client's tolerance to the current.
Turn the current up or down gradually.	There is danger of electric shock if the current is turned up or down suddenly. This is because the sudden surge of current will stimulate the muscles to contract.
Keep the electrode(s) in contact with the skin throughout the treatment. Turn the intensity down before removing it.	There is a danger of shock if the electrode(s) is lifted off the skin during treatment because the circuit will be broken.
Speak to the client throughout the treatment.	You need to ensure they are comfortable and to be alert to contra-actions occurring.

Desincrustation procedure

Preparation of working area

1. Place machine on a suitable stable base on the correct side of the couch.

2. Check plugs, leads and electrodes.

3. Test the machine – Set up the leads and electrodes for a desincrustation treatment. Place the bar electrode on a folded towel covered with tissue. Hold the ball/tweezer electrode, place it on the bar electrode and slide it up and down as you switch on the machine and turn up the intensity slowly. You should see the indicator on the milliammeter increase. Turn the intensity down and switch off the machine.

   Or:

   Place a dampened cover on the bar electrode anode (+) the inactive electrode and hold it in the hand you do not write with. Place the cathode (−) on the flexors of your forearm and stroke up and down on a small area as you switch on the machine and turn up the intensity slowly. As soon as you feel a tingling, prickling sensation turn the intensity down and switch off the machine.

4. Clean the attachments with a disinfecting product.

5. Check intensity controls are at zero.

6. Check the couch is prepared with clean linen and towels.

7. Prepare trolley with:
   ○ petroleum jelly
   ○ desincrustation gel
   ○ dampened cover for inactive electrode
   ○ client consultation record.

Preparation of self

8. Before carrying out treatment ensure you prepare yourself physically and mentally, paying due attention to high standards of professionalism. Adopt a sensitive calm, confident and understanding attitude, as this approach will have a positive effect on your client.

Preparation of client

9. Carry out a consultation, or if a regular client, refer to the notes from their last treatment and discuss the effects and outcomes before proceeding.

10. Check for contra-indications.

11. Check contact lenses and all jewellery have been removed.

12. Place the client in a well-supported and comfortable position.

13. Protect hair and clothing.

14. Explain the treatment to the client. They will feel a tingling sensation and warmth. You will turn down the intensity slightly so they will not experience any tingling but the treatment will still be effective.

WASH YOUR HANDS

15. Carry out a thermal and tactile sensitivity test.

16. Cleanse and tone the skin with suitable products.

17. Carry out a skin analysis.

18. Apply a little petroleum jelly around the eye area.

> **Best practice** B
>
> Position the machine on the left side of the couch if you are right-handed and the right side of the couch if you are left-handed to avoid crossing over or changing hands.

> **Remember**
>
> Warn the client that if they have dental fillings or bridge work they may experience a metallic taste in their mouth during treatment. They should let you know if this is the case, as you will need to turn the intensity down.

> **Be aware** !
>
> If the client has an open cut, blemish or abrasions, cover with petroleum jelly. The broken skin may have a higher water content, which will increase the intensity of the current and cause the client discomfort.

Technique for desincrustation

19. Select the appropriate electrodes and plug them into the machine.

   ↓

20. Place the bar electrode anode (+), the inactive electrode, in a dampened sponge cover and give it to the client to hold or place behind their shoulder.

   ↓

21. Apply a desincrustation product.

   ↓

22. Place the cathode (−), the working electrode, on the client's skin. Choose an area of high sensitivity (e.g. the forehead), and switch on.

   ↓

23. Turn the current up slowly, moving the electrode on the area. Very low current is needed. This must be within the client's tolerance.

   ↓

24. As soon as the client feels a tingling, sensation, turn the current down slightly. The treatment will still be effective.

   ↓

25. Move the electrode(s) slowly and firmly over the area, use a circular movement with the ball or sponge electrode and rhythmical even movements each side of the face with the rollers.

   ↓

26. Keep in verbal contact with the client to monitor progress of the treatment and be alert to contra-actions.

   ↓

27. At the end of the treatment, turn the intensity down slowly and switch off with electrode still in contact with the face.

   ↓

28. *Reverse the polarity* of the machine so that the working electrode is now the anode (+).

   ↓

29. Place the electrode on the forehead again and repeat the procedure for 2–3 minutes. This will restore the natural pH of the skin.

   ↓

30. Turn the intensity down slowly as before, switch off and remove the electrode.

   ↓

31. The skin must be thoroughly wiped over with damp cotton wool.

   ↓

32. Carry out comedone and milia extractions if required (page 296).

   ↓

33. Apply toner and blot with tissue.

   ↓

34. Continue with the facial routine depending on client's needs.

   ↓

35. Update the consultation record with salient points about the treatment for future reference. This will include the outcome of the sensitivity test.

Remember

If the client has a greasy skin rather than greasy areas use the roller electrodes and the ball, tweezer or sponge electrode for congested areas around the nose and chin.

Be aware !

If client is unable or unwilling to remove wedding (or other) rings, ensure the client does not hold the inactive electrode in the hand with rings on as metal is a good conductor of electricity.

Be aware !

It is the tolerance of the client which dictates the maximum current; manufacturers will give guidelines which you must check before commencing treatment.

Remember

Keep the electrode in contact with the skin otherwise the client will experience a small electric shock.

Be aware !

As the treatment progresses sebum, which acts as a barrier, is gradually dissolved reducing the skin's resistance and so the client may feel the current intensifying. If necessary turn the intensity down.

Be aware !

Take care when extracting comedones and milia as too much pressure will result in broken capillaries, bruising and permanent marks on the skin. Over a course of treatment blockages will soften especially if the client follows homecare advice too.

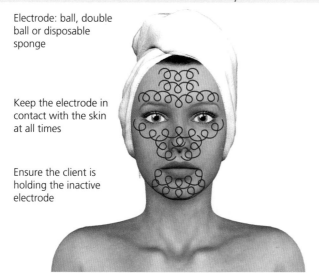

Electrode: ball, double ball or disposable sponge

Keep the electrode in contact with the skin at all times

Ensure the client is holding the inactive electrode

△ **Figure 8.6** Treatment technique for desincrustation

Timing of treatment

○ Greasy skin conditions: 7–10 minutes.

○ Combination skin: 4–6 minutes.

○ Dry, mature skin with congestion: 3–5 minutes.

Refer to manufacturer's instructions for specific guidance.

Contra-actions to desincrustation and iontophoresis

○ Excessive erythema: caused by intensity too high and/or prolonged treatment. Place a cool compress on the skin and apply a suitable product or mask that will help to calm and soothe the tissues.

○ Burns: the danger is minimal as the time of application is short, current intensity low and the electrode is moving continually. However, if a burn occurs apply sterile cold water to the area to prevent the burn getting worse, apply a soothing, healing lotion or cream. Advise the client not to touch the area. In the unlikely event of a galvanic burn, medical attention should be sought.

Remember
Always seek feedback from your client and give appropriate aftercare advice (see pages 73–4).

Recommendations for desincrustation

This is a general cleansing treatment that is of benefit to most skin types. For greasy and congested skins, suggest a course of treatment once a week for the first 2–3 weeks to cleanse and decongest the skin and to help improve the texture and tone. This could be complemented with a direct high frequency treatment using oxygenating cream to refine the pores, help dry the skin and heal blemishes, and/or vacuum suction to increase lymphatic drainage and help with the removal of comedones and blocked pores.

If the skin becomes dehydrated, advise the client to have treatment every 2 weeks. As the secretions become more regulated suggest an iontophoresis treatment after desincrustation. Active ingredients can be chosen in a range of gels, creams and ampoules to hydrate, nourish and revitalise the skin to suit the client's needs.

Cleaning of the electrodes

Wash the metal electrodes in hot soapy water, use a brush to remove any remaining gel, rinse and dry, and wipe the holder with a disinfecting solution. Store electrodes in a sanitiser. Some electrodes can be sterilised in the autoclave. Always refer to the manufacturer's instructions.

Best practice B
Any remaining gel can hardened quite quickly so soak this part of the electrode(s) in water while you complete the treatment.

Facial iontophoresis treatment

This uses a direct current to introduce beneficial products into the skin. The treatment is based on the principle that like charges repel and opposite charges attract.

A source of direct current is applied to the skin and the electrodes are used to repel ions of beneficial substances into the skin.

Manufacturers produce a wide range of gels, ampoules and creams suitable for various skin conditions. The products contain ions, which carry either negative or positive charges. The success of this treatment is dependent upon:

○ correct identification of the skin condition.

○ the selection of the appropriate product for the skin condition.

○ the selection of the appropriate electrode to repel the product.

  ○ If the product is negatively charged, the cathode (−) will be the working electrode. The cathode (−) will repel the anions (−) in the product into the skin.

  ○ If the product is positively charged, the anode (+) will be the working electrode. The anode (+) will repel the cations (+) in the product into the skin.

Remember
The working electrode has to be the same polarity as the product.

Electrodes for iontophoresis

Gels, ampoules and creams that are repelled under electrodes are thought to achieve deeper penetration than manual applications. Penetration is thought to be less than 1 mm, but deeper absorption may be achieved via the capillary circulation and transport through cell membranes.

▽ **Table 8.6** Electrodes for iontophoresis

Electrode	Example	Suggestions for use
Rollers		Working electrodes used over the face and neck
Ball or double ball		Working electrode used on and around the nose area and over the chin. Check manufacturer's instructions to find out if it can be used around the eye area
Bar electrode		Inactive electrode

Learning point (L)

Research has indicated that low level intensity currents and low ionic concentrations may well be as effective as high intensity currents and high ionic concentrations (on the basis that a few ions entering slowly will find it easier to enter the skin than a mass of ions all with the same charge repelling each other as they are forced through). However, some products may require certain intensities for their repulsion, and manufacturers sometimes offer guidelines, which should be carefully followed. When products without guidelines are used, it should be borne in mind that a low current is often effective.

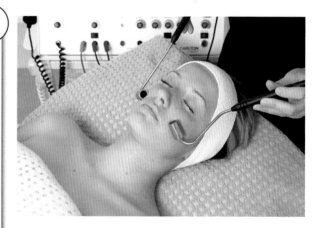

△ **Figure 8.7** Iontophoresis treatment

Benefits of iontophoresis

This form of treatment can be used for a wide variety of skin conditions. A careful skin analysis must be made to diagnose the problem areas. The appropriate product can then be selected to suit the needs of the client.

○ **Hydration** and **moisturising:** many products are manufactured for moisturising and hydrating a dry, dehydrated and mature skin; serums containing collagen, elastin and placental extracts are particularly beneficial.

○ **Regeneration:** products are available for the repair and regeneration of mature skin and of damaged skin, particularly after exposure to the sun and wind.

○ **Stimulating:** products for stimulating a sluggish, sallow complexion include extracts of seaweed and other marine products. Care must be taken not to overtreat with these products.

○ **Improvement of sensitive skins:** gels, ampoules and creams are available for the treatment of the sensitive, couperose skin. Care must be taken when treating these skin types as many conditions can be exacerbated by the direct current. Rosacea and highly vascular conditions would be contra-indicated and should not be treated with galvanic current.

▽ **Table 8.7** Physiological effects and benefits of iontophoresis

Physiological effects	Benefits: Hydration and moisturising	Regeneration	Stimulating	Improve sensitive skin
Different products will give different effects beneath the cathode and the anode, depending on the working electrode and the chemical composition of the product.				
Vasodilation, with hyperaemia and erythema, will increase the circulation to the area, bringing oxygen and nutrients to improve the condition of the skin.	√	√	√	√
Improvement in the colour and texture of the skin, due to an increase in blood flow and an increase in desquamation.	√	√	√	√
Desquamation is aided, due to increased cellular activity of the basal layer.	√	√	√	√
When using iontophoresis the main effect will depend on, and be specific to, the product used. Manufacturers recommend their products for specific skin types and also indicate which electrode should be used for repelling the ions into the skin. Therefore careful skin analysis must be carried out and the appropriate product selected to achieve the most beneficial outcome for the client. Other effects will be due to stimulation by the direct current.	√	√	√	√
Inter-polar effects (effects between the two electrodes)				
Increased blood and lymph flow.	√	√	√	√
Increased permeability of blood vessel walls.	√	√	√	√
Improved cell metabolism.	√	√	√	√

Contra-indications

See pages 161–2.

Dangers of iontophoresis

There is a danger of shock if the:

○ current is turned up or down suddenly

○ electrode(s) are lifted off the skin during treatment.

There is a slight risk of burning:

○ if the equipment is faulty

○ if the intensity of the current is set too high

○ if your technique is poor.

Precautions should be taken to minimise the risk of harming the client and to ensure you give an effective treatment.

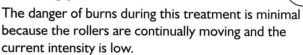

Learning point

The danger of burns during this treatment is minimal because the rollers are continually moving and the current intensity is low.

Be aware

The intensity of the current used for facial work will depend on the tolerance of the client and the erythema reaction produced. Check manufacturer's instructions.

▽ **Table 8.8** Precautions to take with iontophoresis

Precaution	Explanation
Test the machine.	This is to check it is in good working order and ensure it will not cause harm to you or your client.
Carry out thermal and tactile sensitivity test (see page 71).	This is to ensure the client can distinguish between hot and cold sensations and feel the difference between sharp and soft objects so that you know the client will be able to report any discomfort to you.
Use petroleum jelly under the eyes.	This acts as insulation to prevent 'flash', as the skin is delicate under the eyes. This is an uncomfortable sensation and may happen if the electrode moves too near the eye. Always check manufacturer's instructions as some electrodes can be used under the eye area.
Place the rollers/ball electrode on a sensitive area of skin (e.g. the forehead or jaw line) and keep them moving while turning the current up slowly and steadily.	This is to assess client's tolerance. Also, there is a danger of electric shock if the current is turned up or down suddenly or if the intensity is turned up before the electrode is in contact with the face/neck. This is because the sudden surge of current will stimulate the muscles to contract.
Turn the intensity down slightly when the client feels a tingling sensation.	This treatment is more effective with a low-intensity current and low ionic concentrations. Turn the current up only within the tolerance of the client.
Move the rollers/ball electrode slowly over the face without breaking contact with the skin.	This is to prevent the client experiencing a shock if the electric circuit is broken.
Do not knock the rollers together during treatment.	The current will flow from one roller to the other, making the treatment ineffective.
Turn the current down slowly before removing the electrodes.	This is to prevent the client experiencing a shock if the electric circuit is broken.
Speak to the client throughout the treatment.	You need to ensure they are comfortable and to prevent contra-actions occurring.

Iontophoresis procedure
Preparation of working area

1. Place machine on a suitable stable base on the correct side of the couch.

2. Check plugs, leads and electrodes.

3. Test the machine – Set up the leads and electrodes for an iontophoresis treatment. Place the bar electrode on a folded towel covered with tissue. Hold a roller electrode, place it on the bar electrode and slide up and down as you switch on the machine and turn up the intensity slowly. You should see the indicator on the milliameter increase. Turn the intensity down slowly and switch off the machine.
Or:
Place a dampened cover on the bar electrode the inactive electrode and hold it in the hand you do not write with. Place the roller electrode on the flexors of your forearm and slide up and down on a small area as you switch on the machine and turn up the intensity slowly. As soon as you feel a tingling, prickling sensation turn the intensity down slowly and switch off the machine.

4. Clean the attachments with a disinfecting product.

5. Check intensity controls are at zero. Prepare the leads and electrodes, check the polarity of the gel, ampoule or cream you will be using and set the rollers at the same polarity, for example positive (+) product, positive (+) roller electrodes. As like charges repel, the roller electrodes will repel the product into the skin.

6. Check the couch is prepared with clean linen and towels.

7. Prepare trolley with
   ○ petroleum jelly
   ○ gel, ampoule or cream
   ○ dampened cover for the inactive electrode
   ○ client consultation record.

Preparation of self

8. Before carrying out treatment ensure you prepare yourself physically and mentally, paying due attention to high standards of professionalism. Adopt a sensitive, calm, confident and understanding attitude, as this approach will have a positive effect on your client.

Preparation of client

9. Carry out a consultation, or if a regular client refer to the notes from their last treatment and discuss the effects and outcomes before proceeding.

10. Check for contra-indications.

11. Check contact lenses and all jewellery have been removed.

12. Place the client in a well-supported and comfortable position.

13. Protect hair and clothing.

14. Explain the treatment to the client using terminology they will understand. They will feel a tingling sensation and warmth. You will turn down the intensity slightly so they will not experience any tingling but the treatment will still be effective.

WASH YOUR HANDS

15. Carry out thermal and tactile sensitivity test.

16. Cleanse and tone the skin with suitable products.

17. Carry out a skin analysis.

18. Apply a little petroleum jelly around the eye area.

Best practice B

Position the machine on the left side of the couch if you are right-handed and the right side of the couch if you are left-handed to avoid crossing over or changing hands.

Remember

Warn the client that if they have dental fillings or bridge work they should let you know as you will need to turn down the intensity.

Remember

If the client has an open cut, blemish or abrasions, cover with petroleum jelly as the broken skin may have a higher water content which will increase the intensity of the current and cause the client discomfort.

Technique for iontophoresis

19. Place the *inactive* electrode in a dampened sponge cover and give it to the client to hold or place behind their shoulder.

↓

20. Apply the product evenly over the face and neck.

↓

21. Place one roller onto the client's skin, switch on the machine and turn up the current slowly until a tingling sensation is felt, turn down the intensity slightly then place the other roller on the opposite side of the face/neck.

↓

22. Move the rollers over the face and neck, maintain an even pressure and a rhythmical movement.

↓

23. Keep in verbal contact with the client to monitor progress of the treatment and be alert to contra-actions.

↓

24. Remove one roller and turn the current down slowly and switch off the machine before removing the other roller.

↓

25. Apply a little more gel and, repeating the procedure for turning the machine on and off, use the ball electrode for concentrated work on and around the nose, chin, labial nasal folds and lines on the outer eye area and between the brows.

↓

26. *Reverse the polarity* – if required, *check product information* – repeat the procedure for 2 minutes. This will help to restore the natural pH of the skin.

↓

27. Remove excess product, apply toner and blot with tissue.

↓

28. As the products continue to work after the treatment it is recommended to complete the treatment with a suitable face mask, tone and moisturise.

↓

29. Update the consultation record with salient points about the treatment for future reference. This will include the outcome of the sensitivity test.

Remember
Ensure the client does not hold the inactive electrode in the hand with rings on as metal is a good conductor of electricity.

Remember
Place one roller on a sensitive area of skin e.g. the forehead or jaw line and keep it moving while turning the current up slowly and steadily to client's tolerance.

Remember
Do not break contact with the skin and make sure the rollers do not touch each other.

Be aware
It is the tolerance of the client that dictates the maximum current.

Learning point
Some manufacturers recommend a direct high frequency with oxygenating cream to follow iontophoresis as it releases oxygen into the tissues and also has an anti-bacterial and germicidal effect.

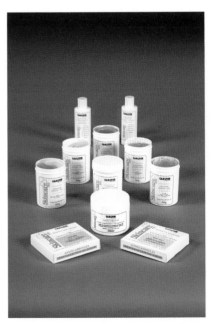

△ **Figure 8.8** Gels, ampoules and cream for iontophoresis treatment

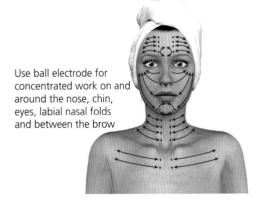

Use ball electrode for concentrated work on and around the nose, chin, eyes, labial nasal folds and between the brow

△ **Figure 8.9** Treatment technique for iontophoresis

Timing of treatment

○ 7–10 minutes, depending on the skin type and condition.

Refer to manufacturer's instructions for specific guidance about the duration of the treatment.

Contra-actions

See page 166.

> **Remember**
>
> Always seek feedback from your client and give appropriate aftercare advice (see page 86).

Recommendation for iontophoresis

Suggest a course of 6 treatments, one every 2–4 weeks, depending on the condition of the skin. A treatment plan might start with desincrustation to deep cleanse the skin, then the iontophoresis treatment to help absorb products suitable for the skin condition, followed by direct high frequency for its anti-bacterial and germicidal effect. Complete the treatment with mask and moisturiser.

For an intensive course of treatment, suggest one treatment per week for 3 weeks. Monitor progress and review the treatment plan.

Cleaning of the electrodes

Wash the metal electrodes in hot soapy water, use a brush to remove any remaining gel, rinse and dry, wipe the holder with a disinfecting solution. Store electrodes in a sanitiser. Some electrodes can be sterilised in the autoclave. Always refer to the manufacturer's instructions.

> **Best practice** ⓑ
>
> Any remaining gel can hardened quite quickly, so soak this part of the electrode(s) in water while you complete the treatment.

Body galvanic treatment

The application of a direct current to the tissues of the body will produce certain effects (see Table 8.1). These effects are thought to soften areas of cellulite and aid its dispersal.

Body galvanic (iontophoresis) treatment uses products in the form of gels and ampoules containing liquid serum preparations specially manufactured to treat cellulite. These preparations contain charged ions of beneficial substances, which are repelled into the skin by use of the appropriate electrode. The product usually carries negatively charged beneficial ions, therefore the cathode (−) is used as the working electrode to repel them into the tissues. This method uses the effects of the product as well as the polar and the inter-polar effects of the current. This form of treatment is known as body iontophoresis.

▽ **Table 8.9** Electrodes for body galvanic treatment

Electrode	Example	Use
Pair of carbon impregnated electrodes		Working and inactive electrodes

Benefits of body galvanic (iontophoresis)

○ To soften areas of cellulite and aid its absorption.
○ To improve the condition of the skin and tissues.
○ To improve areas of stasis.

Learning point Ⓛ

The term 'stasis' means stagnation in the normal flow of bodily fluids.

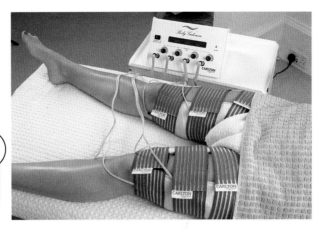

△ **Figure 8.10** A body galvanic treatment

▽ **Table 8.10** Physiological (polar) effects and benefits of body galvanic (iontophoresis)

Physiological (polar) effects	Soften areas of cellulite and aid its absorption	Improve skin tissues	Improve areas of stasis
Effects at the cathode (–)			
The product will form an alkali under the cathode (–), which softens the skin and tissues. Products such as gels and ampoules containing negatively charged ions will be repelled into the skin by the cathode (–).	√	√	√
An *increase* in the water and tissue fluid in the area of the electrode due to increased permeability of vessel walls and to the movement of water molecules away from the anode (+) towards the cathode (–). This will soften the area.	√	√	√
Vasodilation with hyperaemia and erythema; more blood will flow to the area bringing nutrients and oxygen and removing metabolites.	√	√	√
Heat is produced under the electrode; the client should feel an even, comfortable warmth.	√	√	√
Irritation of sensory nerve endings; it *increases* the conductivity of nerves and blood flow to the area.	√	√	√
Effects at the anode (+) working electrode when the polarity is reversed. The anode is usually the inactive electrode in body galvanic. Some products contain substances that utilise the effects of the anode (+) for the last 2–3 minutes of treatment. Always check the instructions on the product.			

(Continued)

(Continued)

Physiological (polar) effects	Benefits		
	Soften areas of cellulite and aid its absorption	Improve skin tissues	Improve areas of stasis
The formation of an acid restores the natural pH of the skin.	√	√	√
The acid tightens and firms the skin refining the pores.	√	√	
The release of oxygen revitalises the skin (oxygen will be a bi-product of the reaction at the anode).	√	√	√
Inter-polar effects (effects between the two electrodes)			
Increased blood and lymph flow.	√	√	√
Increased permeability of blood vessel walls.	√	√	√
Improved cell metabolism.	√	√	√

Contra-indications to body galvanic (iontophoresis)

Learning point Ⓛ

Check the contra-indications listed in the manufacturer's instructions to ensure you do not invalidate your insurance policy should the client be injured during or after treatment.

▽ **Table 8.11** Reasons for contra-indications to body galvanic

Contra-indication	Reason
Body piercing adornments	Avoid the area or cover the adornment as it may be made of material that conducts an electrical current and will cause a shock.
Bruising (extensive)	May cause further damage resulting in increased bleeding. Bruises must be allowed to heal before giving treatment unless they can be avoided.
Chemotherapy, radiotherapy	The client will be under medical supervision. In line with acceptable work ethics and professional code of practice, you must seek medical consent before commencing any treatment.
Cuts and abrasions	The broken skin may have a higher moisture content, which will increase the intensity of the current and cause the client discomfort. Small cuts may be insulated with petroleum jelly.
Diabetes	Clients with diabetes may have impaired sensitivity and poor circulation therefore will not be able to give accurate feedback on the intensity of the current. Healing may also be slow. Great care must be taken to avoid damage to the skin or any other injury. If in doubt seek GP's consent.

(Continued)

(Continued)

Contra-indication	Reason
Epilepsy	Find out as much as possible about the client's condition. If it is controlled epilepsy, the treatment may be safe to carry out but recommend the client seeks medical advice. Do not leave anyone suffering from epilepsy unattended in a room or on the couch.
Heart conditions	The increase in the blood circulation may put too much pressure and stress on the heart. Seek medical consent.
High blood pressure	Blood pressure varies with age, weight and fitness, but some clients have consistently high blood pressure. Treatments can frequently help, especially if the client is worried about a particular part of their body. Medical advice should be sought if the client is not currently on medication.
Lack of skin sensitivity may be due to neurological disorders, injury, scar tissue, etc.	Sensitivity tests are essential for all galvanic treatments as the client must be able to report any build-up of heat (hot spots) and must report if the intensity of the current is too high.
Low blood pressure	The treatment reduces both diastolic and systolic pressure, so the client may feel dizzy or faint if they sit up or get off the couch too quickly following treatment. Always supervise and give assistance if necessary.
Medication in the form of ointments that have been applied to the skin to treat muscular aches and pains	These will sensitise the area. Always wash skin thoroughly to avoid this possibility.
Metal pins or plates in the area to be treated	Metal is a good conductor, so the intensity of the current will increase in the area and may cause the client discomfort. Avoid treating these areas.
Oedema	Treatment may make the condition worse, as blood and lymph is increased in the area. Recommend the client seeks medical advice, as there may be an underlying problem that prevents treatment.
Pacemaker	Do not give treatment, as the current may interfere with the electrical impulses to the heart.
Pregnancy	Do not give treatment, as the current penetrates the tissues there may be a risk to the foetus.
Scar tissue (recent)	Scar tissue is composed of thick fibrous connective tissue that has limited blood circulation and defective sensation. If the scar tissue is recent it must be allowed to heal completely before treatment is given to the area. If treatment is given before healing is complete, there is a danger of further damage to the tissues, delaying the healing process.
Skin diseases	There is a risk of cross-infection.
Skin disorders for example eczema and psoriasis	The skin is red with flaky, dry patches; the treatment will cause more sensitivity in the area and exacerbate the condition.
Varicose veins	Area should be avoided, as the tissues around the vein may be fragile and easily damaged. There is a tendency for the stagnating blood to form clots, which may be dislodged by the treatment.

Dangers of body galvanic (iontophoresis)

There is a danger of shock if the:

○ current is turned up or down suddenly

○ equipment is faulty.

There is a slight risk of burning:

○ if the equipment is faulty

○ if the intensity of the current is set too high

○ if using saline solution, as the solution is too concentrated.

Burns

Burns are often caused by poor technique of application and must be avoided. An awareness of the nature and causes of burns will enable you to develop good technique, thus ensuring that burns do not occur.

An increase in blood flow to an area will result in the production of heat to that area. The amount of heat produced will be directly proportional to the intensity, time and resistance. Because the processes of conduction, convection and radiation are restricted under the pads, there is a build-up of heat.

If the intensity of the current is high, the time during which it flows is too long or if the resistance to the current is high, there is a danger of producing a thermal burn. The intensity and time of current flow must be carefully controlled and careful consideration must be given to avoid areas of high resistance.

> **Learning point** (L)
>
> Areas of hard tissue, such as scars, large freckles or moles can be areas of high resistance. Care should be taken to avoid them.

Burns can result from the following:

○ the current is applied with metal touching the tissues, either in the form of jewellery, or metal plates and pins in tissues. Always remove jewellery and avoid giving treatment to areas around metal plates

○ the electrode or its connections coming into direct contact with the skin

○ the client has defective skin sensation and is unable to feel that the intensity is too high or that the current is concentrating in one spot

○ pads being unevenly saturated, giving rise to dry/moist spots resulting in areas of high resistance (dry) and areas of low resistance (moist)

○ unevenness within the pads preventing good, even skin contact

○ gaps and air spaces allowed between the skin and the electrode. This happens if a stiff electrode does not adapt to the rounded contour of the body

○ the sponge covers are too close together so that current concentrates between them

○ the current concentrates on one area. This may be due to a break in the skin

○ the product has not been washed out of the sponge covers after a previous treatment

○ the treatment has not been explained carefully to the client. (The importance of reporting discomfort and hot spots and the consequences of not doing so must be explained clearly to the client.)

> **Be aware**
>
> Burns may also occur if the client is lying with full body weight on the electrode. This pressure limits the circulating blood and its action of conducting heat away from the area. Therefore, if the posterior aspect of the body is being treated, clients should lie in the prone position (face down) and vice versa.

> **Be aware**
>
> Tight, elasticated straps also restrict the blood flow; they should apply even, firm pressure over the electrode but not be so tight as to restrict the circulation.

Remember

Thermal burns are the result of too much heat. *Galvanic burns*, or electrical burns are the result of too great an intensity of current and affect the tissues below the surface. They can take a long time to heal. *Chemical burns* can be caused by alkalis or acids that are too highly concentrated. These are unlikely when using preparatory products.

Best practice   **B**

Accurate technique and careful application will prevent thermal, galvanic and chemical burns.

Precautions should be taken to minimise the risk of harming the client and to ensure you give an effective treatment.

▽ **Table 8.12** Precautions to take with body galvanic

Precaution	Explanation
Test the machine.	You need to check it is in good working order and ensure it will not cause harm to you or your client.
Check the sponge covers are of even thickness.	Uneven thickness will cause higher current intensity in the area.
Carry out sensitivity test, thermal and tactile (see page 71).	This is to ensure the client can distinguish between hot and cold sensations and feel the difference between sharp and soft objects. The client must be able to give accurate feedback about the intensity of the current.
Check for broken skin.	This will have a low resistance to current and therefore the current would concentrate here and cause a burn. Cover with petroleum jelly.
Cleanse the area thoroughly before treatment.	To remove sweat, sebum, and lotions, as these will form a barrier to the current.
Turn the current up slowly; adjust if necessary and at the end of treatment turn the current down slowly.	A sudden increase or decrease in current intensity gives the client a shock, as the muscles may contract.
Speak to the client throughout the treatment.	This is to check that the treatment is comfortable and there are no hot spots that will cause burns.
Cleanse the area after treatment.	This is to remove any product residue.
Wash the sponge covers in hot soapy water, rinse and dry.	This is not only for hygiene, but importantly, to remove the product residue from the sponge covers as a build-up could cause burns to the next client.

Body galvanic (iontophoresis) procedure

Preparation of working area

1. Place machine on a suitable stable base on the correct side of the couch.

2. Check plugs and leads.

3. Ensure the electrodes and sponge covers are clean.

4. Test the machine:
   ○ Plug the leads into the machine. Place the ends of the positive and negative leads together and turn up the intensity; the milliammeter should indicate the current is flowing.

   Or:
   ○ Place a pair of pads together so that the carbon surfaces meet and turn up the intensity; the milliammeter should indicate the current is flowing.

5. Check intensity controls are at zero. Prepare the leads and electrodes and check the polarity of the product, (this is usually negative). Select the appropriate polarity on the machine.

6. Check the couch is prepared with clean linen and towels.

7. Prepare trolley with:
   ○ petroleum jelly
   ○ gel, ampoule
   ○ warm water (or dilute saline solution) to dampen the sponge covers for the working and inactive electrodes
   ○ elasticated straps
   ○ client consultation record.

Preparation of self

8. Before carrying out treatment ensure you prepare yourself physically and mentally, paying due attention to high standards of professionalism. Adopt a sensitive, calm, confident and understanding attitude, as this approach will have a positive effect on your client.

Preparation of client

9. Carry out a consultation, or if a regular client refer to the notes from their last treatment and discuss the effects and outcomes before proceeding.

10. Check for contra-indications.

11. Check all jewellery has been removed from the area.

12. Place the client in a well-supported and comfortable position.

13. Explain the treatment to the client using terminology they will understand. They will feel a slight tingling sensation, which will give way to *mild* warmth.

WASH YOUR HANDS

14. Carry out sensitivity test, thermal and tactile.

15. Cleanse the area thoroughly to remove sebum, sweat and body lotion.

16. Assess the location and amount of cellulite present and the type of padding that would be most beneficial.

17. Apply petroleum jelly on any broken skin or cover with a waterproof plaster.

Best practice B

Position the machine on the left side of the couch if you are right-handed and the right side of the couch if you are left-handed to ensure you are in control of the dials.

Remember

Some products require the polarity to be reversed for 2–3 minutes at the end of treatment to restore the natural pH of the skin.

Be aware

Always check manufacturer's instructions about the product before carrying out treatment; do not assume all products follow the same format.

Learning point L

Sponge covers may be dampened with water or dilute saline solution (1 teaspoon of salt to 1 pint (600mls) water). Check manufacturer's instructions for guidance. Saline solution is a better conductor of electricity.

Best practice B

If your client has already been for a treatment, you can place the straps on the couch ready for when they arrive to save time.

Remember

If the thighs and hips are to be treated, place the client in the supine position (face up).

If the buttocks or back are to be treated, place the client in the prone position (face down).

Technique for body galvanic (iontophoresis)

18. Position the elasticated straps in the area.

↓

19. Soak the sponge covers in warm water/saline solution, and squeeze out the excess.

↓

20. Place the working electrode – the cathode (–) – in the dampened sponge cover; apply the product with a spatula to the side of the sponge with the active graphite pad facing it and place this on the area of cellulite.

↓

21. Place the inactive electrode anode (+) in a dampened sponge cover and position opposite or parallel to the cathode (–).

↓

22. Secure the electrodes in position with elasticated straps.

↓

23. Make sure the sponge covers and electrodes mould to the body and contain no air spaces and that the elasticated strapping applies even pressure all over.

↓

24. Turn up the intensity control slowly until a tingling, warming sensation is felt.

↓

25. Stay with the client; as the treatment progresses the skin resistance will fall and you may have to decrease the intensity.

↓

26. At the end of treatment turn the intensity control down slowly. Reverse the polarity if required for 2–3 minutes so that the anode (+) becomes the working electrode. This will restore the natural pH of the skin, tighten and firm the tissues.

↓

27. Turn the intensity down slowly as before, then switch off the machine.

↓

28. Remove the elasticated straps, sponge covers and electrodes.

↓

29. The skin should be evenly pink under each sponge cover, and there should be a more marked reaction under the cathode (–).

↓

30. Cleanse the skin to remove any remaining product and apply a soothing lotion.

Best practice B

When possible involve your client by asking them to hold the cathode (-) in place while you prepare the inactive electrode, the anode (+).

Remember

Stress to the client the importance of reporting any discomfort, any concentration of current in one area or any hot spots.

Best practice B

Place your hand lightly on the body part as you increase the current to draw the client's attention to the intensity and their comfort level.

Be aware

The desired intensity will depend on the client's tolerance, the product used and the size of the pad. Check manufacturer's instructions for guidance.

Be aware

If the area of skin under the electrodes is very sensitive, do not carry out further treatments. Allow the tissues to settle down.

Timing of treatment

Maximum 20 minutes. Refer to manufacturer's instructions for specific guidance.

Contra-actions to body galvanic (iontophoresis)

○ Excessive erythema: caused by intensity too high and or prolonged treatment. Place a cool compress on the skin and apply a suitable product that will help to calm and soothe the tissues.

○ Burns: the danger with body galvanic is the risk of burns (see page 176 for information on causes). Apply sterile cold water to the area to prevent the burn getting worse; apply a soothing, healing lotion or cream. Advise the client not to touch the area. If it is a severe burn, recommend the client seeks medical advice.

Remember

Always seek feedback from your client and give appropriate aftercare advice, see pages 73–4.

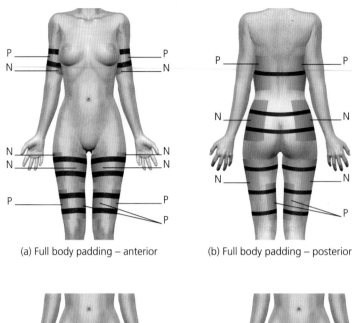

(a) Full body padding – anterior   (b) Full body padding – posterior

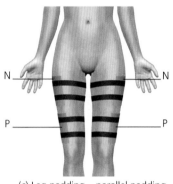

(c) Leg padding – parallel padding   (d) Leg padding – opposite padding

△ **Figure 8.11** Body galvanic padding

Recommendations for body galvanic (iontophoresis)

For most effective results advise the client to book a course of 10–12 treatments and have 2 to 3 treatments per week. Recommend the client has combined treatments:

○ gyratory vibrator to stimulate the circulation to the area and aid the dispersal of fat (if the client is on a reducing diet)

○ vacuum suction, which will improve lymphatic drainage, aiding the removal of toxins and waste from the area

○ micro-current, which will help to firm body contours and skin tone as the client follows a healthier lifestyle under your guidance.

Cleaning of sponge covers and pads

Wash the sponge covers thoroughly in warm soapy water, rinse and leave them to dry. Store in a sanitiser ready for the next client. Wipe the pads with warm soapy water. Avoid scrubbing the carbon facing, rinse and dry thoroughly. Wash straps in warm, soapy water regularly.

Refer to manufacturer's instructions for specific guidance.

Combined systems using body wraps, clays, etc.

Some systems utilise the galvanic current in the treatment of the whole body, via body wraps, clay, etc. These treatments use specially formulated products to achieve the desired results. The current is used for its effect in stimulating the circulation, increasing lymphatic drainage and for stimulating metabolic rate, thus enhancing the effect of the products. These treatments use far lower current intensities than the previous methods, and manufacturer's instructions must be strictly adhered to.

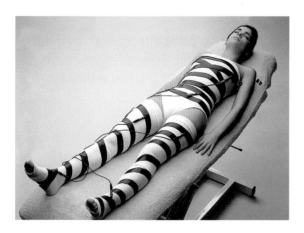

△ **Figure 8.12.** Combined system

SUMMARY

- Galvanic treatments use a low-voltage direct (or constant) current, sometimes called a galvanic current. This current flows in one direction only and has polarity.
- One electrode is negatively charged, called the *cathode (–)*; the other electrode is positively charged, called the *anode (+)*.
- Treatments which use the direct current are:
  - *desincrustation* – facial treatment – cleansing.
  - *iontophoresis* – facial treatment – beneficial ions for various skin types.
  - *body galvanic (iontophoresis)* – body treatment for cellulite using appropriate products.
- The effects produced depend on two scientific principles:
  - the chemistry of electrolysis, and
  - the law of physics, which states that like charges repel and opposite charges attract (i.e. positive repels positive and negative repels negative; and positive attracts negative).
- An electrolyte is a chemical compound that transmits a current. It may be a solution or paste. The compounds making up the solution dissociate (split) into cations (+) and anions (–). These move towards opposite poles because of the attraction of opposite charges: *cations* (+) move towards the *cathode* (–), and *anions* (–) move towards the *anode* (+). Certain reactions take place at the electrodes.

Desincrustation treatment to the face

- This uses the cathode (–) as the working electrode and a preparatory product similar in its chemical make up to saline solution. The alkali formed at the cathode will saponify sebum, break down keratin and relax pores, releasing blockages and sebum, which will soften and cleanse the skin. The alkali in the product does destroy the acid mantle so the polarity is reversed at the end of the treatment to help restore it.

Iontophoresis

- This is the repulsion of ions of beneficial substances into the skin. These substances must be placed under the correct electrode for repulsion to take place. If the product contains negative anions, the negative cathode (–) must be used as the working electrode for repulsion. If the product contains positive cations, the positive anode (+) must be used as the working electrode for repulsion.

> **Remember**
>
> Like charges repel.

- This is a very effective and useful treatment as a wide variety of products are available to treat most skin types.
- There is very little danger with facial work, as the current intensities are low and the electrodes are moving. However, the client will receive a shock if the intensity is turned up or down too quickly, or if the electrode is lifted off the skin with the intensity turned up. This is because the sudden surge of current will stimulate the muscles to contract.
- The intensity of the current used for facial work will depend on the tolerance of the client and the erythema reaction produced. Check manufacturer's instructions for guidance.

Body galvanic (iontophoresis)

■ This uses an anti-cellulite gel or ampoule placed under the working electrode: the cathode (–). This substance will be repelled into the skin to produce the desired effect. The treatment also uses polar and inter-polar effects, such as the softening of tissues and changes in the circulation and metabolic rate of the tissue through which the current passes.

QUESTIONS

Oral questions

Facial galvanic treatment: desincrustation

1. What type of current is used in desincrustation treatment?

2. Give two very important procedures that must be carried out prior to treatment.

3. Why is careful skin analysis important prior to desincrustation treatment?

4. Why is the sensitivity test so important?

5. What products would you use for desincrustation?

6. How is the current applied to the client?

7. Why would you place a sponge cover on the inactive electrode?

8. How does the treatment cleanse the skin?

9. What procedure do you follow before turning the current on?

10. Why is it important to place the working electrode on a sensitive area when turning up the intensity?

11. Why is it important to turn the current intensity up slowly?

12. Why is it necessary to place petroleum jelly under the eye area?

Facial galvanic treatment: iontophoresis

1. What current is used for iontophoresis?

2. How is the current applied to the client?

3. Which electrode would be the working electrode?

4. Why is the selection of the correct electrode important?

5. What type of client would benefit from ionto-phoresis?

6. How does this treatment improve the skin?

7. How would you select current intensity?

8. How long would you give the treatment?

9. If your client experiences excessive erythema, what action would you take?

10. During the consultation you find out your client has high blood pressure. How will you respond?

Body galvanic (iontophoresis) treatment

1. What is body iontophoresis?

2. What type of current is used in body galvanic treatment?

3. What type of client would benefit from this treatment?

4. How is the client prepared for treatment?

5. How is the current delivered to the client?

6. Why is it necessary to cover small cuts with petroleum jelly?

7. What are the reasons for taking great care when giving treatment?

8. Why is it necessary to place the client in a prone lying position when treating the posterior aspect of the body?

9. Why is it important to evenly cover the electrodes?

10. Explain what happens under the cathode as the working electrode.

11. What happens in the tissues between the electrodes/poles (inter-polar effects)?

12. How would you deal with a burn?

Multiple-choice questions

1. What type of current is used for galvanic treatments?

   a Interrupted surged current.
   b Direct current.
   c High frequency current.
   d Alternating current.

2. What effect does alkali have on the tissues?

   a Refines the pores of the skin.
   b Softens the tissues.
   c Increases cell metabolism.
   d Restores the pH balance.

3. What is produced at the anode when using saline solution?

   a Hydrochloric acid.
   b Hydroxyl ions.
   c Hydrogen gas.
   d Sodium hydroxide.

4. The statement that like charges repel and opposite charges attract is:

   a the chemistry of electrolysis
   b the law of inverse squares
   c the effect between the two electrodes
   d a law of physics.

5. A current applied to the face or body by means of two electrodes will be carried through the tissues because tissue fluid contains a high percentage of:

   a water
   b potassium
   c salts
   d calcium.

6. The working electrode used for the majority of a desincrustation treatment is the:

   a cathode
   b anions
   c anode
   d cations.

7. Iontophoresis facial treatment works on the principle that:

   a an alkali is formed
   b the acid mantle is dissolved
   c the product softens the skin's surface
   d like charges repel.

8. Which of the following is an interpolar effect?

   a Increases blood flow.
   b Saponifies sebum.
   c Aids desquamation.
   d Prevents the loss of moisture.

9. Turn the current up or down gradually to:

   a avoid excessive erythema in the area
   b assess the client's tolerance to the current
   c avoid stimulating the muscles to contract
   d prevent the client experiencing a 'flash'.

10. Why is it important to insulate cuts and abrasions?

    a There will be a lack of skin sensitivity in the area.
    b The higher moisture content will increase the intensity of the current.
    c The increase in blood circulation may make the condition worse.
    d The stimulation of lymph may cause swelling in the area.

11. Burns can result from a body iontophoresis treatment if the:

    a sponge pads are dampened in saline solution
    b client touches the area during treatment
    c correct electrode is not placed on the area of cellulite
    d electrode comes into direct contact with the skin.

12. Which of the following will intensify the current during a facial desincrustation treatment?

    a The removal of dead cells from the skin's surface.
    b Increase in sweat on the surface of the skin.
    c The removal of sebum from the area.
    d Insufficient product on the skin.

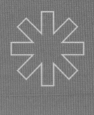

9 Electro-muscle stimulation (EMS) and micro-current

Objectives

After you have studied this chapter you will be able to:

▌ describe the structure of skeletal muscle tissue

▌ differentiate between muscle fibre types and their stimulation by specific frequencies

▌ describe the type of current and wave forms used for muscle stimulation

▌ identify the controls on the machine and explain their effects

▌ describe the benefits and effects of treatments

▌ explain the contra-indications to treatment

▌ explain the dangers and precautions to treatment

▌ explain the contra-actions that may occur during and/or after treatment and the appropriate action to take

▌ carry out treatments, paying due consideration to maximum efficiency, comfort, safety and hygiene.

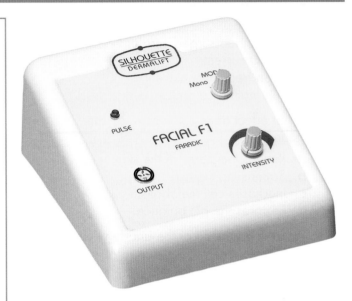

△ **Figure 9.1** Machine for muscle stimulation of the face

Electrical stimulation of muscles

Figures 9.1 and 9.2 show machines used for muscle stimulation. A variety of muscle stimulators are to be found on the market, and they range from simple single outlet machines with pre-set controls to the very complex machines with multi-outlets and a range of variable controls. However, they all produce electrical pulses, which are applied to the body by means of electrodes. When the pulses are applied, they stimulate the motor nerves and result in the contraction of muscles. The muscles are made to contract and relax, simulating active exercise. The treatment is used to improve muscle tone and condition and to maintain muscle strength.

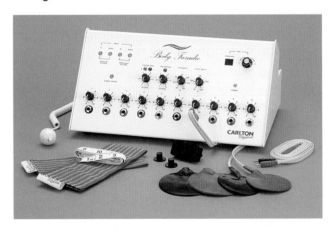

△ **Figure 9.2** Machine for muscle stimulation of the body

The impulses are produced by modifying direct or alternating currents. The current amplitude must be variable and must be of sufficient intensity and duration to produce a contraction.

Normal muscle contraction is brought about when impulses from the brain are transmitted via motor nerves to the muscles. The impulses produced by machines have the same effect as those from the brain. They stimulate the motor nerve directly and this will initiate a contraction in the muscles supplied by that nerve.

> **Be aware**
>
> This treatment will not strengthen muscle. You will need to discuss resisted exercises with the client if they want to improve muscle strength.

Refer back to your anatomy and physiology notes on the nervous system, especially the section on the transmission of nerve impulses, as this will help you understand the principles of EMS and micro-current treatments.

Remember

To produce a contraction, the current must be variable, of high enough intensity and of sufficient duration.

The original current used for muscle stimulation was produced by the Smart-Bristow coil and was known as the **faradic current**. This term is sometimes used today to describe muscle-stimulating treatments (e.g. faradism or faradic treatment). The terms TENS, EMS and NMES (NMS) are also used.

○ TENS stands for transcutaneous electrical nerve stimulation. This type of stimulation is used for pain control and is not generally used in beauty therapy. Modern equipment may include TENS to reduce pain and therefore improve client comfort.

○ EMS stands for electrical muscle stimulation. This term covers stimulation of both *innervated muscle* and *denervated muscle*. Different types of pulses are used for these two types of muscle.

Learning point

Innervated muscle refers to muscle with an intact nerve supply. *Denervated muscle* means lacking in nerve supply due to injury or disease.

○ NMES or NMS stands for neuro-muscular (electrical) stimulation. This term covers the stimulation of *innervated muscle*. The pulse is used to stimulate a nerve and the impulse is transmitted via the nerve to the muscle, initiating a contraction.

Learning point

When using nerve stimulation to produce muscle contraction, it is more accurate to use the terms NMES or NMS when referring to these treatments. However, EMS is commonly used.

○ MES stands for micro-current electrical stimulation. The muscle fibres are stimulated directly by very low amperage current.

Muscle physiology

The voluntary contraction of skeletal muscle is controlled by the brain. Impulses initiated in the brain are transmitted via the spinal cord and peripheral motor nerve to the muscle fibres, causing them to contract. Electrical pulses imitate these impulses.

Skeletal muscle

Skeletal muscle is composed of long, thin, multinucleated cells called muscle fibres. These muscle fibres are composed of myofibrils separated by sarcoplasm, and they have an outer membrane called the sarcolemma. Muscle fibres are grouped together to form muscle bundles, and many bundles make up the complete muscle. Under an electron microscope, light and dark bands can be seen along the length of the fibre; these are known as A and I bands and are composed of two types of protein: actin and myosin. The movement of these bands into each other constitutes muscle contraction.

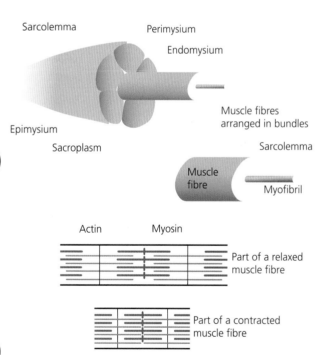

△ **Figure 9.3** The structure of voluntary muscle tissue

Muscles will contract in response to stimuli. Normally, these stimuli originate in the brain and are transmitted to muscle fibres via nerves. Because the stimuli are electrical in nature, a suitable electrical pulse from a machine can be used to initiate a contraction. The electrical pulse can be applied anywhere along the course

185

of a motor nerve, but the best response is obtained if it is applied at the point where the nerve enters the belly of the muscle, known as the motor point.

Muscle fibre types

A muscle is composed of different types of muscle fibres. This enables individual muscles to perform various functions. Research has shown that these differences are imposed upon the fibres by their motor neurones. By imposing a certain pattern of activity on to the fibre, different physiological and biochemical properties develop. All the muscle fibres supplied by one motor neurone have similar properties.

Remember

A motor neurone is a nerve cell that carries impulses away from the brain and spinal cord to muscles.

Impulses from the central nervous system (CNS), which stimulate the different muscle fibres, are discharged at different frequencies.

Learning point

Frequency means the number of pulses per second.

This becomes an important consideration when using electrical stimulation. Selection of the appropriate frequencies must be made for effective stimulation of the whole muscle. Specific frequencies can be used to produce certain characteristics in fibres when training athletes for particular events.

▽ **Table 9.1** Properties of muscle fibres

Slow oxidative fibres (SO): *red fibres or slow twitch fibres*	Fast glycolytic fibres (FG): *white fibres or fast twitch fibres*	Fast oxidative fibres (FOG)
These fibres are capable of sustaining tension for long periods, and are active for nearly 24 hours per day.	These fibres are used intermittently for short periods only. They are recruited when speed, e.g. reflex activity and burst of power are required.	These contain both oxidative and glycolytic enzymes and are recruited for general activities that require neither speed nor endurance.
They have a high level of endurance without fatigue. Containing high levels of oxidative enzymes, they depend mainly on aerobic metabolism.	They have low levels of endurance and fatigue easily. They have high levels of glycolytic enzymes and depend on anaerobic metabolism.	
They are well supplied with blood having a high-density capillary network.	They have a low-density capillary network.	
They are recruited for endurance activities, such as maintenance of posture, swimming and marathon running.		
Certain muscles will have a much higher proportion of these fibres (e.g. the soleus muscle in the lower leg).	Certain muscles will have high proportions of these fibres, e.g. the orbital muscles of the eye, *orbicularis oculi*.	
Impulses are transmitted to these fibres at frequencies of between 6 and 15Hz.	Impulses are transmitted to these fibres at frequencies of between 30 and 80Hz.	Impulses are transmitted to these fibres at frequencies of between 20 and 40Hz.

A muscle will be composed of a mixture of fibres – the percentage of each fibre type will differ for each muscle and will depend on the function of the muscle. Research has shown that electrical stimulation can be used to change muscle properties.

If fast glycolytic muscle fibres are stimulated at frequencies between 6 and 15Hz on a daily basis for a considerable length of time, they contract more slowly and do not fatigue easily. The biochemical characteristics are also changed; there is a decrease in glycolytic enzymes and an increase in oxidative enzymes; capillary density also increases. In this way, fast glycolytic fibres can be changed to slow oxidative fibres (so fibres do not respond in the same way).

Electrical stimulation

As explained above, a muscle will contract in response to an impulse from the brain, reaching it via its motor nerve. Stimuli or pulses of current produced by machines and applied to the motor nerve by electrodes will produce the same result; that is, contraction of muscles supplied by that nerve.

Some foreign units use modified AC, but British units in the main use modified DC. These units produce low frequency, interrupted direct current of between 10 and 120Hz. There are units on the market that offer upper range low frequency current of between 200 and 800Hz. Research has shown, however, that maximal force is developed in human muscle at between 40 and 80Hz. There is, therefore, little purpose in using higher frequencies, and careful consideration should be given to the effects of using these frequencies. Although sensory stimulation is reduced by higher frequencies, and they 'feel more comfortable', their safety and some of the claims made should be questioned as the mode in which they work is unclear.

Although there are a large number of different units available, one basic concept remains common to all – impulses are produced which stimulate the motor nerves resulting in the contraction of muscles supplied by those nerves. The muscles are made to actively contract and then relax, improving their tone and condition and maintaining strength, providing that the treatment is carried out on a regular basis.

Pulses, impulses and stimuli

○ A constant flow of current or a slow, rising electrical pulse will not produce a contraction as the muscle adapts to the current. This is known as *accommodation*.

○ The direct current must be modified to produce pulses, which rise steeply and fall at regular intervals.

○ The intensity must be high enough and the duration of the pulse long enough to produce a contraction.

○ *I* is the *intensity* of the current; on the machine this is controlled by the intensity control to each pair of electrodes.

○ *D* is the *duration* of the pulse or pulse width; this is pre-set on some machines but others have a pulse width control. A pulse width of under 100microamps (μs) is not effective and the best results are obtained with pulse widths of between 200 and 300μs.

○ Some units produce pulses of different shapes.

○ The shape of the pulse is known as the *wave form* (see Figure 9.5).

○ It is the rate of rise of each pulse that determines the response in the muscle. A pulse that rises sharply produces the best response in innervated muscle and the rectangular pulse is generally used in beauty therapy units.

○ A single, adequate pulse will produce a twitch in the muscle. The muscle contracts as the current rises and the contraction diminishes as the current falls; the muscle relaxes completely when the current stops.

○ If a number of pulses are applied to the muscle, the type of contraction produced will depend on the interval between the pulses.

○ If the interval between pulses is long enough for the muscle to relax, then a series of twitches will be produced in the muscle, giving a tremulous contraction.

○ If the pulses follow each other in rapid succession, the muscle has no time to relax and a smooth contraction is produced. A smooth contraction of a muscle is known as a **tetanic** contraction.

○ The number of pulses produced every second is known as the frequency and is measured in Hz.

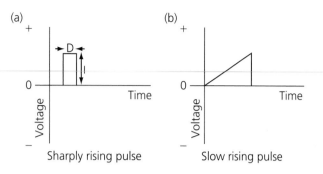

△ **Figure 9.4** Sharp and slow rising pulses

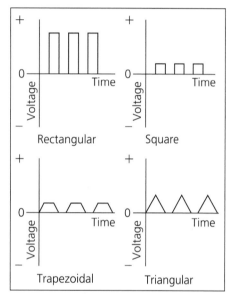

△ **Figure 9.5** Wave form: different-shaped pulses

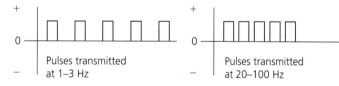

△ **Figure 9.6** Pulses of different frequency

Frequency

○ The frequency of the pulses is an important consideration because the different fibres within a muscle will respond in a different way to various frequencies.

○ Below 20Hz (i.e. pulses per second) only the slow fibres will be showing smooth, fused tetanic contractions; the faster fibres will be showing quivering, trembling contractions.

○ As the frequency is increased to 40Hz, the majority of fibres will be showing fused tetanic contractions, although some fast fibres may require higher frequencies to produce maximum force.

○ At 60Hz, the majority of fast fibres will be showing smooth, fused tetanic contractions and the whole muscle will contract smoothly. This can be represented diagramatically.

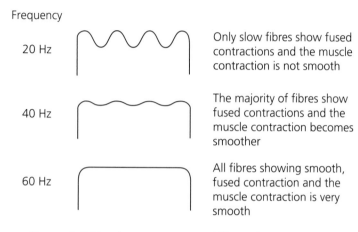

△ **Figure 9.7** Muscle contraction at different frequencies

○ In most human muscle, maximal force is developed in the frequency range of 40–80Hz, and there is nothing to be gained by using higher frequencies. The highest frequency recorded during normal transmission is around 100Hz.

Contraction time

○ The pulses are grouped together in 'trains' or 'envelopes', with a rest period in between. When the current flows, the muscle contracts; when the current stops, the muscle relaxes.

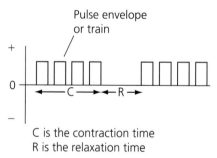

△ **Figure 9.8** Trains or envelopes of pulses

○ On most machines, the contraction and relaxation period can be varied.

○ In order to improve client comfort, the pulse envelope is surged so that the strength of the pulses rises gradually to peak intensity.

○ The current may then stop suddenly on some units, or decrease gradually on others.

○ The rate of rise of the current is known as the *ramp time*.

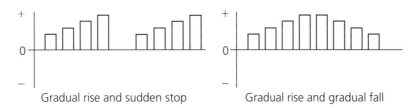

Gradual rise and sudden stop   Gradual rise and gradual fall

△ **Figure 9.9** Surged envelopes

Phasic selection

○ Many units have a phasic control and offer a choice of *monophasic* or *biphasic* current.

○ With monophasic current, the current flows mainly in one direction; that is, electrons flow from the negative electrode (cathode) to the positive electrode (anode) without variation. Consequently, the negative electrode will produce the stronger contraction. This is an important consideration when using duplicate or split padding in body EMS treatments. The negative electrode (cathode) should always be placed on the weaker muscle or weaker side.

○ With biphasic current, each alternate pulse is reversed so that with the first pulse, electron flow is from cathode to anode but with the second pulse, flow is reversed. In this way polarity is cancelled out and even strength contractions are produced under each pad.

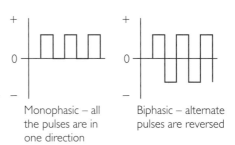

Monophasic – all the pulses are in one direction   Biphasic – alternate pulses are reversed

△ **Figure 9.10** Monophasic and biphasic pulses

Stimulation of the facial muscles

This treatment is used to improve facial contours and delay the appearance of ageing. The units for facial stimulation are very simple units with an on/off switch and an intensity control to one pair of electrodes; some have a surge control. Some of the large body units include a special terminal for facial stimulation.

Method of application

The current is conducted from the machine to the client by means of a lead and an electrode.

▽ **Table 9.2** Block electrode

Electrode	Example	Use
Block electrode		Both the cathode and the anode are set into an insulating holder. This is placed over a group of muscles or a branch of the facial nerve, and these are stimulated six to eight times and repeated three times.

Muscles of the face and neck

▽ **Table 9.3** Muscles of the face and neck

Muscle	Position	Action
Occipito frontalis	Covers top of skull	Wrinkles the forehead, raises the eyebrows and moves the scalp
Temporalis	Situated on the side of the head above and in front of the ear to the lower jaw	Raises the mandible and closes the jaw
Corrugator	Between the eyebrows	Draws eyebrows inwards and down
Procerus	Covers the bridge of the nose and inserts into the frontal bone	Forms horizontal lines on the bridge of the nose
Nasalis	Side of nose	Compresses the nostrils
Orbicularis oculi	Surrounds the eye	Closes the eye gently or tightly
Levators of the upper lip	Above the upper lip	Raises the upper lip
Levator palpebrae	Muscle of the eyelid	Raises the upper eyelid
Zygomaticus	Above the corner of the mouth to the zygomatic bone	Raises the corner of the mouth
Buccinator	Deep, horizontal in the cheek	Draws the cheek towards the teeth when chewing
Risorius	Extends laterally from the corner of the mouth	Draws the mouth sideways and outwards
Masseter	Between mandible and zygomatic arch	Raises the mandible to close the mouth
Depressor anguli oris	Below corner of the mouth	Draws corner of the mouth downwards
Depressor labii inferioris	Covers the side of the chin and inserts into obicularis oris	Pulls down the bottom lip
Mentalis	Centre of the chin and inserts into the lower border of obicularis oris	Protrudes lower lip and wrinkles the chin
Orbicularis oris	Around the mouth	Closes and protrudes the lips
Digastric	Beneath the chin	Protrudes the jaw, depresses the mandible
Platysma	Covers the side and the front of neck	Depresses the angle of mouth, wrinkles the skin of the neck
Levator scapula	Covers the back and side of the neck	Elevates shoulder and rotates scapula
Pterygoids	Lateral cheek area beneath the masseter	Muscles of mastication, move the jaw from side to side
Sternocleidomastoid	Each side of the neck	Flexes neck with both sides working Action of one side: laterally flexes the neck at same side and rotates it to the opposite side

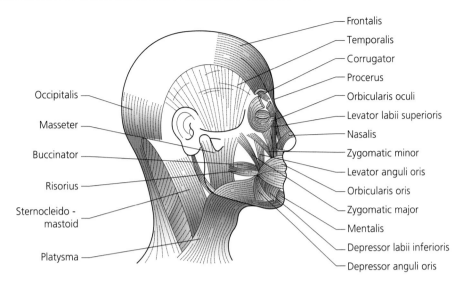

Occipitalis
Masseter
Buccinator
Risorius
Sternocleido - mastoid
Platysma

Frontalis
Temporalis
Corrugator
Procerus
Orbicularis oculi
Levator labii superioris
Nasalis
Zygomatic minor
Levator anguli oris
Orbicularis oris
Zygomatic major
Mentalis
Depressor labii inferioris
Depressor anguli oris

△ **Figure 9.11** Muscles of the face and neck

Benefits of facial EMS

○ To improve condition of ageing skin with poor elasticity and muscle tone.
○ To firm contours of face and neck.
○ As a preventative measure, to delay the effects of ageing and promote cellular function.
○ To reduce slight puffiness around the eyes.

▽ **Table 9.4** Physiological effects and benefits of facial EMS

Physiological effects	Improve ageing skin	Firm contours of face and neck	As a preventative measure to ageing	Reduce slight puffiness around the eyes
It improves muscle tone and the general condition of the muscle. This results in improvement of the contours of the face.	√	√	√	
The pumping action increases the supply of blood to the skin and muscle, thus bringing nutrients and oxygen to the body part and removing waste products. This results in improved condition of skin and muscle.	√	√	√	√
The contraction and relaxation of muscles aids the removal of fluid from the area; it relieves swelling, but this will be temporary.	√	√	√	√
Vasodilation giving erythema.	√	√	√	√
It irritates sensory nerve endings.	√	√	√	√

Contra-indications to EMS for face and body

Learning point

Check the contra-indications listed in the manufacturer's instructions to ensure you do not invalidate your insurance policy should the client be injured during or after treatment.

▽ **Table 9.5** Reasons for contra-indications to EMS

Contra-indication	Reason
Bell's palsy, paralysis, stroke	These conditions may benefit the client but always seek medical advice.
Bony areas (superficial)	As there is no underlying padding the current will be too intense, causing client discomfort. Avoid or work around the area if possible.
Bruising	May cause further damage resulting in increased bleeding. Bruises must be allowed to heal before giving treatment unless they are small and it is possible to work around them.
Cancer	The client will be under medical supervision. In line with acceptable work ethics and professional code of practice you must seek medical consent before commencing any treatment.
Chemotherapy, radiotherapy	The client will be under medical supervision. In line with acceptable work ethics and professional code of practice you must seek medical consent before commencing any treatment.
Cuts and abrasions	The broken skin may have a higher water content, which will increase the intensity of the current and cause the client discomfort. Cover small cuts with petroleum jelly or work around these areas.
Diabetes	The client may have defective sensation, therefore will not be able to give accurate feedback. Some clients can be treated but be aware that the tissues are liable to bruise quite easily, and tissue healing is impaired.
Defective sensation	The client will be unable to give accurate feedback about the contractions and could cause harm or injury to the client. Always carry out a tactile test.
Dysfunction of the nervous system	Muscles may exhibit increased tone (spasticity), which could be made worse by having treatment. Suggest an alternative treatment.
Epilepsy	Find out as much as possible about the client's condition. If it is controlled epilepsy, the treatment may be safe to carry out but recommend the client seeks medical advice. Do not leave anyone suffering from epilepsy unattended in a cubicle or on the couch.
Facial and body piercing adornments	Avoid the area or cover the adornment as it may be made of materials that conduct an electrical current and will cause a shock.
Heart conditions	The increase in blood circulation may put too much pressure and stress on the heart. Seek medical consent.
Headaches or migraine	The stimulation of the blood circulation will exacerbate the condition. The body needs time to heal before having treatment. Client will be too tense and the treatment will be ineffective and uncomfortable for them.

(Continued)

(Continued)

Contra-indication	Reason
High blood pressure	This varies with age, weight and lifestyle of client. Some have consistently high blood pressure. Treatments can frequently help, especially if the client is worried about face or body conditions. Medical advice should be sought if the client is not currently on medication.
Hypersensitive and highly vascular skin conditions	Treatment will exacerbate the condition due to the increase of blood to the area. The use of saline solution as the medium may irritate the skin.
Injectable treatment (recent)	The skin may be red, tender and painful with bruising and swelling. The skin needs time to settle down and heal before having further treatment. Injectables include Botox, which blocks signals to the muscles stopping them contracting, therefore the client will not want you to treat these areas. Fillers plump out lines and wrinkles, adding fullness to the face. Do not give treatment, as the pumping action of the muscles may dislodge the filler.
Low blood pressure	This is not usually an issue. Be aware that the client may feel dizzy or faint if they sit up or get off the couch too quickly following treatment. Always supervise and give assistance if necessary.
Medication causing thinning or inflammation of the skin (for example steroids, accutane, retinol)	The skin will be sensitive, so avoid stimulating treatments as these will exacerbate the condition. The products used for treatments may cause an allergic reaction in some clients.
Metal pins and plates (superficial) – and large number of dental fillings and bridgework	Metal is a good conductor, so the intensity of the current will increase in the area and will cause the client discomfort. Avoid the area or suggest an alternative treatment.
Muscle injury or spasm	Treatment will aggravate the condition and cause more damage to the muscle.
Nervous client	The bleeping or humming of the machine, and the sensation of their muscles contracting may make the client feel too apprehensive. This may result in them tensing their muscles during a body treatment or pulling away from the electrode in mid contraction during a facial treatment. Suggest an alternative treatment.
Pacemaker	The current may interfere with the electrical impulses to the heart. Liaise with their GP.
Pregnancy	This treatment involves the current penetrating the tissues so there may be a risk to the foetus. Suggest an alternative treatment.
Recent dermabrasion/ recent chemical peels/ IPL/laser/epilation	May aggravate the tissues as the skin will still be sensitive and will need time to heal before having treatment.
Scar tissue (recent)	Scar tissue must be allowed to heal completely before treatment is carried out in the area. If treatment is given before healing is complete, there is a danger of further damage to the tissues delaying the healing process. There is also a possibility of loss of skin sensation. Avoid the area or suggest an alternative treatment.

(Continued)

(Continued)

Contra-indication	Reason
Scleroderma, a connective tissue disease that affects the blood vessels and muscles	Treatment will aggravate the condition and cause discomfort to the client.
Sinus congestion	Treatment will be uncomfortable for the client and could also aggravate the condition further. Avoid the area or suggest an alternative treatment.
Skin diseases	There is a risk of cross-infection.
Skin disorders e.g. severe eczema, psoriasis	The skin is red with dry, flaky patches. The treatment will cause more sensitivity in the area and make the condition worse.
Thrombosis or phlebitis	Avoid treatment if a client suffers from either or both of these conditions (known as thrombophlebitis). Dislodging or fragmenting a blood clot is the greatest danger of treatment to the legs as death could result if medical treatment is not administered quickly.
Undergoing medical treatment	In line with acceptable work ethics and professional code of practice, seek medical consent before commencing treatment.
Undiagnosed lumps, swelling and inflammation	Recommend the client seeks medical advice, as there may be an underlying problem that prevents treatment.

Precautions to take with facial EMS

There are no dangers specific to EMS. However, precautions should be taken to minimise the risk of harming the client and to ensure you give an effective treatment.

▽ **Table 9.6** Precautions to take with facial EMS

Precaution	Explanation
Test the machine	You need to check it is in good working order and ensure it will not cause harm to you or your client.
Carry out tactile sensitivity test (see page 71).	This is to ensure the client can distinguish between sharp and soft objects. The client must be able to give accurate feedback about the intensity of the current.
Cleanse the skin.	Cream, oil and sebum will form a barrier to the current.
Ensure the intensity controls are at zero.	If the electrode is placed on the skin with the intensity control turned up, the muscle will immediately contract, causing discomfort to the client.
If there is a surge control, select the correct length of surge to suit the client.	A client with poor muscle tone will need a longer surge so muscles can reach maximum contraction and the potential to achieve beneficial results.

(Continued)

(Continued)

Precaution	Explanation
Dampen the block electrode with saline solution or a conducting solution and ensure it remains moist throughout the treatment. Prepare a saline solution by mixing one teaspoon of salt to one pint/600mls of water.	The purpose of solution is to conduct the current and achieve a good contraction.
Turn up current during the contraction period only when the light is on.	The client must be able to feel the current increasing and tell you if it becomes uncomfortable.
Do not move the electrode from one muscle to another with the intensity turned up.	The amount of intensity required to achieve a contraction will vary from muscle to muscle and may be uncomfortable for the client.
Treat both sides of the face equally.	To ensure a balanced result.
Do not over-treat.	It will cause muscle fatigue and will take longer to achieve an effective outcome.
Speak to the client during treatment.	You need to ensure they are comfortable. Be alert to contra-actions occurring.

EMS facial procedure

Preparation of working area

1. Place machine on a suitable stable base on the correct side of the couch.
   ↓
2. Check plugs, lead and electrode.
   ↓
3. Test the machine. Place the block electrode on your thenar eminence. No saline solution is needed for this as the graphite is a good conductor of current. Switch on the machine and turn up the intensity during the contraction period until you feel a tingling, prickling sensation and a small contraction. Turn down the intensity during the relaxation period. Switch off the machine and wipe the electrode with a disinfecting solution.
   ↓
4. Check intensity controls are at zero.
   ↓
5. Check the couch is prepared with clean linen and towels.
   ↓
6. Prepare trolley with:
   - ○ petroleum jelly to cover small open wounds
   - ○ warm saline solution or suitable conducting solution
   - ○ client consultation record.

Preparation of self

7. Before carrying out treatment ensure you prepare yourself physically and mentally, paying due attention to high standards of professionalism. Adopt a sensitive calm, confident and understanding attitude, as this approach will have a positive effect on your client.

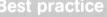

Best practice **B**

Position the machine on the left side of the couch if you are right-handed and the right side of the couch if you are left-handed to avoid crossing over or changing hands.

Be aware

Metal jewellery will conduct the current and therefore increase the intensity causing client discomfort.

Remember

Warn the client that if they have dental fillings or bridge work they may experience a higher intensity of current around this area as metal is a good conductor. If so, you will need to turn the intensity down to client's tolerance.

Preparation of client

8. Carry out a consultation, or if a regular client refer to the notes from their last treatment and discuss the effects and outcomes before proceeding.

↓

9. Check for contra-indications.

↓

10. Check contact lenses and all jewellery have been removed.

↓

11. Protect hair and clothing.

↓

12. Explain the treatment to the client. They will feel a prickling sensation giving way to a contraction. Ask the client to report any discomfort.

WASH YOUR HANDS

13. Carry out a tactile sensitivity test.

↓

14. Cleanse and tone the skin with suitable products.

↓

15. Carry out a skin analysis and assess the condition of the muscles.

↓

16. Place the client in a comfortable semi-reclining position.

Technique for facial EMS

17. Position the *contraction/stimulation/surge* and *relaxation/interval* dials to suit the client's needs.

↓

18. Dampen the block electrode with saline or conducting solution or dampen a square of cotton wool/lint with saline/conducting solution and place it over the electrode.

↓

19. Place the electrode on the muscle.

↓

20. Turn up the intensity control slowly during the *contraction* period until a prickling sensation is felt; continue increasing the intensity until a contraction is obtained.

↓

21. After 6 to 8 contractions turn the intensity down to zero during the *relaxation period*.

↓

22. Move the electrode to the next muscle on the other side of the neck and repeat the procedure. Work systematically covering each side of the neck/face before moving onto the next muscle.

↓

23. Keep in verbal contact with the client to monitor progress and be alert for contra-actions.

↓

Learning point

Use an exfoliator to remove excess sebum and dead skin cells. This will make the skin more receptive to the current.

Remember

If the client has any open blemishes or abrasions cover with petroleum jelly as the moisture will intensify the current.

Learning point

If the client lies flat on the couch the force of gravity can distort their facial features, especially on more mature clients with lack of muscle tone.

24. At the end of treatment, turn the intensity to zero, re-move the electrode and switch the machine off.

↓

25. Remove any medium from the skin using a suitable product.

↓

26. Continue with the facial routine depending on client's needs.

↓

27. Update the consultation record with salient points about the treatment for future reference. This will include the outcome of the tactile sensitivity test.

Be aware

You should be able to see the machine and the client at all times, and be in easy reach of controls.

Learning point

It is difficult to locate the sternocleidomastoid muscle on some clients. Ask your client to turn their head to the left or right, and you will see a strap-like muscle running from the back of the ear to the clavicle. Place the electrode on the motor points and ask the client to turn their head back.

Learning point

The terms 'contraction', 'stimulation' and 'surge' are the various names applied to the dial on the machine that controls the time taken for the muscle to achieve a contraction. The terms *relaxation* and *interval* are the names applied to the dial on the machine that controls the time during which the muscle relaxes. In this book the terms 'contraction' and 'relaxation' are used.

Learning point

Treatment usually starts on the neck as it is easier for you to locate the motor point(s) of a specific muscle and it will also enable the client to get used to the sensation. Placing the electrode on a specific area of the face will stimulate more than one muscle to con-tract as they are more numerous and more compact, being attached to adjacent muscles, to bone and to skin. The client may feel apprehensive when experi-encing a number of muscles of facial expression mov-ing at the same time, so help them to relax by talking through each stage.

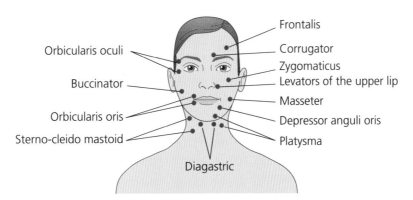

△ **Figure 9.12** Motor points of the superficial muscles of the face

Reasons for poor contractions

Poor contractions may result for the reasons given below.

▽ **Table 9.7** Reasons for poor contractions

Reason	Explanation
The intensity is too low.	Not enough current to initiate a contraction.
The electrode is too dry or dirty.	A wet, clean electrode is a better conductor of current; a dirty electrode offers resistance.
There is grease on the skin.	Grease is a barrier to the current.
The electrode is positioned incorrectly.	Accurate placing of the electrode on the motor point gives the best contraction, as this is the point of maximum excitability.
Contact between the skin and the electrode is poor.	Gaps offer resistance to current.
Terminals are loose or have poor contact.	The current will not flow if the circuit is broken.

Timing of treatment

Specific muscles are stimulated in turn, six to eight contractions per muscle. The procedure is repeated three times approximately 15–20 minutes to complete the treatment.

Refer to manufacturer's instructions for specific guidance.

Contra-actions for facial EMS

○ Muscle fatigue: caused by over-stimulation of muscles. Work over the area with effleurage and lymph drainage movements to aid the removal of toxins and waste. Recommend the client drinks plenty of water to flush out toxins and waste.

○ Excessive erythema in the area: could have been caused by too strong a salt solution or an allergic reaction to an alternative product used on the skin. Apply a cold compress to the area; use a suitable hypoallergenic product to soothe the area.

Remember

Always seek feedback from your client and give appropriate aftercare advice, see pages 73–4.

Recommendations for facial EMS

Suggest a course of 10–12 treatments, 3 times per week. To soften and warm tissues beforehand, recommend a steam treatment or alternatively apply a hot towel over the face and neck, as this will increase the skin's response to the current.

Vacuum suction performed after a facial EMS will complement this treatment, as it will help to increase lymphatic drainage in the area, aiding the removal of toxins and increasing blood circulation to the tissues.

Advise facial exercises for homecare, for example:

○ Obicularis oculi – half close one eye and hold for 2–3 seconds, repeat on other eye. Repeat 3–4 times a day.

○ With mouth closed, press the surface of the tongue against the roof of the mouth. Hold for 2–3 seconds and repeat. Repeat 3–4 times a day.

Activity (A)

Research appropriate firming facial exercises and prepare a homecare information sheet, with diagrams.

Cleaning the electrode

Wipe the electrode with warm soapy water and dry thoroughly.

Always check manufacturer's instructions for specific guidance.

Stimulation of superficial body muscles

This treatment is used to improve body contours and restore muscle tone (see Figure 9.3). The machines for body muscle stimulation are very complex and they have multiple outlets. The controls vary in number and in terminology. You must familiarise yourself with the machines you are using in order to select the settings to suit the client.

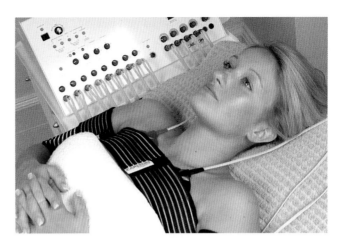

△ **Figure 9.13** Body EMS treatment

Method of application

▽ **Table 9.8** Body electrodes

Electrode	Example	Use
Rubber pads		These are the most common form of electrode. They are made of rubber impregnated with a good conductor, such as graphite. They come in various sizes and may be round or square. Only one side is conductive, the other side is rubber insulated.

Machine controls

○ **On/off switch.** This switches the current on and off; there is usually a light that comes on to show that the current is flowing.

○ **Contraction time/surge control/surge envelope/ stimulation period.** This controls the length of time the current is flowing; that is, the length of the surge envelope or train; it controls the length of time the muscle contracts. While the current flows, the muscle contracts; when the current stops, the muscle relaxes. The surge length should be long enough to produce a good contraction. Muscles with poor tone or with a thick layer of covering fat require a longer surge. The surge control usually varies from ½ second to 2½ seconds.

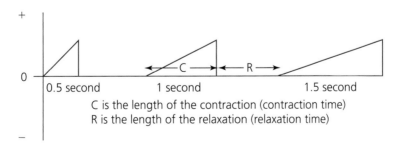

△ **Figure 9.14** Surges of different length

○ **Relaxation control/interval or rest period**. This controls the length of the rest period between the contractions. The rest period should be equal to, or slightly longer than, the surge period; this allows the muscle to relax fully, preventing muscle fatigue and build-up of lactic acid, which would cause pain. It should not be too long as this is a waste of time. Some machines have an inbuilt automatic optimum relaxation time.

○ **Ramp-time**. This controls the rate of rise of the current; individual pulses are inhibited gradually to give build-up to peak flow. Sharp rises give the best response. The rate must not be too slow as the muscle will accommodate.

○ **Frequency control/pulses per second/Hz**. This controls the number of pulses per second. The importance of frequency is discussed fully on page 188. Frequency determines the strength of contraction at the motor unit.

Remember

Different fibre types will respond differently to different frequencies. Up to 20Hz only the slow fibres will be showing smooth contraction. At 40Hz the majority of fibres will be showing smooth contractions, although some fast fibres may require a higher frequency.

By selecting a frequency of 40 to 60Hz, most fibres in the muscle will be contracting smoothly. The frequency within this range can be selected to provide the most comfortable smooth contraction for the client. If there is a tremor in the muscle, a higher frequency is needed.

Remember

There is nothing to be gained by selecting frequencies over 80Hz as near maximal force is developed in human muscle with frequencies between 40 and 80Hz. Some machines offer timed sequences beginning with lower frequencies moving through middle into higher frequencies.

○ **Phase control**. This offers biphasic or monophasic pulses.

  ○ Monophasic/uniphasic/single pulses. The current flows mainly in one direction, therefore the polarity of the pads remains the same for each

contraction. One will be negative (−), the cathode, and the other positive (+), the anode. Leads usually indicate this by one having a groove or being rounded – check with the manufacturer's instructions to establish which is which. As the cathode produces the greatest response, it should always be placed on the weaker muscle.

Remember

Monophasic is useful for split and duplicate motor point padding if one muscle is weaker than another.

  ○ Biphasic/dual pulses. The current behaves like an alternating current (AC) as alternate pulses are reversed: it therefore eliminates polarity. It provides an even current under both pads.

Remember

Biphasic: if muscles are of equal power, and for longitudinal padding, biphasic pulses may be used.

○ **Mode control/programme control**. This controls the rhythms of the contraction and relaxation times.

  ○ Constant. The rhythm of the programme remains the same once selected. The length of contraction and relaxation remain the same throughout treatment.

  ○ Variable/rhythmic/active. The rhythm of the contraction and relaxation vary throughout the treatment. Variable rhythm has the advantage of preventing the client anticipating the contraction and resisting it. This is useful with tense, nervous clients. Most machines have a selection of variable contraction times that will give the muscles thorough, non-repetitive exercise.

○ **Pulse width**. This alters the width of each pulse; when the pulse width is increased, it has a similar effect to increasing the intensity control. This is because additional current is provided as the pulse is on for a longer period.

  ○ Pulse widths under 100μs are not effective; over 300μs can be uncomfortable.

  ○ A medium width of between 200 and 300μs produces a good contraction. Select 150–200μs at the commencement of treatment.

Learning point

If the client cannot tolerate an increase in intensity due to discomfort, increase the pulse width, which may produce a better contraction.

○ **Maximum and minimum gain/master output.** This control increases the current to all the outlets being used – to increase the intensity when the client has got used to the sensation.

Learning point

Maximum and minimum output: this control can be at zero at commencement of treatment, or it can be set midway so that the intensity can be increased or decreased during treatment.

○ **Intensity controls (output controls) and pulse amplitude.** These control the current flowing through each pair of pads. Most machines have an intensity control for one pair of pads.

As the intensity control is turned up, the amount of current flowing through the pad increases. When selecting intensity, 'a good visible contraction within the tolerance of the client' is the best guide. Avoid turning the intensity too high, thinking that a stronger contraction is always better. Muscle fibres obey the 'all or none law', that is once the stimulus is great enough

to produce a contraction, there will be no increase in response by turning up the intensity. However, as the intensity of the current is increased, the strength of contraction is seen to increase. This is because more motor units are stimulated. Some machines have numbers around the intensity control that serve as a rough guide. The intensity control will be turned up to obtain optimum maximum contraction with minimum discomfort.

The placement of pads (electrodes)

The correct placement of pads is very important and will affect the outcome of the treatment. In order to pad effectively, you must understand the methods of padding and know the position of the motor points of the superficial muscles. A pad placed anywhere on the muscle will initiate a response, but may well be uncomfortable. The most effective and comfortable contraction is obtained if a muscle is stimulated at the motor point; that is, where the nerve enters the muscle belly (see page 185). Motor point padding should always be used if possible, as it allows very precise targeting of muscles and enables suitable intensities to be selected for individual muscles. Stimulation here is more effective at lower intensities and is therefore more comfortable for the client.

There three main types of padding: longitudinal, duplicate and split.

Longitudinal padding

In the past, this method used the pads near the origin and insertion of the muscle. However, as muscle function may be impaired by padding off the motor points, longitudinal padding must now mean *padding on the upper and lower motor points of a muscle.* This is only possible on long muscles with more than one motor point. This is an excellent method of motor point padding as all the current is applied to one muscle and the intensity is controlled to gain maximum contraction of the muscle. Also as the current from one pair of pads is applied to one muscle, a lower intensity will produce the desired contraction, which will be more comfortable for the client. This would always be the method of choice for muscles with two motor points. The next pair of pads is applied to the same muscle on the other side of the body. Muscles that may be padded longitudinally include: rectus abdominus, rectus femoris, gracilis, trapezius, triceps.

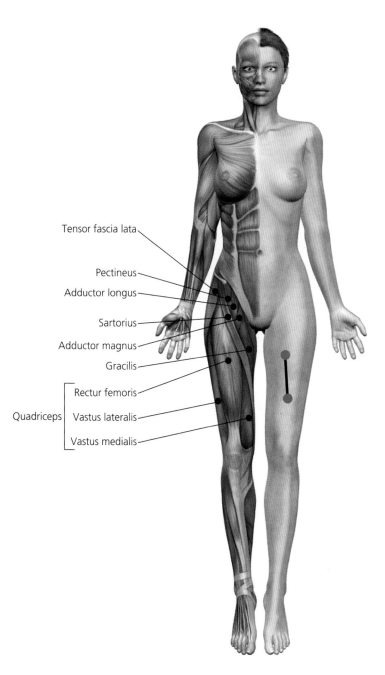

Tensor fascia lata

Pectineus

Adductor longus

Sartorius

Adductor magnus

Gracilis

Rectur femoris

Quadriceps { Vastus lateralis

Vastus medialis

△ **Figure 9.15** Longitudinal padding to rectus femoris

Duplicate padding

A pair of pads is placed on the *motor points of two adjacent muscles*; the next pair is placed on the same two muscles on the other side of the body. This method has the disadvantage that the intensity cannot be controlled to individual muscles, and muscles may require different intensities if one is weaker than another. The use of monophasic pulses will help if the cathode is placed on the weaker muscle. As the current is divided, a higher intensity may be required to produce the desired contraction and will be less comfortable for the client. When using duplicate motor point padding, always try to pad muscles with the same or similar action.

Muscles which are suitable for duplicate padding include: gluteus medius and tensor fasciae latae (abductors); adductor longus and gracilis (adductors); external oblique and rectus abdominus (abdominals).

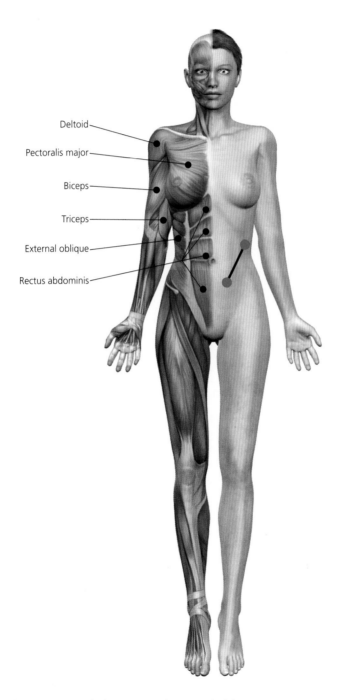

Deltoid

Pectoralis major

Biceps

Triceps

External oblique

Rectus abdominis

△ **Figure 9.16** Duplicate padding to rectus abdominus and external obliques

Split padding

One pair of pads is split and placed on the motor point of the same muscle, but on opposite sides of the body. Again, the current is divided between two muscles, which prevents individual control. If one side of the body is weaker than the other, monophasic pulses should be used and the cathode placed on the weaker muscle. If muscles are of equal strength, biphasic pulses should be used. This is a useful method for using up the last pair of pads. Muscles suitable for split padding include: right and left pectorals; right and left triceps; right and left gluteus maximus.

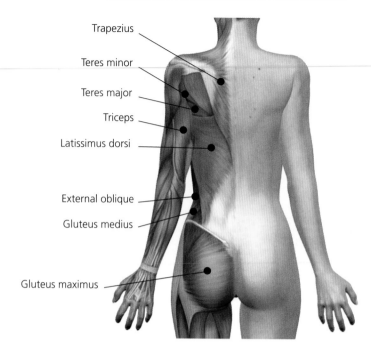

Trapezius
Teres minor
Teres major
Triceps
Latissimus dorsi
External oblique
Gluteus medius
Gluteus maximus

△ **Figure 9.17** Split padding to the triceps

Factors to bear in mind when padding

▽ **Table 9.9** Factors to bear in mind when padding

Factor	Reason
Thoroughly cleanse the skin to remove sebum and dirt, using a suitable cleansing product.	To remove all barriers from the skin.
Pre-heat the muscles with some form of heat treatment, for example infra-red, sauna, or steam bath.	This will increase the response. The steam bath is particularly effective as it also moistens the skin.
Always pad on motor points, if possible, and ensure the placing of the pads is accurate.	This will ensure an effective and comfortable contraction.
Use longitudinal padding if a muscle has more than one motor point.	The intensity can be selected to obtain maximum contraction of that muscle.
Place a muscle in its relaxed mid-range position.	This will give optimum contraction.
The brain does not register individual muscle movement, but rather patterns of movement. During normal body movement, antagonistic muscles do not contract together. When the prime mover contracts, the antagonist relaxes.	The padding of opposite muscles should be avoided. In practice it is not always possible to adhere rigidly to this rule, and providing there is no movement at the joint, opposing muscles are sometimes padded, e.g. the adductors and abductors of the hip joint.
Consider the phase control when padding.	With *biphasic* current the contractions are even under both pads. With *monophasic* current the cathode is stronger and should therefore be used where one muscle of a pair may be weaker than the other very useful for duplicate and split padding.
Select appropriate control settings.	To suit the needs of the client and to ensure a comfortable and effective muscle contraction.

Learning point ⓛ

When using duplicate padding, do not use one pair on antagonistic muscles, as one is likely to be weaker than the other and the intensity to each group cannot be individually controlled; for example biceps and triceps.

Factors that influence the strength of the contractions

Many factors influence the strength of contractions. Output controls regulate the amount of current flowing to the tissues, but do not give much indication as to the strength of contraction that will result. This varies and depends on many factors, as shown below.

▽ **Table 9.10** Factors that influence the strength of contractions

Factor	Reason
The condition of the muscle	Well-toned muscles respond to lower intensity of current.
The depth of the muscle	EMS is effective on superficial muscles only.
The amount of covering fat	Fat is an insulator; therefore, current will not pass through.
Warm muscles contract more readily	The tissues are more receptive to the current and also the client will feel relaxed and will not anticipate the contraction and tense their muscles.
Moist skin offers less resistance to the current	Water is a good conductor.
The selection of appropriate padding for the size of the muscle	This will ensure an effective contraction and positive results.
Firm, even padding giving good surface contact	This will ensure maximum effect.
The number of motor units activated	A motor point is where the nerve enters the belly of the muscle. Activating more than one motor point will ensure a good contraction at lower intensity and therefore this will be more comfortable for the client.
The rate of rise of the current	A sharp rise produces a contraction, a slow rise allows for accommodation of the muscle fibres.

Motor points of the superficial body muscles

The motor points are shown in Figures 9.18 and 9.19.

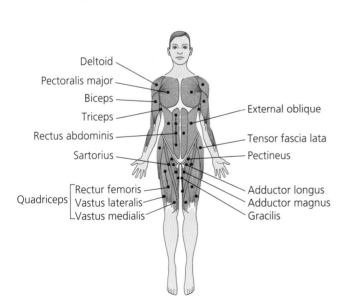

△ **Figure 9.18** Superficial muscles and motor points (anterior)

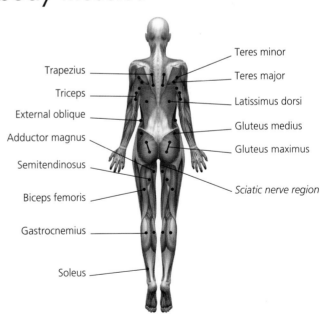

△ **Figure 9.19** Superficial muscles and motor points (posterior)

Suggested methods for body padding

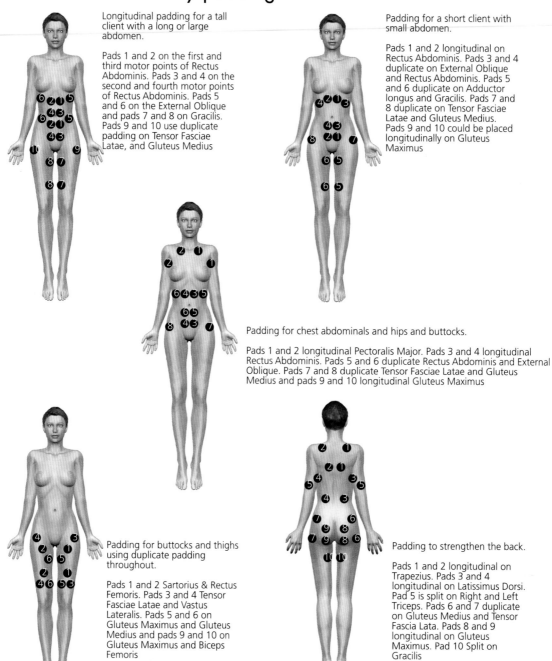

Longitudinal padding for a tall client with a long or large abdomen.

Pads 1 and 2 on the first and third motor points of Rectus Abdominis. Pads 3 and 4 on the second and fourth motor points of Rectus Abdominis. Pads 5 and 6 on the External Oblique and pads 7 and 8 on Gracilis. Pads 9 and 10 use duplicate padding on Tensor Fasciae Latae, and Gluteus Medius

Padding for a short client with small abdomen.

Pads 1 and 2 longitudinal on Rectus Abdominis. Pads 3 and 4 duplicate on External Oblique and Rectus Abdominis. Pads 5 and 6 duplicate on Adductor longus and Gracilis. Pads 7 and 8 duplicate on Tensor Fasciae Latae and Gluteus Medius. Pads 9 and 10 could be placed longitudinally on Gluteus Maximus

Padding for chest abdominals and hips and buttocks.

Pads 1 and 2 longitudinal Pectoralis Major. Pads 3 and 4 longitudinal Rectus Abdominis. Pads 5 and 6 duplicate Rectus Abdominis and External Oblique. Pads 7 and 8 duplicate Tensor Fasciae Latae and Gluteus Medius and pads 9 and 10 longitudinal Gluteus Maximus

Padding for buttocks and thighs using duplicate padding throughout.

Pads 1 and 2 Sartorius & Rectus Femoris. Pads 3 and 4 Tensor Fasciae Latae and Vastus Lateralis. Pads 5 and 6 on Gluteus Maximus and Gluteus Medius and pads 9 and 10 on Gluteus Maximus and Biceps Femoris

Padding to strengthen the back.

Pads 1 and 2 longitudinal on Trapezius. Pads 3 and 4 longitudinal on Latissimus Dorsi. Pad 5 is split on Right and Left Triceps. Pads 6 and 7 duplicate on Gluteus Medius and Tensor Fascia Lata. Pads 8 and 9 longitudinal on Gluteus Maximus. Pad 10 Split on Gracilis

△ **Figure 9.20** Suggested methods for body padding

Benefits of body EMS

○ Figure reshaping, particularly when used in conjunction with active exercise.

○ To re-educate muscles with poor tone due to prolonged disuse (e.g. adductors and triceps).

○ To restore muscle tone of abdominals after pregnancy.

○ To firm the pectoral muscles, which may correct breast sag.

○ To firm body contours and maintain an attractive figure, while losing body weight through dieting.

▽ **Table** 9.11 Physiological effects and benefits of body EMS

Physiological effects	Figure reshaping	Re-educate muscles with poor tone	Restore muscle tone of abdominals	Firm the pectoral muscles	Firm body contours
The stimulation of motor nerves resulting in muscle contraction. The selection of an appropriate frequency will produce contraction of most fibres of a muscle. (This differs from active movement when only a percentage of fibres contract: it therefore improves muscle tone.)	√	√	√	√	√
It improves the circulation due to the pumping action of the contracting muscles. This increases the nutrients and oxygen brought to the body part and speeds up the removal of waste products.	√	√	√	√	√
It increases the metabolic rate, which improves the condition of the muscle.	√	√	√	√	√
It stimulates the sensory nerve, giving the prickling sensation.	√	√	√	√	√
It produces vasodilation and erythema under the pads.	√	√	√	√	√

Contra-indications to body EMS (see pages 192–4).

Remember

EMS is effective on superficial muscles only. It will not penetrate the deeper layers nor a covering of fat.

Remember

EMS will restore muscle tone but will not strengthen muscles. Resisted exercises must be given to improve muscle strength.

Precautions to take with body EMS

There are no dangers specific to EMS. However, precautions should be taken to minimise the risk of harming the client and to ensure you give an effective treatment.

▽ **Table 9.12** Precautions to take with body EMS

Precaution	Explanation
Examine and test the machine.	You need to check it is in good working order and ensure it will not cause harm to you or your client.
Carry out tactile sensitivity test (see page 71).	This is to ensure the client can feel the difference between sharp and soft objects and therefore able to give accurate feedback on the depth of contractions.
Cleanse the skin.	Cream, oil and sebum will form a barrier to the current.
Select appropriate points on all controls.	To meet the needs of the client so muscles can reach maximum contraction with the potential to achieve beneficial results.
Dampen the electrodes with saline or conducting solution and ensure they remain moist throughout the treatment.	The purpose of saline solution is to conduct the current and achieve a good contraction.

(Continued)

(Continued)

Precaution	Explanation
Strap the pads securely.	To ensure a good contraction the pads need to contour the area.
Ensure the intensity controls are at zero.	The muscles will immediately contract causing great discomfort to the client.
Turn up during the *contraction period* only.	The client must be able to feel the current increasing and tell you if it becomes uncomfortable.
Ensure that: ○ the intensity is not too high ○ pads are over motor points ○ pads are not over bony points ○ pads are not covering open abrasions.	This is to avoid discomfort being caused to the client.
If the intensity: ○ is too high ○ the rest interval too short the treatment is prolonged.	Muscle fatigue can result.
Avoid heavy padding of chest region: pad anterior or posterior but not both.	Stimuli may interfere with the heart rhythm.
Turn down and switch off during the relaxation period at the end of treatment.	This is to avoid causing the client discomfort by turning off the machine mid-contraction.
Speak to the client during treatment.	You need to ensure they are comfortable and be alert to contra-actions occurring.

Body EMS procedure

Preparation of working area

1. Place machine on a suitable stable base on the correct side of the couch.
   ↓
2. Check plugs and leads.
   ↓
3. Ensure the electrodes are clean.
   ↓
4. Test the machine – Set up the leads and pads for an EMS treatment. Test each pair of pads. Overlap the 2 pads and place the graphite surface of each pad against your thenar eminence; no saline solution is needed. Switch on the machine and turn up the intensity during the contraction period until you feel a tingling, prickling sensation and a small contraction. Turn down the intensity during the relaxation period. Switch off the machine. Repeat for all sets of pads. Wipe pads with a suitable solution.
   ↓
5. Check intensity controls are at zero.
   ↓
6. Check the couch is prepared with clean linen and towels.
   ↓

Best practice B

Position the machine on the left side of the couch if you are right-handed and the right side of the couch if you are left-handed to ensure you are near to and in control of the dials.

Best practice B

If it is a regular client you can save time by positioning the straps on the couch ready for treatment rather than sorting them out when the client is already on the couch.

7. Prepare trolley with:
   ○ petroleum jelly to insulate small cuts, abrasions and bruises
   ○ warm saline or conducting solution to conduct the current
   ○ selection of straps of varying lengths
   ○ client consultation record.

↓

Preparation of self

8. Before carrying out treatment ensure you prepare yourself physically and mentally, paying due attention to high standards of professionalism. Adopt a sensitive calm, confident and understanding attitude, as this approach will have a positive effect on your client.

Preparation of client

9. Carry out a consultation, or if a regular client refer to the notes from their last treatment and discuss the effects and outcomes before proceeding.

↓

10. Check for contra-indications.

↓

11. Check all jewellery has been removed from the area.

↓

12. Place the client in a well-supported and comfortable position.

↓

13. Explain the treatment to the client; that is, a prickling sensation followed by contraction; reassure the client and encourage them to relax.

WASH YOUR HANDS

14. Carry out tactile sensitivity test: sharp and soft.

↓

15. Cleanse the skin with suitable products.

↓

16. Assess the condition of the muscles and the type of padding that will be effective.

Technique for body EMS

Patterns of padding for use on the body

In order to pad accurately, you must understand the three methods of padding and the position of the motor points of the superficial body muscles.
Padding should then be selected to suit the client. Some suggestions are shown in Figure 9.20.

↓

17. Select the appropriate controls, frequency, mode, etc.

↓

18. Select a suitable padding layout and make a note of it on the record card.

↓

19. Secure the straps around the area to be treated.

↓

20. Moisten the surfaces of the pads evenly with saline or a conducting solution and place them accurately over the identified motor points; ensure a firm even contact.

↓

21. Check that the intensity controls are at zero.

↓

Be aware

Depending on client's needs use pillows or rolled towels for client comfort; for example place under the knees if the client has a back problem.

Learning point

Placing the client in a low half-lying position will achieve better abdominal contractions as the muscles are relaxed and will contract in mid-range.

Be aware

Failure to carry out a tactile sensitivity test may cause injury to the client and result in legal action.

Learning point

Recommend a pre-heat treatment using steam, sauna, infra-red/radiant heat lamps or shower – heat improves muscle action and moistens the skin, thus lowering its resistance.

Remember

Do not position the pads over bony points or too near muscle tendons as this will result in poor contractions.

Best practice B

When turning up each pair of pads place your hand lightly over them so the client's attention is focused on achieving a comfortable and effective contraction.

22. Switch the machine on and turn each intensity control up slowly until the client feels a tingling, prickling sensation in each pair of pads. Increase the intensity to all pads until a good visible contraction is obtained.

↓

23. Cover the client and keep them warm.

↓

24. Check the intensity of contractions after 10 minutes, increase if required. Adjust the pulse width as required.

↓

25. Keep in verbal contact with the client to monitor progress of the treatment and be alert for contra-actions.

↓

26. As the client grows accustomed to the sensation, and as pads dry out slightly, the intensity may be increased.

↓

27. At the end of treatment switch off the machine during the relaxation period and turn all dials to zero.

↓

28. Remove the pads in reverse order to avoid tangling.

↓

29. Cleanse the treated area as the medium may cause skin irritation.

↓

30. Continue with the body routine depending on client's needs.

↓

31. Update the consultation record with salient points about the treatment for future reference. This will include the outcome of the tactile sensitivity test.

Reasons for poor contractions

Poor contractions may result for the reasons given below.

▽ **Table 9.13** Reasons for poor contractions

Reason	Explanation
The intensity is too low	Not enough current to initiate a contraction.
The pads are too dry or dirty	Wet, clean pads are better conductors of current; dirty pads offer resistance.
Grease on the skin	Grease is a barrier to the current.
Treating over a depth of fat	Fat impedes the flow of current.
Incorrect positioning of the pads	Accurate placing of the pads on the motor point gives the best contraction as this is the point of maximum excitability.
Poor contact between the skin and the pads	Gaps offer resistance to current. Avoid bony points as it is difficult to obtain even contact; the current will concentrate at the bony point.
Poor contact or loose terminals	The current will not flow if the circuit is broken.

Be aware !

To avoid causing the client any discomfort turn the intensity down slowly to zero during the relaxation period before performing any of the following:

○ moving the pads

○ applying pressure to the pads

○ pushing the terminals into the socket.

Remember

The intensity can be increased by turning up individual intensity dials or increasing the 'maximum and minimum gain/master output' dial.

Remember

If a client is finding the treatment uncomfortable try increasing the pulse width dial as this helps to produce a better contraction.

Timing

Approximately 30–45 minutes. Book the client in for an hour's treatment. The extra 15 minutes is to greet the client and enquire about the effects of the previous treatment and to give aftercare and homecare advice at the end of treatment.

Refer to manufacturer's instructions for specific guidance.

Contra-actions for body EMS

○ Muscle fatigue: caused by over-stimulation of muscles. Work over the area with effleurage and lymph drainage movements to aid the removal of toxins and waste. Recommend the client drinks plenty of water to flush out toxins and waste.

○ Excessive erythema in the area: may have been caused by too strong a salt solution, an allergic reaction to an alternative product used on the skin or a reaction to graphite pads. Apply a cold compress to the area followed by a suitable hypoallergenic product to soothe the area. If the client is allergic to the graphite pads place a dampened sponge/envelope on the area before positioning the pads.

Remember

Always seek feedback from your client and give appropriate aftercare advice (see pages 73–4).

Recommendations for body EMS

The treatment can be carried out 2–3 times per week for 6–8 weeks, as required. It would be more beneficial for the client to purchase a course of 10–12 treatments: they usually receive one treatment free and there is a strong possibility that a course will ensure commitment.

Gyratory vibrator prior to EMS warms and prepares the tissues, especially if a preheat treatment is not an option. A vacuum suction treatment could follow EMS to aid lymphatic drainage of the area and prevent a build-up of toxins and waste.

The client should be taught exercises to carry out at home to increase the effectiveness of the treatment (see page 78).

Cleaning

Wipe the pads with warm soapy water. Avoid scrubbing the carbon facing, rinse and dry thoroughly. Wash straps in warm, soapy water regularly.

SUMMARY OF EMS

- Electrical impulses produced by machines will stimulate motor nerves, resulting in the contraction of muscles supplied by those nerves.
- Muscles are composed of bundles of muscle fibres.
- The motor point is the point where the motor nerve enters the belly of the muscle.
- Each muscle is made up of different types of muscle fibre, that is:
  - slow oxidative fibres
  - fast glycolytic fibres
  - fast oxidative glycolytic fibres.
- These fibres respond in different ways to different rates of frequencies of impulses: slow fibres contract smoothly to low frequencies up to 20Hz; fast fibres contract smoothly to higher frequencies up to 80Hz.
- Smooth muscle contraction is obtained at frequencies of between 40 and 80Hz.

Electrical stimulation

- Pulses must be of sufficient duration and intensity to produce a contraction (high frequency currents have pulses of short duration and will not stimulate motor nerves).
- A sharply rising pulse produces the best contraction; slow rising pulses allow the muscle to accommodate. Pulses are grouped together in trains or envelopes with rest periods in between.
- When the current flows, the muscles contract; when the current stops, the muscles relax.
- Pulses are surged so that each pulse increases in intensity to peak value and then decreases. The rate of rise of the current is known as the ramp time. The frequency of the current is the number of pulses per second. Different muscle fibres respond differently to different frequencies. Only slow fibres will contract smoothly to

frequencies under 20Hz; the fast fibres require frequencies of around 60–80Hz to produce smooth contractions.

■ Frequencies in the range of 40–80Hz will produce good smooth contractions when using EMS. A few minutes at the lower range of 20Hz, moving into middle range of 40–60Hz and then to 80Hz and back to middle gives a thorough treatment.

■ The intensity selected should produce 'a good visible contraction' within the tolerance of the client.

Phasic controls

■ Monophasic selection means that one pad is slightly stronger than the other; the cathode (–) is stronger than the anode (+). This may be used for duplicate or split padding if one muscle is weaker than the other when the cathode (–) would be used on the weaker muscle.

■ Biphasic selection means that alternate pulses are reversed, which eliminates polarity; the current is even under both pads. This may be used with longitudinal padding or with other methods if the muscles are of equal strength.

■ The pulse width selected is between 200 and 300μs.

■ Always use motor point padding.

■ Three methods are used on the body:

● longitudinal: a pair of pads are on one muscle, one on the upper motor point, the other on the lower motor point. Repeat this on the other side of the body.

● duplicate: a pair of pads are on two adjacent muscles, one on the motor point of one muscle, the other on the motor point of the other muscle. Repeat this on the other side of the body.

● split padding: a pair of pads are on the same muscle, but on opposite sides of the body, one on the motor point of the right muscle, the other on the motor point of the left muscle.

Micro-current treatment

Micro-current is very low intensity, direct current, which is modified to produce low frequency pulses of differing wave forms. The current is delivered in microamps (μA), which is of lower intensity than the previous direct current used in galvanic treatments and the modified/pulsed direct current used in muscle stimulating treatments, which was delivered in milliamps (μA). One milliamp equals one thousand microamps.

Micro-current therapy has been used in the medical field for many years to promote tissue healing: these very low-intensity electrical currents stimulate the cells' metabolic processes. Micro-currents are more closely related to the body's own bio-electrical activity and augment the body's own healing process. Research indicates that weak stimuli increase physiological activity, whereas very strong stimuli inhibit, therefore these small pulses of current are more effective and beneficial in improving the condition of the tissues than the previously used stronger stimuli.

Micro-current is used in beauty therapy to maintain a youthful appearance, combat the effects of ageing on the skin, improve the condition of muscles of the face and body, enhancing face and body contours. It can also improve the

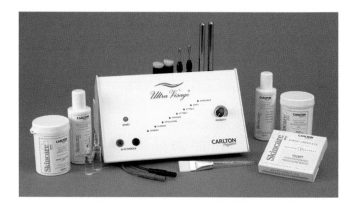

△ **Figure 9.21** A micro-current unit for face and body

appearance of scar tissue, cellulite and stretch marks.

The current:

○ increases circulation of blood and lymph

○ accelerates intracellular processes and the exchange of substances across cell membranes

○ improves the metabolic rate and is thought to normalise the activity within the cells; stimulates myofibrils thus improving muscle function

○ can be used for its polar effects under the cathode or anode depending on the electrode connections (in the same way as the galvanic treatments).

Being of low intensity, the current is not as irritating to sensory nerves. It produces lower grade sensations and is therefore less painful for the client and can be tolerated for a longer time. Some machines are battery powered and not connected to the mains, which eliminates the danger of mains electric shock.

If the machine is mains operated, then the transformer is used to step down the voltage and isolate the output, which also eliminates the danger of mains shock.

These treatments are becoming very popular as they are effective and feel more comfortable than those previously available. They are well advertised by the manufacturers and clients are aware of their effects, uses and advantages. Demand is increasing and more and more businesses are offering these treatments.

Machines

Micro-current machines produce direct current of very low amperage, which is modified to produce low frequency pulses of current with different wave forms.

Micro-current machines deliver current flow in micro-amps.

1 milliamp = 1/1000 of an amp

1 microamp = 1/1000 of a milliamp

Micro-current machines for the beauty market vary widely in design and cost. Basically they all use the latest electronic microchip technology to produce similar small pulses of current. However, they differ in their design and application and in the number and type of programmes offered. Most of the machines available offer multiple preset programmes for different conditions and different areas of the face and body.

The direct current is used for desincrustation and iontophoresis. Other treatments are possible because electronic devices in the machine modify the direct current. The flow is made to start and stop at regular intervals; to rise sharply or gradually, producing a selection of wave forms of different duration and frequency.

Examples of wave forms:

○ sine wave

○ square or rectangular wave

○ triangular

○ trapezoidal

○ ramp.

Sine wave/alternating wave form

Alternating current has no polarity and will not produce muscle contraction; it is used for its stimulating effects on metabolism, blood circulation and lymphatic drainage. Some machines have an auto build-up setting, where the intensity varies within each cycle from minimum to maximum values.

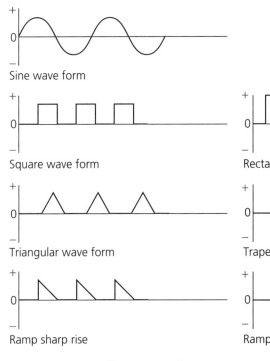

Sine wave form

Square wave form

Triangular wave form

Ramp sharp rise

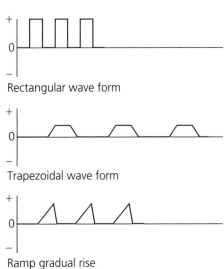

Rectangular wave form

Trapezoidal wave form

Ramp gradual rise

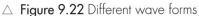

△ **Figure 9.22** Different wave forms

213

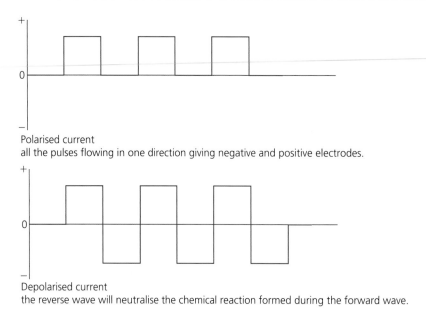

Polarised current
all the pulses flowing in one direction giving negative and positive electrodes.

Depolarised current
the reverse wave will neutralise the chemical reaction formed during the forward wave.

△ **Figure 9.23** Polarised and depolarised current

Interrupted/pulsed direct current

The type of pulses offered on the machine will vary: some systems offer a wider variety than others. They may be pre-programmed, or a wave form control may be available, allowing selection. The indications for use will be explained in the instruction manual for your machine.

As explained earlier, interrupted direct current can be used to stimulate motor nerves, which will result in a contraction of the muscles supplied by that nerve. However, if the current intensity is insufficient to stimulate the motor nerves, a muscle contraction may still be produced through direct stimulation of the muscle fibres. Micro-current is low-intensity current, too low to stimulate the motor nerves, but providing the intensity of the current and the duration of the impulses are adequate, the muscle fibres will be stimulated directly and will contract. The contraction will be weaker and not as visible as the contraction produced by the nerve stimulating higher amperage faradic-type currents. With micro-current treatment there is no visible contraction of the muscle. However, some systems are designed to produce adequate higher intensity pulses that will stimulate the muscle fibres in this way.

Research indicates that when an adequate interrupted current is applied to a muscle, a contraction of the fibres

and shortening of the muscle will result. However, claims are made that micro-current will stimulate the sensory receptors within the muscles and their tendons. These include **muscle spindles**, which control the degree of stretch and **Golgi organs**, which affect the degree of tension within the muscle. By adapting the technique of application, micro-current may be effective in tightening slack muscles and stretching tight muscles. The beneficial physiological changes that occur in the muscle will improve its condition and function but will not increase strength.

A course of 10–12 treatments 2–3 times per week is required to bring about this improvement. Visual observation of facial and body contours before and after treatment will indicate improvement.

Although pulsed, the current will be polarised, as each pulse is flowing in the same direction and will produce galvanic effects. One electrode will be positive and the other negative depending on the electrode connections and as with galvanic current, chemical changes/reactions will take place under the electrodes. This current can therefore be used for its chemical polar effects and to repel beneficial ionized preparations into the skin (iontophoresis). It is also used by some systems for the moisturising phase of the programme.

When the effects at the cathode are required, the negative electrode must be the working (active) electrode, the other electrode, the anode, must be stationary and away from the area. When the effects at the anode are required, the positive electrode must be the active electrode and the cathode will be stationary and away from the area.

If this polar effect is not required, some systems reverse the current between impulses to give depolarised current. The chemicals produced at the poles during the forward impulse are neutralised by the reverse wave.

Controls

These will vary depending on which machine you are using. The instruction manual will explain the function of each control and their mode of action. If you are in doubt ask the manufacturer.

Examples of machine controls

○ **On/off switch/button**: this switches on the power to the unit.

○ **Intensity switch/button/dial:** this increases or decreases the current flow. Some units have a dial that is turned up to increase the amount of current flowing and turned down to decrease the current. Other systems have buttons for selecting low, medium, high. The intensity selected will depend on the area being treated and the tolerance of the client.

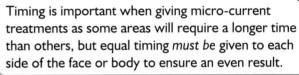

Learning point

Micro-current treatments should always be comfortable: a very, very mild tingling sensation should be felt.

○ Some areas such as around the eyes will be more sensitive than others and will require lower intensity. Current values can vary from around 10μA up to around 600μA and even higher up to and above 1000μA into the milliamp range.

○ Wave form: most machines produce a selection of wave forms (as explained earlier in the chapter). The method in which they generate these may differ but the effects they produce will be similar. The training manual will indicate selection.

○ Frequency: some machines allow selection of frequency, that is the number of pulses per second, but this is usually pre-programmed.

○ Polarity switch/button: this allows selection of negative or positive electrode (depending on the electrode connections). Selection will depend on whether the effects under the cathode or anode are required.

○ Programme selector: this allows the programme to be selected depending on the effect required and the part of the body being treated. Different machines offer different pre-set programmes, so read the instruction manual thoroughly to ensure that you select the most suitable for the client.

○ Timer: this allows the time to be set for each area. A tone, bell or buzzer will sound when the treatment of each area is complete.

Learning point

Timing is important when giving micro-current treatments as some areas will require a longer time than others, but equal timing *must be* given to each side of the face or body to ensure an even result.

Application of current

The current may be applied manually using probe or roller electrodes or may be applied automatically using small adhesive electrodes placed on appropriate points on the skin. Most of the systems are designed for use by a trained therapist but a few of the simple to operate pre-programmed units are on sale to the general public.

Before purchasing a system make sure that you thoroughly investigate the market. Look at as many systems as possible, ask for a demonstration, read the training manual thoroughly and you can then make an informed choice and select the most suitable machine to meet your needs. *You must then receive product training from the manufacturer.* This is essential because the treatment procedure will be specific to the system you choose. Systems vary widely in design, the number and type of programmes offered, the terminology used and the complexity of operation. You must always closely follow the instruction manual that accompanies your particular machine.

Types of electrodes for the face and body

The current is delivered to the client by means of two or more electrodes. The current flows from one, through the skin, to the other, the client completing the circuit. The electrodes vary in design depending on the system.

▽ **Table 9.14** Electrodes used to apply micro-current

Electrode	Example	Use
Rollers		These are small metal rollers, which move easily over the surface of the skin and are attached to handles with a terminal lead connection. The recommended product must be spread evenly over the part to be treated and the rollers moved slowly and evenly over the entire area. **Learning point** (L) Always keep a space between the rollers when working; if the rollers touch, the current will flow from one to another and not through the client's skin.
Probes		These are long, pencil-like electrodes that are thicker in diameter for the body, with a lead connection to one end with a metal head or socket on the other. Cotton buds are sometimes inserted into facial probes, which have sockets for this purpose. Some probes have only one socket for one cotton bud while others have two sockets for two cotton buds (i.e. twin buds in each electrode). This gives greater coverage. Probes are used in pairs, the current flowing from one to the other through the tissues. They may be moved at the same time, either towards or away from each other, or one may be held stationary while the other moves away or towards it. Some machines have both electrodes in one holder, making it easier to use. Both electrodes must be in contact with the skin for the current flow. The skin must be kept moist throughout, usually with a specific preparation supplied by the manufacturer depending on the treatment being carried out.
Small adhesive electrodes		These are small, round or square electrodes that are attached to leads that have terminal connections to the machine. They have a conductive adhesive side and a non-conductive rubberised side. They are applied to the skin at specific points to provide automatic treatment. This method of application frees you to do other things, for example a hand or foot massage, or mini manicure or pedicure. The pattern of application depends on the required effect; follow the diagrams in the instruction manual.
Gloves		Some systems have gloves that are attached to leads. You wear the gloves and move your hands over the moistened part in massage-type movements. This is a good way of covering large areas.

Benefits of micro-current to the face and body

○ Maintains a youthful appearance.

○ Improves the appearance of lines on ageing skin.

○ Improves the colour and texture of the skin.

○ Improves muscle condition and function. It is claimed that by adapting the technique, lax muscles may be toned and shortened or tight muscles stretched.

○ Improves the contours of the face and body.

○ Reduces the appearance of scar tissue and stretch marks.

○ Improves areas of cellulite.

Best practice   B

Low intensity current and good technique may produce a general relaxing effect for the client.

Micro-current also produces reactions under the electrodes (poles), similar to those produced by galvanic treatments. These can be used to improve the condition of the skin and to aid the absorption of beneficial products.

▽ **Table 9.15** Physiological effects and benefits of micro-current for the face and body

Physiological effects	Maintain a youthful appearance	Improve the appearance of ageing skin	Improve the colour and texture of the skin	Improve the condition of muscles	Improve contours of the face and body	Reduce the appearance of scar tissue and stretch marks	Improve areas of cellulite
Increases the circulation to the skin, bringing more oxygen and nutrients to the cells and speeding up the removal of metabolites (waste products).	√	√	√	√	√	√	√
Improves lymphatic drainage thus reducing puffiness.	√	√	√	√	√	√	√
Improves the permeability of the cell membrane, allowing easier passage of substances in and out of the cells.	√	√	√	√	√	√	√
Increases cell metabolism, which will improve the condition of the skin.	√	√	√	√	√	√	√
Increases the production of ATP (adenosine triphosphate), the breakdown of which provides the energy for cellular activity.	√	√	√	√	√	√	√
Improves protein synthesis, which improves the condition of the tissues.	√	√	√	√	√	√	√
Stimulates activity of the basal layer and cell mitosis which enhances skin renewal.	√	√	√	√	√	√	√
Improves ion exchange, which normalises the activity of deficient cells and aids the repair of damaged cells thus helping the body's own healing processes.	√	√	√	√	√	√	√
Stimulates the fibroblasts, which improves the production of collagen and elastin.	√	√	√	√	√	√	√
Stimulates myofibrils, improving muscle condition and function. It is claimed that by adapting the technique, a slack, atrophied muscle can be toned and shortened, or a tight muscle can be stretched, but the mode in which this is achieved is unclear.	√	√		√	√		

▽ **Table 9.16** Effects of cathode and anode as active electrode

Effects when the cathode is used as the active electrode	Effects when the anode is used as the active electrode
The alkali produced at the **cathode** will saponify sebum and soften the skin. This will have a deep cleansing effect. It will also break down keratin in the superficial layers of the skin, aiding desquamation.	The acid formed at the anode tightens and hardens the skin and has an astringent effect.
Water is drawn towards the cathode, which produces a temporary hydrating effect. This softens the skin and any scar tissue.	Water moves away from the anode.
Produces vasodilation with hyperaemia and erythema.	Vasodilation with hyperaemia and erythema but not as great as under the cathode.
Increases conductivity and excitability of nerves.	Decreases the conductivity and excitability of nerves.
Products containing negatively charged ions will be repelled into the skin.	Products containing positively charged ions will be repelled into the skin.

Contra-indications to micro-current for face and body

▽ **Table 9.17** Reasons for contra-indications to micro-current for face and body

Contra-indication	Reason
Bruising	May cause further damage resulting in increased bleeding. Bruises must be allowed to heal before giving treatment unless they are small and it is possible to work around them.
Chemotherapy, radiotherapy	The client will be under medical supervision. In line with acceptable work ethics and professional code of practice you must seek medical consent before commencing any treatment.
Cuts and abrasions	The broken skin may have a higher water content, which will increase the intensity of the current and cause the client discomfort. Small cuts may be insulated with petroleum jelly.
Diabetes	The client may have defective sensation therefore will not be able to give accurate feedback. Some clients can be treated but be aware that the tissues are liable to bruise quite easily, and tissue healing is impaired.
Defective sensation	The client will be unable to give accurate feedback about the contractions and could cause harm or injury to the client. Always carry out a tactile test.
Epilepsy	Find out as much as possible about the client's condition. If it is controlled epilepsy, the treatment may be safe to carry out but recommend the client seeks medical advice. Do not leave anyone suffering from epilepsy unattended in a room or on the couch.
Eyes: avoid passing the current through the eyeball	The skin of the eyelid is thin so the client may experience 'flash' and also discomfort if too firm a pressure is applied with the electrode. Avoid the eye area and forehead if the client suffers with headaches and migraine.
Heart conditions	The increase in the blood circulation may put too much pressure and stress on the heart. Seek medical consent.
High blood pressure	Blood pressure varies with age, weight and fitness, but some clients have consistently high blood pressure. Treatments can frequently help, especially if the client is worried about a particular area of their body. Medical advice should be sought if the client is not currently on medication.

(Continued)

(Continued)

Contra-indication	Reason
Hypersensitive skin	Clients with very sensitive skin must not receive stimulating treatments as these will exacerbate the condition.
Malignant tumours	An electrical current penetrates deeper into the tissues, which may have an adverse affect on malignant tumours that metastasise (spread to other parts of the body).
Metal pins, plates, extensive dental fillings and bridge work	Metal is a good conductor, therefore the intensity of the current will increase in the area and will cause the client discomfort. Avoid the area or suggest an alternative treatment,
Muscle injury or spasm	This will aggravate the condition and cause more damage to the muscle.
Pacemaker	The current may interfere with the electrical impulses to the heart.
Skin diseases	There is a risk of cross-infection.
Skin disorders, for example eczema and psoriasis	The skin for both conditions is red with flaky dry patches. The treatment will cause more sensitivity in the area and exacerbate the condition.
Spastic muscles	Treatment will exacerbate the condition as the muscles already have a high degree of muscle tightness.
Undiagnosed lumps, swelling and inflammation	Recommend the client seeks medical advice as there may be an underlying problem that prevents treatment.

Remember

If these polar effects are not required, some systems offer the possibility of reversing the current between impulses to give depolarised current. The chemicals produced at the electrodes during the forward impulse are neutralised by the reversed wave.

Learning point

Check the contra-indications listed in the manufacturers' instructions to ensure you do not invalidate your insurance policy should the client be injured during or after treatment.

Precautions to take with micro-current

There are no specific dangers to micro-current treatments as the current values are very low. However, precautions should be taken to minimise the risk of harming the client and to ensure you give an effective treatment.

▽ **Table 9.18** Precautions to take with micro-current for face and body

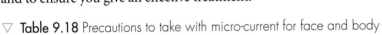

Precaution	Explanation
Examine and test the machine.	You need to check it is in good working order and ensure it will not cause harm to you or your client.
Carry out sensitivity tests, thermal and tactile in the area to be treated (see page 71).	This is to ensure the client can distinguish between hot and cold sensations and feel the difference between sharp and soft objects so that you know the client will be able to report any discomfort to you.
Check that all jewellery has been removed from the area.	Metal is a good conductor of electricity and may cause the client discomfort.
Check contact lenses have been removed, if appropriate.	As the eye area is included in the facial treatment the lenses may become dislodged.
Check hearing aids have been removed, if appropriate.	The current may have an adverse affect on the battery and cause the client discomfort.
Cleanse the area.	To remove creams, lotions, sweat and excess sebum as these will form a barrier to the current.

(Continued)

(Continued)

Precaution	Explanation
If using cotton buds in the probes, only use those recommended by the manufacturer.	Some cotton buds with plastic holders will be non-conductors of electricity.
Apply the gel or lotion liberally according to the manufacturer's instructions.	To conduct the current.
Use a lighter pressure around the eye area.	Too firm a pressure around the delicate eye area will cause client discomfort. Also, the client may experience flashing of lights.
When working over the face, ensure that you give equal treatment to both sides.	To ensure a balanced result.
Follow the manufacturer's instructions carefully. Always make sure that they are specific to the system that you are using.	To ensure an effective treatment.
Speak to the client during treatment.	You need to ensure they are comfortable. Be alert to contra-actions.

Micro-current to the face and body procedure

Preparation of working area

1. Place machine on a suitable stable base on the correct side of the couch.

   ↓

2. Check plugs, leads and electrodes.

   ↓

3. Test the machine – Set up the leads and appropriate electrodes for treatment. Refer to manufacturer's instructions for information on how to test the machine.

   ↓

4. Clean the electrodes or change the cotton buds ready for treatment.

   ↓

5. Check intensity controls are at zero.

   ↓

6. Check the couch is prepared with clean linen and towels.

   ↓

7. Prepare trolley with:
   - petroleum jelly to cover small open cuts and abrasions
   - conducting solution
   - client consultation record.

   ↓

Preparation of self

8. Before carrying out treatment ensure you prepare yourself physically and mentally, paying due attention to high standards of professionalism. Adopt a sensitive, calm, confident and understanding attitude, as this approach will have a positive effect on your client.

   ↓

Preparation of client

9. Carry out a consultation, or if a regular client refer to the notes from their last treatment and discuss the effects and outcomes before proceeding.

   ↓

10. Check for contra-indications.

    ↓

11. Check jewellery has been removed and contact lenses/hearing aid, if applicable.

    ↓

Best practice B

Whether you are treating the face or body, position the machine so you can easily access the controls without leaning across the client or crossing over hands.

Best practice B

Take a before and after photograph to reinforce the positive results of this treatment. It is also a useful marketing tool if the client is willing to participate.

Remember

Metal jewellery will conduct the current and therefore increase the intensity, causing client discomfort.

Best practice B

For facial work, if a client lies flat on the couch the force of gravity can distort the facial features (especially on more mature clients with lack of muscle tone). Place in a semi-reclining position.

12. Position client comfortably depending on area to be treated.

↓

13. Protect hair and clothing as appropriate.

↓

14. Explain the treatment to the client. They will feel a very mild tingling, pulsating sensation.

↓

WASH YOUR HANDS

15. Carry out a thermal and tactile sensitivity test.

↓

16. Cleanse the skin with suitable products.

↓

17. Carry out a skin analysis and assess the condition.

↓

Technique for micro-current to the face or body

18. Select the electrodes, prepare them as instructed in the manual and secure them into the machine.

19. Check you have selected the correct polarity, if required.

↓

20. Apply suitable product, for example gel, to the area.

↓

The technique will be specific to the part of the body being treated, the effect required and the system you are using. Carefully adhere to the instructions issued by the manufacturer as these will give a step-by-step guide to the selection of current intensity, frequency, waveform, duration and the movements to perform.

↓

Common themes for micro-current technique to the face and body include:

○ Circulation phase: using the electrodes to increase the blood circulation, bringing oxygen and nutrients to the area; warming the skin and stimulating cell metabolism, which will improve the condition of the tissues.

○ Lymph drainage phase: using the electrodes to draw lymph towards the lymph nodes, aiding the removal of toxins and waste from the area.

○ Lifting phase: focussing on the muscles to improve condition and contour; to tighten and tone; to firm and shorten; to relax and restore length. The probes are used as a pair to move at the same time, either towards or away from each other or one may be held stationary while the other moves away from or towards it.

↓

21. Keep in verbal contact with the client to monitor progress of the treatment and be alert to contra-actions.

↓

Remember

Warn the client that if they have dental fillings or bridge work they may experience slight discomfort as metal is a good conductor. If using the facial pads place them above or below these areas.

Remember

If the client has any open blemishes or abrasions cover with petroleum jelly as the moisture in the tissues will intensify the current.

Be aware

As the treatment progresses you may have to apply more gel, as it absorbs into the skin, leaving the surface dry. The purpose of the gel is to conduct the current so ensure there is always sufficient on the skin.

22. At the end of treatment remove the product, unless it is recommended to leave it on for its beneficial effects.

23. Continue with the routine depending on client's needs.

24. Update the consultation record with salient points about the treatment for future reference. This will include the outcome of the thermal and tactile sensitivity test.

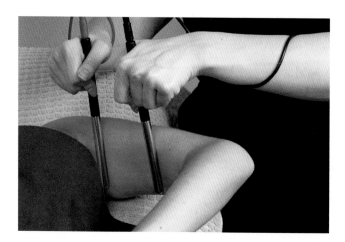

△ **Figure 9.24** Micro-current treatment

Timing of treatment

This will depend on the area being treated, client needs and the choice of programme selected. It will also vary from one machine to another. Refer to manufacturer's instructions for specific guidance.

The procedure is similar for treating other parts of the body and treatment is effective for a range of conditions such as bust firming and lifting, anti-cellulite treatment, improving stretch marks and scar tissue, improving the tone and contours of the upper arm (especially the triceps).

Contra-action to micro-current

○ Muscle fatigue: overstimulation of muscles; caused by incorrect wave form, frequency and intensity. Work over the area with effleurage and lymph drainage movements to aid the removal of toxins and waste. Recommend the client drinks plenty of water to flush out toxins and waste.

Remember

Always seek feedback from your client and give appropriate aftercare advice. See pages 73–4.

Recommendations for micro-current

Clients should be encouraged to book a course of 10–12 treatments, 2–3 times per week for the first few weeks, reducing to once per week as the result becomes evident. The number of treatments depends on the condition being treated, client's age and lifestyle. The timing and cost of treatment will depend on the condition. Treatment sessions are usually available from 30–90 minutes. Once results have been achieved the client should be advised to book maintenance treatments.

Cleaning

Dispose of cotton buds if used in a lined bin; use a suitable disinfecting solution to clean the electrodes. Always refer to manufacturer's instructions for specific guidance.

SUMMARY OF MICRO-CURRENT TREATMENT

- Micro-current is low-intensity direct current that is modified to produce low-frequency pulses of differing wave forms.
- Micro-current is measured in microamps.
- One microamp is equal to 1/1000 of a milliamp.
- Micro-currents are more closely related to the body's own bio-electrical activity and help to normalise and repair damaged cells. This helps the body's own healing process.
- Current intensity is low therefore there is less stimulation of the sensory nerves. This makes the treatment less painful and more comfortable for the client.
- Machines operated from the mains have a transformer that steps down the voltage and isolates the output current, eliminating the danger of shock.
- The direct current is interrupted to produce different shaped pulses of variable duration and frequency.
- The pulse shape may be sine wave, square/rectangular, trapezoidal, triangular, ramp.
- Sine wave is an alternating wave form and is used for its stimulating effect on metabolism, the circulation of blood and lymph.
- Micro-current does not produce muscle contraction through stimulation of its motor nerve as the intensity is too low. The contraction is produced through direct stimulation of the muscle fibre, providing the intensity and duration are adequate.

- The current may be applied anywhere along the length of the fibre.
- Interrupted/pulsed current is used for muscle fibre stimulation, for its polar effects under the electrodes and for the metabolic and circulatory effects listed.
- Stimulation of a muscle with pulsed current will produce a muscle contraction.
- Pulsed current will also produce polar effects under the electrodes if the pulses are flowing in one direction. Chemical reactions will occur at the cathode and anode and these effects are used in some treatments. When these effects are not required the current may be reversed between impulses, producing depolarised current.
- If the current is depolarized the chemicals formed at the electrodes during the forward wave are neutralised by the reverse wave.
- Machine controls will vary with each system. Look at the controls on the machine and make sure that you understand what each one does and how to operate it correctly. Follow the instructions in the training manual.
- Types of electrodes: roller electrodes, probes, adhesive electrodes, gloves.
- See text for effects, uses, contra-indications, precautions, treatment technique.
- Recommended course of treatment: 10–12 treatments, 2–3 treatments per week.

QUESTIONS

Oral questions

Micro-current

1. What type of current is micro-current?

2. Why is micro-current treatment more comfortable for the client?

3. When would you select micro-current treatments?

4. How does the treatment bring about its effects?

5. What factors determine the selection of wave forms?

6. How often would you recommend treatment?

EMS questions

1. What type of current is used to stimulate facial muscles?

2. When would the use of muscle stimulation be indicated?

3. How is the current applied to the client?

4. What is meant by the motor point?

5. How would you test the machine?

6. **a** Which muscle(s) would you work on if the client had a double chin?

   b Which muscle produces horizontal wrinkles over the bridge of the nose?

   c What is the action of masseter?

7. Are there any specific safety factors that you must consider with this treatment?

8. How many contractions would you give each muscle?

9. What contra-actions may occur either during or after treatment?

10. How long is the treatment?

11. What type of current is used?

12. How is the current applied to the client?

13. Why would you suggest EMS for a client?

14. Where should the pads be placed?

15. How many ways/methods of padding are there?

16. Explain the method of padding you would use for long muscles.

17. Name the method of padding where a pair of pads are placed on adjacent muscles with similar action and repeated on the other side of the body.

18. What is the main disadvantage of split padding?

19. If the contractions were poor what action would you take?

20. How would you prevent muscle fatigue?

21. What precautions should you take prior to treatment?

22. Why must you cover open wounds with petroleum jelly or a waterproof plaster?

23. What treatment would you suggest prior to EMS? Give reasons why.

24. What is the benefit of preheating the tissues?

25. How long would the treatment last?

Multiple-choice questions

1. Muscle fibres are composed of:

   a myofibrils
   b sarcoplasm
   c epimysium
   d sarcolemma.

2. Fast oxidative glycolytic (FOG) fibres are used for:

   a short periods only, when speed is required
   b sustaining tension for long periods
   c reflex activities and when power is required
   d general activities that do not require speed.

3. The action of the risorius muscle is to:

   a raise the upper lip
   b draw the mouth sideways and outwards

c   raise the corner of the mouth

d   draw the cheek towards the teeth.

4. What muscle depresses the angle of the mouth?

a   Platysma.

b   Digastric.

c   Depressor labii inferioris.

d   Mentalis.

5. During facial EMS why should you turn down the intensity after working a muscle before moving onto the next muscle?

a   To talk to the client about the contraction.

b   The outcome of the treatment will be more effective.

c   The intensity will vary for each muscle.

d   To give the client time to relax before continuing.

6. Why should you ensure the block electrode remains moist throughout a facial EMS treatment?

a   To maintain the same level of intensity for each muscle.

b   To help dissolve excess sebum.

c   To prevent the client receiving an electric shock.

d   To achieve a good contraction.

7. When padding an area of the body, where should you place the pads for an effective and comfortable contraction?

a   At the origin and insertion.

b   On the motor points.

c   On the belly of the muscle.

d   Depends on the type of muscle fibres.

8. Monophasic pulses means the:

a   current flows mainly in one direction

b   frequencies should be between 40 and 80Hz

c   current is even under both pads, ensuring maximum results

d   anode is placed on the weaker muscle.

9. The strength of contraction depends on the:

a   area being treated

b   phasic control

c   amount of adipose tissue

d   skin being dry to conduct the current.

10. During treatment you notice the connection to one of a pair of pads is loose, what should you do?

a   Leave it as the muscle appears to be contracting slightly.

b   Turn down the intensity dial to the pair of pads during the rest period and fix it.

c   Push the connection into the socket of the pad during the rest period.

d   Turn off the machine at the main switch during the rest period and fix the connection.

11. What should you do if a client is allergic to the graphite pads?

a   Apply a body cream to the area before placing the pads.

b   Suggest an alternative treatment, for example galvanic.

c   Place a dampened sponge on the skin prior to placing the pads.

d   Prepare a stronger saline solution to protect the skin from the graphite.

12. To pad the abductors of the thigh you will need to place a pad on:

a   gluteus maximus and gluteus medius

b   hamstrings and gluteus maximus

c   sartorius and tensor fascia lata

d   tensor fascia lata and gluteus medius.

10 Micro-dermabrasion

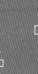

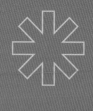

Objectives

After you have studied this chapter you will be able to:

▮ explain the two types of mechanical micro-dermabrasion

▮ identify the controls on the machine and explain their effects

▮ describe the benefits and effects of treatment for different face and body conditions

▮ explain the contra-indications to treatment

▮ explain the dangers and precautions of micro-dermabrasion treatments

▮ explain the contra-actions that may occur during and/or after treatment and the appropriate action to take

▮ carry out micro-dermabrasion treatments, paying due consideration to maximum efficiency, comfort, safety and hygiene.

Skin physiology

Before you begin to learn about micro-dermabrasion, you need to know about the skin and how it works.

The skin forms a tough, waterproof protective covering over the entire surface of the body; it is continuous with the membranes lining the orifices. It covers a surface area of approximately two square metres, and varies in thickness from 0.05 mm to 3 mm, being thickest on the soles of the feet and palms of the hands and thinnest on the lips, eyelids, inner surfaces of the limbs and on the abdomen. The skin includes hair, nails, glands and various sensory receptors.

Healthy skin is smooth, soft and flexible and has a good colour. A grey, ashen or yellow tinge may indicate health problems.

Skin structure

The skin is composed of two main layers with a subcutaneous fatty layer underneath. The two main layers are:

○ epidermis

○ dermis.

These layers may be further subdivided, as follows.

Epidermis

The epidermis is composed of five layers of stratified squamous epithelium. The living cells of the two deepest layers contain nuclei; the dead cells of the upper three layers lose their nuclei and become filled with a protein called keratin. As the cells of the stratum basale multiply they push upward, forming the next layer. The dead cells gradually slough off the surface of the skin to allow the new layer to form.

> **Learning point** ⓛ
>
> Skin cells regenerate, push to the surface and dead cells fall from the skin naturally. Micro-dermabrasion assists this process by removing the dead cells and thereby encourages the growth of new cells.

Stratum basale (Stratum germinativum)

This is the deepest layer of the epidermis. It is composed of a single layer of cuboidal or columnar-shaped cells on a basement membrane and lies directly on the papillary layer of the dermis. The capillary network of the dermis provides nutrients for these living cells.

The cells have a nucleus and multiply by mitosis (cell division).

Approximately one in ten of these basal cells are specialised cells called melanocytes. They produce the pigment melanin from the amino acid tyrosine. Melanin is produced to protect the cells against the damaging effect of ultraviolet radiation. It gives the skin its brown colour.

This layer also contains the nerve endings sensitive to touch (Merkel's discs).

Stratum spinosum

This is composed of eight to ten layers of living cells. Granules of melanin pass into this layer.

The cells begin to lose their shape and have projections or spines, which join the cells together.

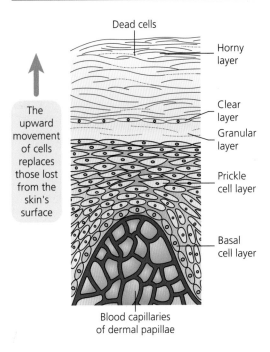

Dead cells

Horny layer

Clear layer

Granular layer

Prickle cell layer

Basal cell layer

The upward movement of cells replaces those lost from the skin's surface

Blood capillaries of dermal papillae

△ **Figure 10.1** Layers of the epidermis

Stratum granulosum

This consists of three to five layers of flattened cells. Enzymes break down the nucleus and the cells die. Keratohyaline is laid down in the cytoplasm, giving the first stages of keratinisation. The protein keratin protects the skin from injury and invasion of micro-organisms and makes it waterproof.

Stratum lucidum

This is composed of several layers of clear, flat, dead cells that are translucent and filled with keratin. This layer is found only on the palms of the hands and soles of the feet, where it provides extra protection.

Stratum corneum

This is the superficial layer and is the layer most affected by micro-dermabrasion treatment. It is composed of many rows of flat, dead, scaly cells filled with keratin, which are constantly shed and replaced (this shedding of cells is known as desquamation).

> **Learning point** ⓛ
> The ageing process naturally leads to an overproduction of the callous cells that make up the stratum corneum. This is referred to as hyperkeratosis.

Sebum secreted by the sebaceous glands helps to keep this layer soft and supple. Rubbing or friction of the skin will increase the rate of desquamation.

> **Learning point** ⓛ
> It takes approximately 28 days for the live cells in the basal layer to reach the horny layer as dead plaques of keratin.

Dermis

The dermis lies under the epidermis and is composed of two layers: the upper papillary layer and the lower reticular layer.

The surface of the papillary layer is ridged, forming an uneven surface. These finger-like projections increase the surface area and are called dermal papillae.

They produce the pattern known as fingerprints. The blood capillary loops of the dermis transport nutrients and oxygen to basal layer cells and remove waste products.

The reticular layer is composed of dense irregular connective tissue with more collagen and elastin fibres. This gives the skin strength, extensibility and elasticity.

The skin's ability to stretch and recoil is necessary during pregnancy and obesity. The ground substance or matrix retains water, helping the skin to remain firm and turgid.

Many structures are found in the dermis. They include blood vessels, lymphatic vessels, sebaceous glands, sweat glands, nerves and nerve endings, hair in hair follicles, erector pili muscles, fibres (white fibres and yellow elastic fibres) and mast cells.

> **Remember**
> The epidermis has *five* layers:
> ○ stratum corneum (horny layer – the superficial layer)
> ○ stratum lucidum (clear layer)
> ○ stratum granulosum (granular layer)
> ○ stratum spinosum (prickle cell layer)
> ○ stratum germinativum (basal layer – this is the deepest layer).
> The dermis has *two* layers:
> ○ papillary layer
> ○ reticular layer.

Cells

Fibroblasts are cells that synthesise the following fibres.

○ White fibres are formed from non-elastic fibres of the protein collagen, lying in layers. They give the skin tensile strength and flexibility, and they bind structures together. They also attract water to keep the skin hydrated.

○ Yellow elastic fibres are formed from the protein elastin. They are scattered throughout the matrix. These highly elastic fibres are capable of stretch and recoil. They give the skin elasticity, enabling it to stretch and return to normal. This is important for pregnancy and obesity. If the skin is over-stretched small tears occur in the dermis. These can be seen as white lines called 'stretch marks'. With ageing, the skin loses elasticity.

Mast cells release histamine following injury or reaction to an allergen. Histamine initiates an inflammatory response, causing dilation of capillaries and increasing the permeability of cell walls. This process aids tissue repair.

Sebaceous glands

These glands secrete an oily substance called sebum. (It consists mainly of waxes, fats and fatty acids, and dehydrocholesterol, which forms vitamin D in sunlight.)

The function of the sebum is to coat the skin and hair and keep the surface smooth and supple. It prevents loss of water from the skin. It also has antiseptic and anti-fungal properties, protecting the skin from bacterial and fungal infections.

Sebum is gradually lost by washing and desquamation but is continually replaced. Massage stimulates the glands to produce more sebum.

> **Learning point** Ⓛ
>
> Together with the sweat secreted by sweat glands, sebum forms a coating on the skin known as the acid mantle because the secretions have a pH of between 5.5 and 5.6 (acidic). This is neutralised when the skin is washed with an alkaline product, but the acid mantle is restored after a few hours.

Micro-dermabrasion

Micro-dermabrasion is the mechanical removal of the surface layer of dead skin cells in order to encourage the regeneration of the skin through the growth of new skin cells. It enhances the appearance of the skin and can be used to target a range of face and body conditions. The treatment aids the process of desquamation either by firing tiny abrasive particles at the surface of the skin, or by the application of rotating heads, which have particles of real or manufactured diamonds encrusted into them.

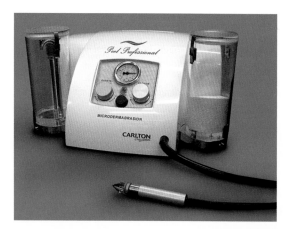

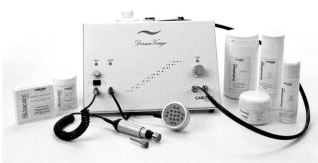

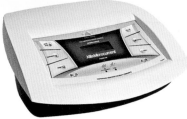

△ **Figure 10.2** Machines on the market that are used for micro-dermabrasion. A variety of types of machines are available. Some use either crystal or diamond technologies and some use both.

Crystal micro-dermabrasion

As explained above, the superficial layer of the skin constantly sheds and renews. Dull, dead, keratinised cells are replaced by new, healthy cells, giving a clear, glowing complexion. Micro-dermabrasion contributes to this process, speeding it up and stimulating the production of even more new cells.

The treatment involves the application of very fine abrasive crystals to the skin via a specially designed hand-piece or nozzle, which uses vacuum suction to create a circuit of air. This is used to 'blow' the crystals at pressure onto the skin's surface and to suck up the dead skin cells and 'used' crystals back into a storage container in the machine, for later disposal.

Machines allow you to control the amount of vacuum pressure and some also allow you to control the flow rate of the crystals. Disposable tips are applied to the end of the nozzle to avoid the risk of contamination between clients.

Following micro-dermabrasion, the smooth, unprotected skin underneath the stratum corneum is better able to absorb any beneficial products applied to the skin to complete the treatment. In addition to this, the skin registers the desquamation of the stratum corneum as an injury and rushes to produce new skin cells to replace those that have been removed. The aim of the treatment is to achieve a healthy balance between the new,

functioning cells and the keratinised cells that form a protective layer to the skin.

The crystals used may be manmade or naturally sourced minerals such as aluminium oxide, or may be made from ground up plant sources, such as nut kernels or shells. Aluminium oxide is capable of being made into the finest, most regular crystals and because it is not water soluble, it will not be absorbed into the skin. It is a naturally occurring mineral and there is little risk of allergic reaction. Plant-sourced crystals are likely to have rougher surfaces and therefore to be more abrasive and potential less comfortable for the client.

Because the particles used are so fine, any moisture in the atmosphere will be readily absorbed and will cause the particles to clump together. As well as the danger of clogging the machine, the clumps of particles will attack the skin more aggressively and will slough off chunks of the surface layer rather than just the dead cells. It is vital that the machine is not used or stored in a humid atmosphere and that your hands and the skin of your client are completely dry during treatment.

Machines have a canister into which fresh crystals are poured for each treatment. Most have a separate canister to collect the used crystals.

The vacuum action of the nozzle on the skin has four main functions:

- It pulls and raises a small section of skin to work on.
- It causes slight oedema and brings some impurities to the surface.
- It shoots a stream of crystals across the targeted skin patch.
- It collects the used crystals and dead skin for disposal.

The nozzle, with its disposable tip is connected to the machine via a piece of tubing. You must ensure this is correctly and securely attached at both the nozzle end and at the machine, or the vacuum will not work.

Most machines will have a vacuum intensity dial showing pressure readings in pressure per square inch (PSI).

The dial reading may well show negative numbers (–) because in a vacuum, the pressure is negative. It is vital that you refer to manufacturer's instructions for their recommendations for different treatments.

> **Learning point** (L)
> Client comfort is the definitive determiner of the pressure setting. Allow the client to feel the vacuum on their arm before commencing treatment.

> **Be aware** (!)
> Some areas of the skin will be more sensitive than others such as the thinner skin around the eyes or the nerve-rich skin of the neck. Be more gentle in these areas.

The treatment should be preceded by the application of a suitable pre-peel lotion to disinfect the skin and help to loosen the bonds between the cells of the stratum corneum. This may then be followed by the application of a paste or mask to further breakdown these bonds. This will make the mechanical process of the treatment more effective.

Although most of the crystals and loosened skin particles are sucked back into the machine by the nozzle, a fine dust of crystals and dead skin cells may remain on the skin, especially around the hairline and eyebrows when treating the face. These should be gently wiped away with a suitable post-peel lotion. The lotion will also calm and soothe the skin.

Any products now applied to the skin will penetrate more deeply and be more readily absorbed, giving maximum benefit. These should be selected to suit your client. Check manufacturer's instructions for specific recommendations.

Diamond micro-dermabrasion

This treatment offers a similar effect but instead of using loose crystals as the abrasive substance, uses rotating steel heads encrusted with minute fragments of real, or manmade diamonds. Real diamonds are the hardest known substance. In some machines, different heads of varying sizes are available and may be encrusted with different grades of diamond fragments; coarse, medium or fine. Because diamond is a naturally sourced, inert substance it is unlikely to cause an adverse reaction.

The treatment is gentle. You have control over the amount of pressure you use on the client's skin, so you are able to reduce this for sensitive areas such as the neck and around the eye area. Many machines also offer you control over the speed and direction of rotation of the heads. The slower the speed of rotation, the more abrasive the treatment; the faster the speed, the less abrasive and more superficial the treatment. Because of friction, the skin may look red and feel warm.

In some machines, the dead cells are sucked away by a vacuum within the handpiece, while in others, the cells have to be wiped away after treatment.

The benefits, physiological effects, contra-indications, dangers and precautions, timing, homecare, and recommendations are all common to both methods. There are differences in the treatment technique and cleaning of equipment for each.

Benefits of crystal and diamond methods

- Suitable for most skin types.
- Reduces the appearance of fine lines on ageing skin.
- Over time, helps to improve elasticity of ageing skin.
- Minimises appearance of pigmentation, such as age spots.
- Reduces appearance of scarring and stretch marks.
- Brightens the complexion.
- Refines the skin and reduces appearance of enlarged pores.
- Reduces puffiness.
- Removes hard skin from feet.
- Smooths elbows and knees.

▽ **Table 10.1** Physiological effects of crystal and diamond methods

Physiological effects	Ageing skin with fine lines: improves elasticity	Minimises the appearance of pigmentation	Reduces the appearance of scarring and stretch marks	Brightens the complexion	Refines the skin and reduces the appearance of enlarged pores	Reduces puffiness	Removes hard skin from the feet; smooths elbows and knees
The friction increases the supply of blood to the skin, thus bringing nutrients and oxygen to the area. This results in improved condition of skin.	√	√	√	√	√	√	√
Aids lymphatic drainage removing waste products, and reducing oedema.	√				√	√	
Vasodilation giving erythema.	√		√	√	√	√	
It irritates sensory nerve endings stimulating regeneration of cells in the basal layer.	√	√	√	√	√		√
Aids the process of desquamation by sloughing off superficial layer of stratum corneum. Suitable for most skin types.	√	√	√	√	√		√
The removal of the protective layer of the skin allows beneficial products to penetrate more deeply and to be more readily absorbed.	√	√	√	√	√	√	√
Over a course of treatments, the increase in the number of new cells will help to restore some of the lost elasticity of the skin.	√		√		√		

Contra-indications to crystal and diamond methods

Learning point (L)

Check the contra-indications listed in the manufacturer's instructions to ensure you do not invalidate your insurance policy should the client be injured during or after treatment.

Precautions to take with crystal and diamond methods

There are no dangers specific to crystal or diamond micro-dermabrasion. However, precautions should be taken to minimise the risk of harming the client and to ensure you give an effective treatment.

▽ **Table 10.2** Reasons for contra-indications to crystal and diamond methods

Contra-indication	Reason
Botox injections	Vacuum action and rotary friction may interfere with the injected chemicals, causing an adverse reaction. Wait at least 8 weeks before treatment.
Cuts and abrasions (extensive) (small cuts may be easily avoided)	Skin could become irritated and inflamed and cause the client discomfort.
Dermal fillers	Vacuum action and or/rotation movements may move fillers under the skin. Wait at least 12 weeks before treatment.
Diabetes – Insulin controlled	A number of skin conditions associated with diabetes can be made worse by micro-dermabrasion.
Eczema	Avoid specific areas to reduce risk of irritation.
Glycolic peels	Stratum corneum has already been removed in these treatments. Micro-dermabrasion would act on next layer of epidermis. Wait at least 12 weeks.
Hypersensitive and highly vascular skin conditions	The treatment may irritate the skin further.
Loose skin	Where skin is very loose the process may pinch the skin, causing discomfort to client.
Medication causing thinning or inflammation of the skin (for example steroids, accutane, retinol)	Treatment will be uncomfortable for the client and may also cause an adverse reaction.
Moles – raised and skin tags	Avoid the area. May cause discomfort or bleeding.
Neuro-dermatitis	This condition generates a scratch-itch cycle leading to an eventual thickening of the skin in patches. Treatment could excacerbate the condition and there may be a risk of cross-infection.
Pregnancy	Can make skin hypersensitive.
Psoriasis	This condition is an auto-immune disease in which the skin cells are stimulated into over-production of new cells. Treatment will exacerbate the condition.
Skin diseases	To avoid cross-infection.
Tattoos on area being treated	May irritate skin, if recent. May cause tattoo to fade over time.

▽ **Table 10.3** Precautions to take with crystal and diamond methods

Precaution	Explanation
Examine and test the machine.	You need to check it is in good working order and ensure it will not cause harm to you or your client.
Carry out a tactile sensitivity test (see page 71).	This is to ensure the client can feel the difference between sharp and soft objects so that they can give accurate feedback on treatment.
Ensure crystal flow is functioning.	If crystals have got damp and are clumping together, the machine could clog and the large clumps of crystal could damage the skin.
Ensure skin is completely dry.	To avoid crystals clogging.

(Continued)

(Continued)

Precaution	Explanation
Adjust pressure for sensitive areas according to manufacturer's guidelines but within client tolerance.	The client should tell you if it becomes uncomfortable.
Do not work back and forward over the same area but work in lines in the same direction from one starting point.	To avoid excessive abrasion of one area.
When working on the face, treat both sides equally.	To ensure a balanced result.
Do not over-treat.	It could cause damage to the skin.
Speak to the client during treatment.	You need to ensure they are comfortable. Be alert to contra-actions.
Additional precautions for diamond method	
Adjust your use of pressure for sensitive and normal areas according to manufacturer's guidelines but within client tolerance.	The client should tell you if it becomes uncomfortable.
Move rotating head in a circular motion over the skin following the direction of rotation of the head.	If you move against the rotation the head will drag the skin, causing discomfort and possible damage.
Do not work back and forward over the same area but keep the head moving.	To avoid excessive abrasion of one area.

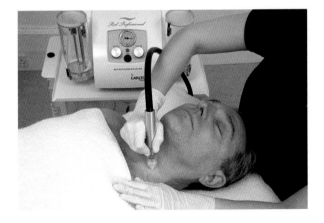

△ **Figure 10.3** Crystal micro-dermabrasion treatment

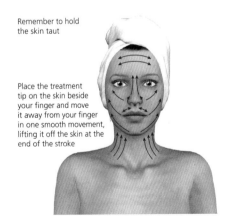

Remember to hold the skin taut

Place the treatment tip on the skin beside your finger and move it away from your finger in one smooth movement, lifting it off the skin at the end of the stroke

△ **Figure 10.4** Direction of crystal treatment

Crystal procedure – face

Preparation of working area

1. Place machine on a suitable stable base on the correct side of the couch.

   ↓

2. Check plugs, leads and connection of the nozzle to the machine. Ensure you have selected crystal micro-dermabrasion option for multi-function machines.

   ↓

3. Fill the fresh crystal canister with the recommended amount of crystals.

   ↓

4. Test the machine. To test the vacuum pressure, cover the hole of the treatment tip and turn up the vacuum intensity dial to its maximum. The intensity gauge should indicate maximum pressure. When you uncover the hole, the reading should drop to zero. To test crystal flow, repeat the above procedure, but observe the crystals in the canister; if flow is functioning properly, they should bounce around the canister.

   ↓

5. Check controls are at zero.

   ↓

6. Check the couch is prepared with clean linen and towels.

   ↓

7. Prepare trolley with:
   - suitable pre-treatment products to prepare the skin
   - suitable post treatment products
   - client consultation record.

   ↓

Preparation of self

8. Before carrying out treatment ensure you prepare yourself physically and mentally, paying due attention to high standards of professionalism. Adopt a sensitive calm, confident and understanding attitude as this approach will have a positive effect on your client.

   ↓

Preparation of client

9. Carry out a consultation, or if a regular client refer to the notes from their last treatment and discuss the effects and outcomes before proceeding.

   ↓

10. Check for contra-indications.

    ↓

11. Check contact lenses and all jewellery have been removed if appropriate.

    ↓

12. Protect hair and clothing as appropriate.

    ↓

13. Explain the treatment to the client saying that they may feel a slight stinging sensation and they should let you know if this becomes too uncomfortable.

    ↓

WASH YOUR HANDS

14. Carry out tactile sensitivity test.

    ↓

15. Cleanse and tone the skin – allow the skin to dry completely.

    ↓

16. Carry out a skin analysis.

    ↓

17. Apply pre-peel product(s) to disinfect the skin and start to loosen the cell bonds. Allow skin to dry completely.

    ↓

Best practice **B**

It is best to become accustomed to working with either hand so that the hand holding the skin taut does not block your view and you can always see what you are doing regardless of which side of the face or body you are working on.

Be aware **!**

Note any open blemishes or abrasions so that you can avoid them.

Technique for crystal method – face

18. Put on non-latex gloves.

> ### Learning point
>
> Gloves should be worn so that:
>
> ○ any moisture from your hands does not come into contact with the crystals
>
> ○ crystal residue does not adhere to your hands and then abrade the client's skin when applying post-treatment products.

↓

19. Set vacuum pressure to between -0.5 and -3 PSI (according to manufacturer's guidelines). Test the pressure on the client's arm so that they know how it feels. Adjust if necessary.

↓

20. Place a finger on the skin to one side of the area to be treated. This is to hold the skin taut, so that it is not pushed along by the treatment tip. Place the treatment tip gently on the skin beside your finger and move it away from your finger in one smooth movement, lifting it off the skin at the end of the stroke.

> ### Remember
>
> Do not push down on the skin, but glide along the surface using a firm but gentle pressure. Pressing too hard will be uncomfortable for the client and has no impact on the effectiveness of the treatment.

↓

21. Keep in verbal contact with the client to monitor progress and be alert for contra-actions.

↓

22. Continue working away from the finger holding the skin in a series of regular steady strokes, gradually working up one side of the face. Then repeat on the other.

> ### Be aware
>
> Do not work in circles or move the nozzle backward and forward over the area as this will lead to over-treatment and irritation of the area.

> ### Be aware
>
> Areas of pigmentation or scarring may require a deeper treatment. This can be achieved by:
>
> ○ increasing the vacuum intensity to between -3.5 to -7.5 PSI (See manufacturer's guidelines and refer to client comfort.)
>
> ○ going over the area a number of times (within client tolerance)
>
> ○ running the treatment tip back and forth between two fingers placed on the skin
>
> ○ moving the treatment tip slowly over the area.

↓

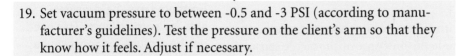

> ### Learning point
>
> Treatment usually starts on the neck but remember that this is one of the most sensitive areas so you may need to alter pressure on the machine.

> ### Remember
>
> The more sensitive the skin, the less vacuum pressure should be used. Refer to manufacturer's instructions for guidelines but always use client comfort as the main determining factor.

> ### Be aware
>
> It is important to turn the dial up slowly to allow the reading to adjust and settle in order to get an accurate reading.

> ### Be aware
>
> You should be able to see the machine and the client at all times, and be in easy reach of controls.

23. When you have evenly covered the whole area, with treatment tip no longer in contact with the skin, turn down the vacuum pressure and switch off the machine.

↓

24. Brush away any remaining crystal dust and dead skin cells.

↓

25. Apply an appropriate post-peel lotion. Allow to dry.

↓

26. Remove gloves.

↓

27. Complete treatment with the application of appropriate products selected for the client's needs.

↓

28. Update the consultation record with salient points about the treatment for future reference. This will include the outcome of the tactile sensitivity test.

Be aware !
Erythema may be considerable for some clients. This need not be a cause for concern; be guided by your client's comfort.

The procedure is the same for treating other parts of the body and treatment is effective for a range of skin conditions such as: age spots on the hands; stretch marks; scarring; for smoothing skin, especially on elbows and knees, prior to tanning treatment; and for the removal of calluses on the feet or hands. Refer to manufacturer's instructions for details of vacuum pressure and specific procedures.

Diamond procedure – face

Preparation of working area

1. Place machine on a suitable stable base on the correct side of the couch.

↓

2. Check plugs, leads and connection of the handpiece to the machine. Ensure you have selected diamond option for multi-function machines.

↓

3. Select the appropriate diamond head for the area you are treating, following manufacturer's guidelines.

↓

4. Test the machine – so that you know which way the head is rotating.

↓

5. Check controls are at zero.

↓

6. Check the couch is prepared with clean linen and towels.

↓

7. Prepare trolley with:
   ○ suitable pre-treatment products, according to manufacturer's guidelines
   ○ soft brush or gauze to remove dead skin cells
   ○ suitable post treatment products
   ○ client consultation record.

↓

Best practice B
It is best to become accustomed to working with either hand so that the hand holding the skin taut does not block your view and you can always see what you are doing regardless of which side of the face or body you are working on.

Preparation of self

8. Before carrying out treatment ensure you prepare yourself physically and mentally, paying due attention to high standards of professionalism. Adopt a sensitive calm, confident and understanding attitude, as this approach will have a positive effect on your client.

↓

Preparation of client

9. Carry out a consultation, or if a regular client refer to the notes from their last treatment and discuss the effects and outcomes before proceeding.

↓

10. Check for contra-indications.

↓

11. Check contact lenses and all jewellery have been removed if appropriate.

↓

12. Position client comfortably depending on area to be treated.

↓

13. Protect hair and clothing as appropriate.

↓

14. Explain the treatment to the client, saying that they may feel a slight prickling sensation and they should let you know if this becomes too uncomfortable.

↓

WASH YOUR HANDS

15. Carry out tactile sensitivity test.

↓

16. Cleanse and tone the skin. Allow skin to dry completely.

↓

17. Carry out a skin analysis.

↓

Technique for diamond method – face

18. Ensure speed control is at minimum and select direction of rotation if applicable to your machine. Place rotating head onto the neck and gently increase speed control.

↓

19. Place a finger on the skin to one side of the area to be treated. This is to hold the skin taut, so that it is not dragged along by the rotating head. Work in small circular movements away from the supporting finger so that the skin is lifted upwards and outwards.

↓

20. Keep in verbal contact with the client to monitor progress and be alert for contra-actions.

↓

21. Continue working upwards and outwards over half the face. Change the direction of rotation to work up the other side of the face. Cover the whole of the face and neck once or twice (no more than three times), according to manufacturer's instructions.

↓

22. When you have covered the whole area the desired number of times, reduce the speed to zero and switch off the machine.

↓

23. Brush away any remaining dead skin cells.

↓

Remember

Note any open blemishes, abrasions, raised moles or skin tags so that you can avoid them.

Learning point L

Treatment usually starts on the *neck* but remember that this is one of the most sensitive areas so you may need to start with lighter pressure.

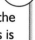

Be aware

You should be able to see the machine and the client at all times, and be in easy reach of controls.

Remember

Make sure your movements follow the rotation of the head.

24. Complete treatment with the application of appropriate products selected for the client's needs.

↓

25. Update the consultation record with salient points about the treatment for future reference. This will include the outcome of the tactile sensitivity test.

The procedure is the same for treating other parts of the body and treatment is effective for a range of skin conditions such as: age spots on the hands; stretch marks; scarring; for smoothing skin, especially on elbows and knees, prior to tanning treatment; for the removal of calluses on the feet or hands. Refer to manufacturer's instructions for details of specific procedures.

Timing of treatment

This will depend on the area being treated. It will also vary from one product to another, as there will be recommendations for suitable absorption times for different products.

> **! Be aware**
>
> Erythema may be considerable for some clients. This need not be a cause for concern; be guided by your client's comfort.

> **! Be aware**
>
> Do not push down too hard on the skin, but glide along the surface using a firm but gentle pressure. Pressing too hard will be uncomfortable for the client and has no impact on the effectiveness of the treatment.

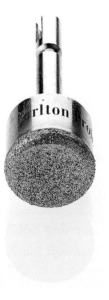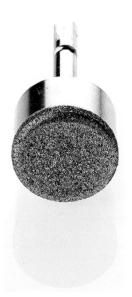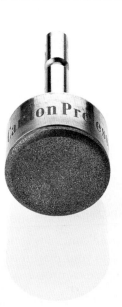

△ **Figure 10.5** Diamond heads

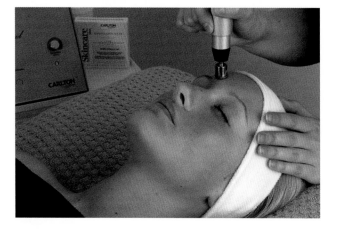

△ **Figure 10.6** Micro-dermabrasion treatment diamond

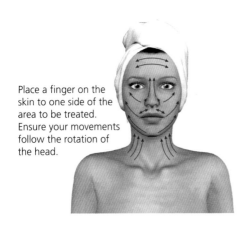

Place a finger on the skin to one side of the area to be treated. Ensure your movements follow the rotation of the head.

△ **Figure 10.7** Direction of diamond treatment

Contra-actions to crystal and diamond methods

This is a gentle treatment and erythema and taut, tingly skin is a normal reaction to it. Skin should be soothed by the application of preparatory post-treatment products.

○ Excessive erythema in the area: place a cool compress on the skin and apply a suitable product or mask that will help to calm and soothe the tissues.

○ Skin prone to flushing later in day following treatment: advise the client to apply a cold compress to the area followed by a suitable hypoallergenic product to soothe the area.

Homecare advice for crystal and diamond methods

Clients should be advised to:

○ avoid exfoliation for 7 days

○ apply a minimum SPF 15/30 moisturising product;

○ avoid products containing retinol during the course of treatments

○ avoid sunbathing, sunbed, or heat treatments 24 to 48 hours prior to next micro-dermabrasion session.

> **Remember**
> Always seek feedback from your client and give appropriate aftercare advice (see pages 73–4).

Recommendations for crystal and diamond methods

The treatment is most effective on skin that is completely dry, so it is best if it does not follow heating or steaming treatments.

The length of the course of treatment and the amount of time between treatments will vary according to the condition being treated: the sensitivity of the skin and the skin's reaction to treatment.

A course of between 10 and 15 weekly treatments is recommended to give maximum benefit without risking damage to the skin. A maintenance programme of a treatment every 4–6 weeks is then recommended to best maintain the skin's condition. Because it takes 28–32 days for the epidermis to renew itself, and this treatment stimulates that process, 4–6 weeks is a good guide to frequency of maintenance treatment.

Cleaning – crystal method

Remove and dispose of treatment tip. Empty used crystal canister at least every day.

> **Remember**
> Avoid getting any part of the machine wet. If parts do require washing, ensure that they are completely dry (48 hours in a drying chamber) before use.

Refer to manufacturer's instructions for specific guidelines.

Cleaning – diamond method

Brush excess skin cells from the diamond head. Refer to manufacturer's instructions for information on cleaning and sterilising of the head.

Multiple-choice questions

1. Skin cells are regenerated in the:
   a horny layer
   b granular layer
   c basal layer
   d clear layer.

2. Melanin is produced to protect the cells against:
   a the damaging effect of ultraviolet radiation
   b invasion by bacteria
   c dehydration
   d ageing.

3. Sebum is produced to:
   a help to heal cuts and abrasions
   b give the skin strength
   c remove dead skin cells
   d keep the surface of the skin smooth and supple.

4. Keratin is a protein that:
   a protects the skin from injury
   b causes the skin to tan
   c reduces the signs of ageing
   d helps new skin cells to multiply.

5. The natural process of shedding dead skin cells is known as:
   a dermabrasion
   b exfoliation
   c desquamation
   d epilation.

6. The main advantage of micro-dermabrasion over chemical peeling is:
   a it is cheaper
   b it is safer for the therapist

   c it is not as time consuming
   d it is easier to control the depth of treatment.

7. Aluminium oxide crystals used for micro-dermabrasion must not come into contact with any moisture because they will:
   a dissolve and be absorbed by the skin
   b stick together and damage the skin
   c cause the machine to rust
   d dissolve and therefore be ineffective.

8. The intensity of the vacuum pressure used for crystal micro-dermabrasion is determined by:
   a the type of crystals used
   b the thickness of the client's skin
   c the area being treated
   d client tolerance.

9. A pre-peel lotion is used to:
   a moisturise the client's skin
   b loosen the bonds between the dead skin cells
   c form a protective layer over the area being treated
   d numb the area being treated.

10. You should wear protective gloves when giving a crystal micro-dermabrasion treatment:
    a to protect your hands from the crystals
    b to protect your hands from the pre-peel lotion
    c to protect your client from infection
    d so that crystals do not stick to your hands and scratch client.

11. Micro-dermabrasion is **not** suitable for:
    a clients who have had recent fillers
    b clients who have enlarged pores

c ageing skin with fine lines

d scar tissue or stretch marks.

12. When giving a diamond micro-dermabrasion treatment you should:

   a work in straight lines, away from the centre

b move the rotating head in a circular motion over the skin, following the direction of rotation of the head

c move the rotating head in a circular motion over the skin, against the direction of rotation of the head

d work back and forth over the same area.

11 Infrared and ultraviolet treatments

Objectives

After you have studied this chapter you will be able to:

▪ explain the terms wavelength and frequency

▪ state the range wavelengths of infrared and ultraviolet rays

▪ understand the principles and scientific laws relating to radiation

▪ describe the benefits and effects of infrared and ultra-violet rays on body tissues

▪ explain the contra-indications to infrared and ultraviolet treatments

▪ explain the dangers and precautions of infrared and ultraviolet treatments

▪ explain the contra-actions that may occur during and/or after treatment and the appropriate action to take

▪ carry out infrared and ultraviolet treatments, paying due consideration to maximum efficiency, comfort, safety and hygiene.

Infrared (IR) rays for heating body tissues and ultraviolet rays for promoting tanning of the skin are the radiation treatments used in beauty therapy. Infrared lamps and radiant heat lamps may both be used to warm the body and soften the tissues in preparation for further treatment. Both infrared rays and ultraviolet rays are part of the electromagnetic spectrum.

The electromagnetic spectrum

Before you begin to learn about infrared and ultraviolet treatments, you need to know about the electromagnetic spectrum and how it works.

Electromagnetic energy is given off by (radiates from) the sun. 'Radiates' means that the energy travels in straight lines, or rays. Some of the electromagnetic rays are perceived as visible light (daylight), enabling us to see. Others are invisible, such as infrared rays, which we experience as heat from the sun and ultraviolet rays, which cause the skin to tan, but which also have the potential to damage skin when over-exposed to these rays.

Harmful rays from the sun are, mostly, filtered out by the earth's atmosphere, but some do get through which is why over-exposure to the sun causes us to burn. The amount of electromagnetic radiation hitting the earth also depends on factors such as the angle of the sun and the amount of cloud cover. This is why countries around the equator, where the sun is directly overhead are hotter than those at the two poles. It is also why the sun feels most intense at midday when it is directly overhead. The water vapour in cloud absorbs some of the infrared rays, reducing the heat, but the ultraviolet rays can still get through, which is why it is still possible to burn on overcast days.

The electromagnetic spectrum is made up of bands of radiation with differing wavelengths and frequencies, each of which will have different physiological effects on body tissues. It is thought that all electromagnetic rays are similar in form, being particles in motion. They are transverse waves, which travel through space without the need of a conductor.

The speed, or velocity, at which they travel is the same for all the bands, being 300,000km/sec (the speed of sound).

Wavelength

The bands of the electromagnetic spectrum have different wavelengths. The wavelength is the distance between a point on one wave and the same point on the next wave.

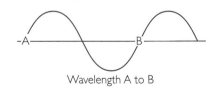

Wavelength A to B

△ **Figure 11.1** Wavelength

Wavelengths of each band emitted from the spectrum

The wave band ranges are shown below, but there is some overlap.

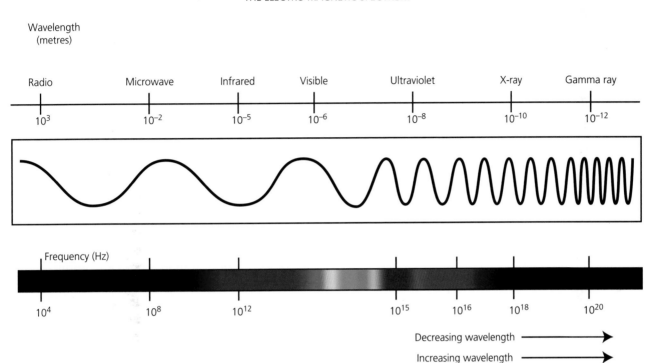

THE ELECTRO MAGNETIC SPECTRUM

Type of wave	Wavelength
Cosmic	up to 0.002 nm
Gamma	0.002 nm to 0.14 nm
X-rays	0.14 nm to 13.4 nm
Ultraviolet	10 nm to 400 nm
Visible	400 nm to 770 nm
Infrared	770 nm to 400,000 nm
Radio	100,000 nm upwards

The shortest wavelength rays are cosmic rays and the longest are radio waves. The distance from A to B is the wavelength. This wavelength varies from the very short wavelength of cosmic rays, measured in nanometres, to the very long wavelength of radio waves measured in metres or kilometres. (One nanometre is a very small measurement, being one millionth of a millimetre. It is written as nm.)

Frequency

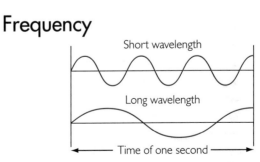

△ **Figure 11.2** Rays of different wavelength will have different frequencies

The bands of the spectrum also have different frequencies. Frequency is the number of complete waves that pass a point in one second. Many more waves of short wavelength will pass the point in one second than those of long wavelength.

The rays of shorter wavelength will have a higher frequency than the rays of longer wavelength. In other words, as the wavelength increases, the frequency decreases.

> **Learning point** (L)
> The term 'frequency' is familiar to us when tuning the radio: programmes are transmitted on the radio at different frequencies.

Units of frequency

Frequency is measured in hertz (Hz). The number of waves past a point in one second is the number of hertz, for example 50 waves passing a point per second = 50Hz. For higher frequencies the units become:

1 kilohertz (kHz) = 1000Hz

1 megahertz (mHz) = 1000kHz

Infrared rays

Infrared rays are electromagnetic waves with wavelengths between 770 nm and 400,000 nm. They are given off by the sun and by any hot object, for example electric fires, gas and coal fires, hot packs and various types of lamps.

The lamps that produce infrared (IR) rays can be divided into two main types:

❍ The non-luminous type (called infrared lamps).
❍ The luminous type (called radiant heat lamps).

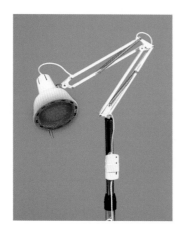

△ **Figure 11.3** A radiant heat lamp

Both these types of lamp emit infrared rays. The difference lies in their wavelength. The non-luminous type emit rays of longer wavelength, around 4,000 nm, while the luminous type emit rays of shorter wave, around 1,000 nm and include waves from the visible spectrum and UVL. The differing wavelengths produce slightly different effects when absorbed by body tissues.

> **Remember**
> Infrared lamps and radiant heat lamps give off (emit) infrared rays. The difference is the wavelength of the rays, which produce different effects.

The non-luminous lamps (infrared lamps)

Many types of non-luminous lamps are produced, but they all have a non-glowing source that emits infrared rays. A common type uses a coil of wire embedded in fireclay, which is placed in the centre of a reflector. When the lamp is switched on, the wire gets hot and heats the fireclay; the rays are then emitted from the hot fireclay, they pass through the air and are absorbed by a body placed in their path. The rays from non-luminous lamps are of longer wavelength, are invisible, are less irritating and less penetrating than the short rays from luminous lamps. They may feel hotter at equal distances and power due to increased absorption in the top layers of the skin. These wavelengths are further from visible light and are consequently called **'far IR'**.

The luminous lamps (radiant heat lamps)

These lamps give off infrared rays from glowing or incandescent sources, such as hot wires or powerful bulbs. These are also placed in the centre of a reflector. When the lamp is switched on, the wire glows, giving off infrared and visible rays and small amounts of ultraviolet rays. Some bulbs have filters to cut out some visible rays and ultraviolet rays; these bulbs are usually red in colour.

The rays produced by these lamps have a shorter wavelength, include some visible rays, are more penetrating (down to the subcutaneous layer) and are more irritating than the rays from non-luminous lamps. These wavelengths are nearer visible light and are consequently called **'near IR'**.

▽ **Table 11.1** Comparisons of infrared and radiant heat lamps

Non-luminous (infrared)	Luminous (radiant heat)
Rays emitted from a heated wire embedded in clay	Rays emitted from glowing wires and bulbs
Long wavelength	Shorter wavelength
Includes no visible rays	Includes some visible rays and a small amount of UVL
Penetrates approximately 1 mm of skin to the epidermis	Penetrates approximately 3 mm of tissue to the dermis/subcutaneous layer
Less irritating	More irritating
May feel hotter at equal power and distance	Will feel less hot at equal power and distance
Takes 10–15 minutes to heat up	Heats up quickly, approximately 2 minutes

Be aware !

These days the majority of lamps used are the radiant heat type as opposed to infrared lamps. This is because they heat up more quickly and it is easy to tell by looking whether or not they are on, which is a feature for safety.

Properties and laws of radiation for infrared treatments

In order to give the most effective and safe treatment, you should be aware of certain laws and principles that govern the behaviour of rays/waves. Infrared light rays will travel in straight lines until they meet a new medium, where they may be *refracted, reflected* or *absorbed*.

Refraction

This is the bending of rays when they meet a new medium. A good example is looking at a stick held in water – it appears to bend. Refraction occurs when rays pass from one medium to another, for example from air through water or glass.

Reflection

This is the reflection of rays when they meet a surface. Shiny or white surfaces reflect more rays than dark surfaces, which absorb rays; a greater proportion of light rays will be reflected by snow than by soil. A mirror is designed to reflect rays.

The law of reflection states the *angle of incidence* is *equal* to the *angle of reflection*. What this means is that light rays bounce off a surface at the same angle as they hit the surface. The greater this angle, the less the concentration in some of the rays. In order to achieve the greatest concentration of light rays hitting a surface, the light source must be perpendicular to that surface, that is: directly above it.

Best practice B

When positioning an infrared lamp for treatment you should ensure that the lamp is angled to point directly at the part to be treated in order to maximise the concentration of light rays hitting the part. It is not a good idea to position the lamp directly above the client as there is a risk of the lamp falling on and burning the client. Position the client and the lamp to maximise the effect of the treatment and minimise the risk of burning (see pages 252 and 256).

The angle of incidence is *one* of the factors governing the proportion of rays absorbed by the medium which the rays strike. This is an important consideration when giving IR treatment, as the effectiveness of the treatment will depend on the number of rays absorbed.

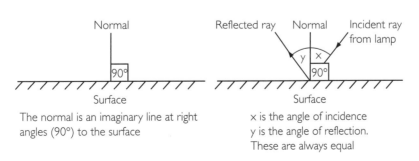

Normal

The normal is an imaginary line at right angles (90°) to the surface

Surface

Reflected ray Normal Incident ray from lamp

x is the angle of incidence
y is the angle of reflection.
These are always equal

Surface

△ **Figure 11.4** Reflection

Absorption

The law of Grotthus states that: 'rays must be absorbed to produce an effect'.

The amount of absorption and consequently the effect depends on the following.

1. The wavelength and frequency of the rays:
   - infrared (non-luminous or invisible rays) is absorbed by body tissues to a level of approximately 1mm below the surface of the skin.
   - radiant heat (luminous or visible rays) is absorbed by body tissues to a level of approximately 3mm below the surface of the skin.

2. The type of medium. Different substances will absorb some wavelengths while allowing others to pass through. Body tissues absorb certain wavelengths to certain levels, but allow others to pass through.

3. The angle at which the rays strike the part also affects absorption. Where the maximum concentration of rays hit the surface, the maximum amount of absorption will take place. The greatest possible concentration of rays hit the surface when the source is perpendicular to the surface.

> **Learning point** (L)
> Sunlight is made up of infrared and ultraviolet rays. Because the sun is perpendicular to the earth's surface at noon, the maximum concentration of rays are hitting the surface, and the sun feels at its hottest. This is why you are most likely to suffer sunburn at this time.

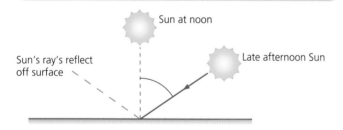

△ **Figure 11.5** Showing sun's rays striking a surface

Intensity of radiation

The intensity of radiation will depend on three factors:
- the intensity of the lamp
- the distance between the lamp and the skin
- the angle at which the rays strike the part.

The intensity of the lamp

Lamps can vary in output and therefore, intensity; all lamps have control dials for increasing and decreasing intensity. If the client feels the intensity is too high, the distance can be increased or the lamp turned down.

The distance between the lamp and the skin

The law of inverse squares is illustrated in Figure 11.6.

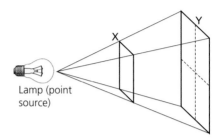

△ **Figure 11.6** Radiation from a point source, showing the law of inverse squares

Law of inverse squares

The intensity of rays from an infrared lamp is also affected by the distance the lamp is placed from the part being treated. The *law of inverse squares* governs this. The law of inverse squares states that 'the intensity from a point source varies inversely with the square of the distance from the point source'. That is to say: the further away the lamp is from the part, the less intense the rays are at the part.

> In simple terms, this means that if the distance of the lamp from the part is doubled (i.e. twice as far away), then the intensity is quartered. If the distance is halved (i.e. the lamp is nearer), the intensity is quadrupled.

> **Be aware** !
> Because the lamp's rays are more intense when it is closer, the *time* the client can spend under the lamp is less, so if the intensity is quadrupled, the time must be halved. If the intensity is quartered, the time spent under the lamp can be doubled, but check manufacturer's instructions for guidance.

> **Remember**
> In order to ensure the most effective treatment, the rays of the infrared lamp must strike the part at an angle of 90°; this will ensure maximum intensity, absorption and effect.

Infrared treatment of the body

Infrared is used to heat body tissues. It may be used to treat localised areas or the body in general.

Benefits of infrared treatment to the body

○ As a general heating treatment to promote relaxation.

○ As a localised treatment for relief of pain and muscle tension.

○ As a preheating treatment, either generally or locally, to increase the circulation and thus make following treatments more effective.

Physiological effects of infrared treatment to the body

Heating of body tissues

When infrared rays are absorbed by the tissues, heat is produced in the area. The rays from luminous generators penetrate more deeply than those from non-luminous lamps. Penetration is approximately 3mm of tissue, therefore superficial and deeper tissues are heated directly.

With non-luminous lamps (which have infrared rays only) the top 1mm of skin is heated directly, but the deeper tissues are heated by conduction.

> **Learning point**
> Conduction is the transfer of heat energy through matter from particle to particle. In the body tissues heat can be conducted from cell to cell.

Increased metabolic rate

Van't Hoff's law states that a chemical reaction capable of being accelerated will be accelerated by heat.

Metabolism involves chemical reactions, which will be accelerated by heat. The increase in metabolic rate will be greatest where the heating is greatest, that is in the superficial tissues; therefore more oxygen and nutrients are required and more waste products and metabolites are produced.

Vasodilation with increase in circulation

Heat has a direct effect on the blood vessels producing vasodilation and an increase in blood flow in an attempt to cool the area. Vasodilation is also produced by stimulation of sensory nerve endings, which causes reflex dilation of arterioles.

Vasodilation is also produced as a result of the increase in metabolic rate and increase in waste products. The metabolites act on the walls of capillaries and arterioles causing dilation.

The heat-regulating centre of the brain will be stimulated as body heat rises. This will result in general dilation of superficial vessels to ensure that the body is not overheated.

> **Learning point**
> **Hyperaemia** is the term used to describe an increase in the flow of blood to the area due to vasodilation. **Erythema** means reddening of the skin due to hyperaemia and vasodilation.

Fall in blood pressure

If the superficial blood vessels dilate, the peripheral resistance is reduced and this will result in a fall in blood pressure. When blood flows through vessels with small lumen, it exerts a certain pressure on the walls. If the lumen is increased by the vessels' dilating, the pressure on the walls will be reduced.

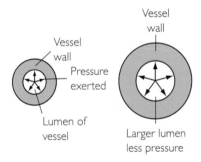

△ **Figure 11.7** Pressure on vessel walls

> **Learning point**
> A fall in blood pressure is due to the blood vessels dilating.

Increase in heart rate

The increased metabolism and circulation means that the heart must beat faster to meet the demand; therefore the heart rate increases.

General rise in body temperature

When one area of the body is heated for a prolonged time, there is a general rise in body temperature by *conduction* and *convection*.

Conduction is the transfer of energy (e.g. heat) between two solid materials that are physically touching each other (warmed skin cells pass heat to surrounding cells). **Convection** is the transfer of heat energy in a gas or liquid by the movement of the warmed matter (in this case, blood). The heat will spread through surrounding tissues and will be carried by the blood circulating through the area.

Increased activity of sweat and sebaceous glands

As the body temperature rises, the heat regulating centres in the brain are affected. The sweat glands are then stimulated to produce more sweat in order to lose body heat. This increases the elimination of waste products.

Stimulation of sebaceous glands causes them to release more sebum.

Effects on muscle tissue

Muscle tissue is affected in two ways:

○ The rise in temperature produces muscle relaxation and relieves tension and pain.

○ When muscles are warm, they contract more efficiently than when they are cold. The increase in circulation provides the nutrients and oxygen necessary for muscle action and the removal of waste is speeded up.

Effects on sensory nerves

Heat has a soothing effect on sensory nerve endings. However, intense heat has an irritating effect.

Pigmentation

Repeated and intense exposure to infrared produces a purple or brown mottled appearance on the area.

Be aware !

Pigmentation may be due to destruction of blood cells and release of haemoglobin.

Learning point (L)

Check the contra-indications listed in the manufacturer's instructions to ensure you do not invalidate your insurance policy should the client be injured during or after treatment.

Contra-indications to infrared treatment for the body

▽ **Table 11.2** Reasons for contra-indications to infrared for the body

Contra-indication	Reason
Bruising (extensive)	The stimulation of blood circulation may increase bleeding. Bruises must be allowed to heal before treatment. Avoid the area.
Defective skin sensation	The client must be able to feel the sensation of heat to be able to give accurate feedback about the intensity of the lamp as the skin could burn.
Deficient circulation	Could cause overheating or burning of the area. Do not treat.
Diabetes	A client with diabetes may have impaired sensitivity and poor circulation. This may cause overheating or burning of the area. Find out more about their condition and if in doubt seek GP's consent.
Headaches and migraines	The heat and the stimulation of the blood circulation will exacerbate the condition. The body needs time to heal before having treatment.
Heart conditions	The increase in the blood circulation may put too much pressure and stress on the heart; seek medical consent.
Heavy colds and fevers	May aggravate the condition.

(Continued)

(Continued)

Contra-indication	Reason
High blood pressure	Blood pressure varies with age, weight and fitness, but some people have consistently high blood pressure. Treatment can frequently help. Medical advice should be sought if the client is not currently on medication.
Hypersensitive skin	A client with hypersensitive skin must not receive treatments that stimulate the blood circulation, as these will exacerbate the condition.
Low blood pressure	The client may feel dizzy or faint if they sit up or get up too quickly or if they receive too long a treatment. Monitor their treatment carefully.
Medium (any area where liniments or ointments have been applied)	These may contain products that heat more rapidly (such as oil or alcohol), and so cause the skin to burn.
Menstruation	Do not advise treatment during the first 2–3 days of a period as it may cause a heavier blood flow. Also blood loss contributes to feelings of faintness.
Metal pins and plates	Metal is a good conductor therefore the intensity of the current will increase in the area and may cause the client discomfort. Avoid treating these areas.
Oedema	The cause may be associated with high blood pressure, kidney conditions or other systemic problems. Seek medical advice to establish the cause.
Phlebitis	Phlebitis is a painful condition where the lining of the vein becomes inflamed and may result in a clot forming on the vein wall, known as thrombosis. Any pressure applied to the vein or increase in the force of the circulation may dislodge the clot. The embolism will then be carried in the blood stream, with potentially fatal consequences. **Do not treat**.
Pregnancy (avoid the last four months)	As blood circulation is stimulated and hormone levels are erratic, treatment should not be advised.
Scar tissue (recent)	Scar tissue must be allowed to heal completely before treatment is given to the area. If treatment is given before healing is complete, there is a danger of further damage to the tissues delaying the healing process. Also skin sensation will be defective in the area, so the client will not be able to give accurate feedback about the intensity of the heat.
Skin diseases	There is a risk of cross-infection.
Skin disorders, for example eczema and psoriasis	The skin for both conditions is red with flaky dry patches. The treatment will cause more sensitivity in the area and exacerbate the condition.
Soft tissue injury (recent)	This requires treatment with ice applications to constrict the capillaries and reduce tissue swelling.
Sunburn	Treatment will make the condition worse, as it will increase the sensitivity of the tissues.
Thrombosis	This is a blood clot in a vein, usually found in the calf muscle. An increase in circulation could cause the blood clot to be transported in the blood stream to the lungs and heart, with fatal consequences. **Do not treat**.

Dangers of infrared treatment to the body

Burns may be caused if:

○ the heat is too intense

○ the client is too near the lamp and fails to report overheating

○ the skin sensation is defective and the client may not be aware of overheating

○ the client touches the lamp

○ the lamp falls and touches the client, or the bedding; overheating of pillows and blankets can cause fire and burns.

Electric shock may result from faulty apparatus or from water in the treatment area producing a short circuit.

Precautions should be taken to minimise the risk of harming the client and to ensure you give an effective treatment.

▽ **Table 11.3** Precautions to take with infrared treatment to the body

Precaution	Explanation
Ensure that the lamp is in good working order and that there are no dents in the reflector.	Dents will cause 'hot spots' on the area, increasing the intensity of rays and so causing burns.
Ensure the flexes are sound and not trailing in a walking area.	To minimise risk of electric shock and to prevent anyone tripping over the flex.
Ensure that the head of the lamp is positioned over a foot if the lamp has three or five feet.	To ensure stability and prevent the lamp from falling.
Ensure that the angle-poise joints are tight and secure.	To minimise risk of the lamp collapsing onto the client.
Do not place the lamp directly over the client.	It may fall and cause burns.
Ensure a safe distance of the lamp from the client.	The distance depends on the client's tolerance and the output of the lamp (18–36 inches, 45–90 cm).
Carry out a thermal sensitivity test (see page 71).	If the client cannot tell the difference between hot and cold, they have defective sensation and the treatment should not be carried out.
Protect the back of the neck with a towel.	Excessive heat on the back of the neck may cause feelings of nausea or a headache.

Infrared treatment procedure – body

Preparation of working area

1. Switch on the lamp to warm up, making sure the lamp is away from all surfaces and directed at the floor for safety.

   ↓

2. Check the couch is prepared with clean linen and towels.

   ↓

3. Prepare trolley with suitable products
   - Tape measure
   - Towel or protective gloves.

   ↓

Preparation of self

4. Before carrying out treatment ensure you prepare yourself physically and mentally, paying due attention to high standards of professionalism. Adopt a sensitive calm, confident and understanding attitude, as this approach will have a positive effect on your client.

   ↓

Preparation of client

5. Carry out a consultation, or if a regular client refer to the notes from their last treatment and discuss the effects and outcomes before proceeding.

   ↓

6. Check for contra-indications.

   ↓

7. Check all jewellery has been removed.

   ↓

8. Place the client in a well-supported and comfortable position.

   ↓

9. Explain the treatment to the client: Warn the client that warmth from the lamp should be comfortable and to alert you if the heat becomes too intense. The client should also be instructed not to touch the lamp or move closer to it.

   ↓

WASH YOUR HANDS

10. Cover the areas not receiving treatment with towel/blanket.

    ↓

11. Carry out a thermal sensitivity test.

    ↓

12. Cleanse the area.

    ↓

Technique for infrared body

13. Protect the client's eyes with damp eye pads if required or protective eye-wear.

    ↓

14. Position the lamp ensuring stability.

    ↓

15. Measure an appropriate distance between 45–90 cm (18–36 inches) and position the lamp. The selected distance depends on two factors:
    - the intensity of the lamp
    - the client's tolerance. 60 cm is a good average, but check manufacturer's instructions.

    ↓

Remember

Infrared lamps take 10–15 minutes to reach maximum output. Radiant heat lamps take around 2 minutes.

Remember

When treating areas of the back, use side lying or the recovery position, well supported by pillows.

Remember

Make sure that the face of the lamp is parallel with the part so that the rays strike the part at an angle of 90° for maximum penetration, absorption and effect. Do *not* place the lamp directly above the client.

Remember

The head of the lamp will be hot. Use a towel or gloves to protect your hands when moving or adjusting the position of the lamp.

16. Observe the client throughout the treatment and be alert to contra-actions.

↓

17. Monitor the effect of heat on the client's skin.

↓

18. At the end of treatment, turn off the lamp and place in a safe place to cool down.

↓

19. Follow with massage or electrical treatments to the area.

↓

20. Update the consultation record with salient points about the treatment for future reference. This will include the outcome of the thermal sensitivity test.

> **Remember**
>
> The client should not rise suddenly after infrared treatment, as the blood pressure is lowered and the client may feel faint.

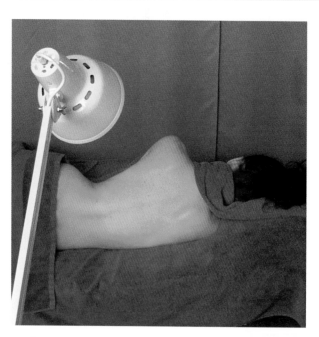 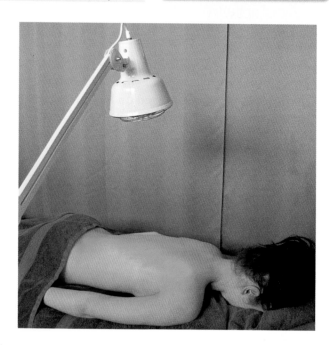

△ **Figure 11.8** Correct positioning and incorrect positioning

Timing of treatment

Treatment time is 15–20 minutes (check manufacturer's instructions), until the desired effect is obtained.

Contra-actions for infrared treatment to the body

○ Headache: irradiating the back of the neck and head or overheating by prolonged exposure may cause headache. Place a cool compress on client's forehead; offer a glass of water and discuss options to continue, cut down or stop the treatment.

○ Faintness: overheating or extensive irradiation may cause a fall in blood pressure, which may cause faintness. Raise the client's legs to improve the blood flow to the brain, make sure there is a flow of fresh air, give the client time to recover.

○ Damage to the eyes: infrared exposure of the eyes can cause cataracts. Clients should close their eyes and turn away from the lamp, wear protective eye-wear or place damp cotton wool over their eyes.

> **Learning point** (L)
>
> Damage to the eyes would occur over a number of treatments rather than instantly, but it is important that clients cover their eyes for each one.

○ Constipation: this may occur following prolonged exposure and if water loss through sweating is not replaced by water intake. Advise the client to drink plenty of water to hydrate the body.

> **Remember**
>
> Always seek feedback from your client and give appropriate aftercare advice. See pages 73–4.

Recommendations for infrared treatment to the body

Infrared radiation can be used as a preheat treatment to a specific area to soften and warm the tissues prior to gyratory vibrator, vacuum suction, electrical muscle stimulation and galvanic.

Remember

Do not use infrared before using tanning equipment, as the reaction to UVL will be intensified. Infrared may, however, be used after over-exposure to UVL to reduce the reaction.

Infrared treatment of the face

Infrared irradiation of the face is used as a preheating treatment to prepare the skin for further treatments and aid the absorption of creams, oils and masks. Very mild heat should be given and particular attention must be paid to totally covering the eyes.

Benefits of infrared treatment to the face

○ To soften and prepare the skin for further treatments.
○ To aid the absorption and enhance the effects of creams, oils and masks.
○ To improve dry and mature skins.

Contra-indications of infrared treatment to the face

Learning point

Check the contra-indications listed in the manufacturer's instructions to ensure you do not invalidate your insurance policy should the client be injured during or after treatment.

Dangers of infrared treatment to the face

Burns may be caused if:

○ the heat is too intense
○ the client is too near the lamp and fails to report overheating

▽ Table 11.4 Physiological effects and benefits of infrared treatment to the face (see also page 247 for more detailed information)

Physiological effects \ Benefits	Soften and prepare the skin for further treatments	Aid the absorption and enhance the effects of creams, oils and masks	Improve dry and mature skins
Heat raises the temperature of the area and increases the metabolic rate.	√	√	√
Increase in circulation due to vasodilation.	√	√	√
Improvement of skin colour due to hyperaemia and erythema.	√		√
Stimulation of sweat glands to produce more sweat, releasing impurities.	√		√
Stimulation of sebaceous gland, releasing sebum to soften and lubricate the skin.	√		√
Relaxation of facial muscles.	√		

○ the skin sensation is defective and the client may not be aware of overheating
○ the client touches the lamp
○ the lamp falls and touches the client, or the bedding; overheating of pillows and blankets can cause fire and burns.

Damage to the eyes: infrared exposure of the eyes can cause cataracts. Place damp cotton wool pads over the client's eyes.

Electric shock may result from faulty apparatus or from water in the treatment area producing a short circuit.

Precautions should be taken to minimise the risk of harming the client and to ensure you give an effective treatment.

▽ **Table 11.5** Reasons for contra-indications to infrared treatment to the face

Contra-indication	Reason
Bruises (extensive)	May be further damaged by the treatment resulting from increased blood flow to the area. Bruises must be allowed to heal before treatment.
Claustrophobic or highly tense, nervous clients	This may not be the most appropriate treatment for the client as the face and neck will be covered with gauze. May cause discomfort and, in extreme cases, trigger a panic attack.
Cuts, abrasions and chapped skin	There is a risk of cross-infection. Avoid the area.
Defective skin sensation	The client must be able to feel the sensation of heat to be able to give accurate feedback about the intensity of the lamp as the skin could burn. Carry out a thermal sensitivity test.
Heavy colds or fever	Risk of cross-infection. May aggravate the condition. Do not treat.
Hypersensitive skin (vascular, florid, couperose skin, rosacea)	A client with hypersensitive skin must not receive treatments that stimulate the blood circulation as these will exacerbate the condition.
Headaches and migraines	The heat and the stimulation of the blood circulation will exacerbate the condition. The body needs time to heal before having treatment.
Scar tissue (recent)	Scar tissue must be allowed to heal completely before treatment is given to the area. If treatment is given before healing is complete, there is a danger of further damage to the tissues delaying the healing process. Also skin sensation will be defective in the area, so the client will not be able to give accurate feedback about the intensity of the heat.
Skin diseases	There is a risk of cross-infection.

▽ **Table 11.6** Precautions to take with infrared treatment to the face

Precaution	Explanation
Ensure that the lamp is in good working order and that there are no dents in the reflector.	Dents will cause 'hot spots' on the area, increasing the intensity of rays and so causing burns.
Ensure the flexes are sound and not trailing in a walking area.	To minimise risk of electric shock and to prevent anyone tripping over the flex.
Ensure that the angle-poise joints are tight and secure.	To minimise risk of the lamp collapsing onto the client.
Ensure that the head of the lamp is positioned over a foot if the lamp has three or five feet.	To ensure stability and prevent the lamp from falling.
Carry out a thermal sensitivity test (see page 71).	If the client cannot tell the difference between hot and cold, they have defective sensation and the treatment should not be carried out.
Do not place the lamp directly over the client.	It may fall and cause burns.
Ensure a safe distance of the lamp from the client.	The distance depends on the client's tolerance and the output of the lamp (18–36 inches, 45–90 cm). Refer to manufacturer's instructions for guidance.
Protect the eyes with damp cotton wool or protective eye-wear.	Infrared rays can damage the eyes.

Infrared treatment procedure – face

Preparation of working area

1. Switch on the lamp to warm up, making sure it is away from all surfaces and directed at the floor for safety.
   ↓
2. Check the couch is prepared with clean linen and towels.
   ↓
3. Prepare trolley with suitable products:
   - gauze
   - 2 bowls for warming the oil
   - tape measure
   - towel or protective gloves.
   ↓

Preparation of self

4. Before carrying out treatment ensure you prepare yourself physically and mentally, paying due attention to high standards of professionalism. Adopt a sensitive calm, confident and understanding attitude, as this approach will have a positive effect on your client.
   ↓

Preparation of client

5. Carry out a consultation, or if a regular client refer to the notes from their last treatment and discuss the effects and outcomes before proceeding.
   ↓
6. Check for contra-indications.
   ↓
7. Check contact lenses and all jewellery have been removed.
   ↓
8. Place the client in a well-supported and comfortable position.
   ↓
9. Protect hair and clothing.
   ↓
10. Explain the treatment to the client. The heat from the lamp will warm the oil on the gauze. This should feel comfortable and they should let you know if it becomes too intense.
    ↓

WASH YOUR HANDS

11. Carry out a thermal sensitivity test.
    ↓
12. Prepare sufficient gauze to cover the client's face and neck. Cut out holes for the nostrils and mouth.
    ↓
13. Warm the selected oil.
    ↓
14. Cleanse and tone the skin using suitable products.
    ↓
15. Carry out a skin analysis.
    ↓

Remember

Infrared lamps take 10–15 minutes to reach maximum output. Radiant heat lamps take around 2 minutes.

Best practice **B**

Fill the larger of two bowls with hot water. Pour sufficient oil in the small bowl, add the gauze and place this in the large bowl to heat through.

Technique for infrared – face

16. Protect the client's eyes with damp cotton wool pads or protective eye wear.

    ↓

17. Place the saturated gauze over the face and neck and move the client's head over to one side to face the lamp.

    ↓

18. Position the lamp ensuring stability.

    ↓

19. Measure an appropriate distance (between 45–90 cm/18–36 inches.) The selected distance depends on two factors:
    ○ the intensity of the lamp
    ○ the client's tolerance (60 cm / 24") is a good average, but check manufacturer's instructions.

    ↓

20. Make sure that the face of the lamp is parallel with the client's face and neck so that the rays strike the part at 90° for maximum penetration, absorption and effect. Do *not* place the lamp directly above the client.

    ↓

21. Observe the client throughout the treatment and be alert to contra-actions.

    ↓

22. Monitor the effect of the heat on the client's skin.

    ↓

23. At the end of the treatment turn off the lamp and place in a safe place to cool down.

    ↓

24. Remove the gauze and follow with a massage routine using the excess oil.

    ↓

25. Continue with the facial routine depending on client's needs.

    ↓

26. Update the consultation record with salient points about the treatment for future reference. This will include the outcome of the thermal sensitivity test.

Best practice **B**

Always dampen the cotton wool pads to prevent wisps of cotton wool irritating the eyes.

Be aware

Warn the client that damp cotton wool pads are placed over their eyes and gauze over the face and neck this is important if they are tense and apprehensive.

Be aware !

The head of the lamp will be hot. Use a towel or gloves to protect your hands when moving or adjusting the position of the lamp.

Be aware !

If the client finds the heat too intense turn down the lamp or move it further away from the client.

Be aware !

It is important to explain to the client that they must remain in this position for the duration of the treatment, so make sure that they are comfortable before commencing treatment. The client should also be instructed not to touch the lamp or move closer to it.

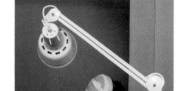
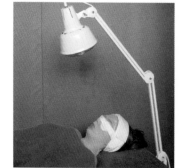

△ **Figure 11.9** Correct and incorrect positioning of lamp

Timing of treatment

Treatment time is 15–20 minutes (check manufacturer's instructions), until the desired effect is obtained.

Contra-actions

○ Headache: caused by over-heating or prolonged exposure. Advise the client to place a cool compress on their forehead and to drink plenty of water to hydrate the body.

○ Damage to the eyes: infrared exposure of the eyes can cause cataracts over a period of time. Always place damp cotton wool pads over the client's eyes.

Ultraviolet irradiation

Ultraviolet rays are part of the electromagnetic spectrum: with wavelengths of between 10 nm and 400 nm, they lie between the end of the visible spectrum and X-rays. Ultraviolet rays are divided into three bands according to their wavelength:

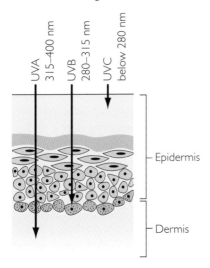

△ **Figure 11.10** Penetration of rays into the skin

○ UVA with the longest wavelength – 315–400 nm
○ UVB the middle band with wavelength – 280–315 nm
○ UVC the shortest wavelength – below 280 nm.

The wavelength determines the penetration and effects of the rays. The skin acts as a protective layer, which absorbs ultraviolet rays, preventing damage of deeper tissues.

Sources of ultraviolet radiation

○ **Natural sunlight** emits all ultraviolet rays. The intensity of UV reaching the earth's surface will vary with the time of year, the time of day, with altitude, latitude and variations in cloud cover and shade. The intensity of radiation will also increase with reflection from light surfaces, such as snow and rippling water. The destructive and harmful UVC rays are absorbed and screened out as they travel through the atmosphere; they do not reach the earth's surface. The effects of natural sunlight are therefore due to UVA and UVB.

> **Be aware**
> There is growing concern that the harmful UVC rays will reach the earth as the ozone layer is becoming thinner and holes are developing.

○ **Artificial sunlight** is produced by high- or low-pressure tubes and lamps. In hospital departments, sun lamps are used to treat a wide variety of medical conditions. These emit UVA, UVB and some UVC rays.

Sunbeds are used for tanning the body. All the harmful UVC rays and most, if not all, of the burning UVB rays are filtered out of sunbeds. However, there are dangers associated with their use and operators who use them should be aware of these.

▽ **Table 11.7** The effects of ultraviolet rays

Ultraviolet rays	Penetration	Function	Potential negative effects
UVA	Down to the capillary loops in the dermis	This causes superficial tanning as it causes the melanin to brown.	Can damage elastin and collagen fibres. May increase risk of skin cancer.
UVB	To the lower levels of the epidermis – the stratum basale	This causes darker, longer lasting tanning because it stimulates production of melanin.	Responsible for sunburn. Over-exposure will cause skin cancer.
UVC	The upper layer of the epidermis stratum corneum	UVC rays are abiotic, they destroy bacteria.	If these rays reach the skin surface, they will damage cells and cause skin cancer.

Sunbeds

These come in various forms:

- a single over-head canopy horizontal sunbed to irradiate one side of the body

- a double canopy horizontal sunbed to irradiate both sides simultaneously. Sunbeds are slightly curved to irradiate the sides of the body as well as front and back.

- vertical sunbeds are available for treatment in the standing position. The timing for vertical tanning treatment is usually greatly reduced because maintaining a standing position can be tiring.

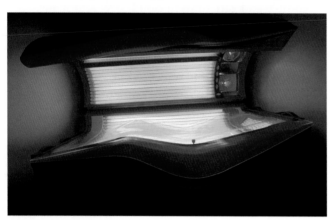

(a)

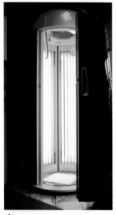

(b)

△ **Figure 11.11** Sunbeds (a) double canopy and (b) vertical

The construction of all sunbeds is similar but the emission intensities and percentages of UVA and UVB rays differ. Sunbeds are made up of a collection of fluorescent tubes closely packed together. These are sometimes referred to as lamps or bulbs. The tubes are around 120 cm in length and usually made of vita glass, which is coated on the inside with a phosphorus lining. This lining is designed to absorb UVC rays and most, if not all, UVB rays. The tubes contain argon gas and some mercury with electrodes sealed at either end.

When the current is switched on, the argon ionises and electrons flow through the tube. The mercury ionises and vaporises and UVL is emitted. The phosphorus coating absorbs unwanted harmful rays.

Learning point

Some sunbeds emit only UVA and tan slowly, while others emit mainly UVA (96–98 per cent) and a small amount of UVB (2–4 per cent). These sunbeds tan more quickly and the tan lasts longer.

Learning point

There are also high pressure tubes on the market that are made of quartz and contain mercury and metal halides. The tubes are filled at a higher pressure than regular ones. The significant difference is that these tubes emit harmful UVC radiation as well as UVA and UVB. The UVC has to be filtered out, as does much of the UVB. Filters are fitted to these sunbeds. It is vital to check the filters regularly for cracks, as they will be ineffective if damaged.

The tubes are packed together side by side. There may be reflectors behind the tubes or tubes may have inbuilt reflectors so that more rays are directed down onto the client rather than spreading over a wider area. This means that tubes can be closer together in the sunbed giving a higher intensity of radiation.

Learning point

Tubes that have a reflective coating painted onto them are referred to as RUVA tubes, where 'R' stands for 'reflective'.

The distance between the tubes and the client is fixed and the sunbeds are designed to produce a certain effect in a set time. The time of exposure will vary, depending on the sensitivity of the client.

Learning point

You should never assume that one sunbed is the same as another. Exposure times may be different and will depend on:

- the intensity of the radiation
- skin type.

Always refer to manufacturer's instructions.

Some features are common to all sunbeds:

○ an on/off switch
○ a timer control
○ an emergency button for quick release.

This should always be explained to the client and they should be able to reach the emergency button from the exposure position. In addition, some sunbeds have a fan to cool the body during treatment, a facial unit to boost facial tanning, ear phones and music.

Health and safety requirements related to sunbeds

The Sunbeds (Regulation) Act 2010 introduced in April 2011 states that children and young people under 18 years are not permitted to have sunbed treatments on commercial business premises.

> **Be aware**
>
> If a young person presents a signed consent form from their parent or guardian you must refuse them treatment.

The Act also requires you to provide clients with information about the health risks of using sunbeds and clients must use protective eye-wear when having treatment.

Best practice B

If a new client arrives for their sunbed treatment and you suspect they may not be 18 years old, ask for proof of age; for example, a student union card or driving licence, or the Proof of Age Standards Scheme (PASS) card.

Under the Health and Safety at Work Act 1974 and the Management of Health and Safety at Work Regulations you must carry out a risk assessment on the sunbed treatment to include exposure of ultraviolet radiation to staff, clients, maintenance operatives and identify the control measures that need to be implemented.

The following points should be applied to all sunbed treatments:

○ Instructions for use should be clearly written and displayed.

○ A sunbed should always be positioned in a well-ventilated room to prevent build-up of ozone, which is damaging to the respiratory system and also to dissipate the heat generated by the sunbed.

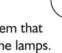

> **Learning point**
>
> Some sunbeds incorporate a cooling system that kicks in at the end of treatment to cool the lamps. The sunbed cannot be used until this process has finished.

○ The sunbed should be isolated in its own room or behind a full-length partition so that all rays are contained and cannot irradiate other clients.

○ The sunbed should be wiped over before and after treatment with a disinfecting detergent.

> **Be aware**
>
> Appropriate detergents supplied by the sunbed manufacturer must be used, as other detergents may:
>
> ○ damage or form a film on the acrylic surfaces
> ○ be toxic or inflammable
> ○ sensitise the skin of the client.

○ Sunbeds require little maintenance, but they should be regularly inspected for electrical and mechanical safety, and any faulty or exhausted tubes replaced immediately, with identical tubes supplied by the manufacturer. Servicing and repair should be carried out by a qualified electrician in accordance with information supplied by the manufacturer.

○ The running time of the sunbed must be recorded as the tubes wear out with use and the intensity is reduced.

> **Be aware** !
>
> Always check the manufacturer's instructions as the working life of tubes will vary from sunbed to sunbed. The intensity of the tubes can be reduced after between 400–800 hours.

○ Always replace tubes with the exact same model as the power of tubes will vary; they must be replaced by tubes of equal power and design in order to maintain radiation output.

> **Be aware**
>
> If you fit your sunbed with the incorrect tubes, it may be operating outside the standard specified by the manufacturer. This means that guidelines given for timings will not be correct. This could lead to damage to the client's skin.

○ A sunbed that has been re-tubed will emit ultraviolet radiation at a higher intensity. Check manufacturer's instructions about reducing session times and also ensure you clearly explain to the client the need for a reduction in exposure time.

Exposure to ultraviolet light

The effects of excessive exposure to UVL are much publicised. We are increasingly aware that too long spent in the sun, and especially allowing skin to burn, can lead to the development of skin cancers. Artificial UVL carries similar risks.

The effects of UV radiation on the skin will depend on the intensity of radiation and on the skin type. The Fitzpatrick Classification Scale is used to classify skin types and reaction to ultraviolet light. It takes into account:

○ your genetic disposition

○ how your skin reacts to the sun

○ how your skin tans.

Under this classification scale there are six skin types.

Learning point ⓛ

A dermatologist called Thomas Fitzpatrick MD, PhD of Harvard Medical School, developed The Fitzpatrick Classification Scale in 1975. It is a useful tool for dermatologists and other medical professionals to assess which cosmetic or medical procedure would benefit the client or patient.

Benefits of ultraviolet irradiation

○ **Tanning:** This is the most common use. It enhances appearance and gives a feeling of wellbeing.

○ **Tonic effect:** UVL is thought to have a general tonic effect, improving appetite and sleep while reducing irritability and nervousness. It is particularly beneficial for sufferers of Seasonal Affective Disorder (SAD), which is thought to be caused by a lack of sunlight.

▽ **Table 11.8** The Fitzpatrick Classification Scale

Skin type	Skin colour	Hair colour	Eye colour	Exposure to UV light
1	White, freckles, very sensitive	Red/blond	Blue, green	Always burns, never tans
2	White, moderately sensitive	Blond/fair	Blue, brown	Burns frequently, tans with difficulty
3	White, moderately insensitive	Light/dark brown	Blue, brown	Unlikely to burn, tans well
4	Olive, Mediterranean, southern Europe	Dark brown, black	Brown	Hardly burns, tans very easily
5	Brown, Middle Eastern descent. Wide variety of undertones	Dark brown, black	Brown	Rarely burns, tans quickly
6	Black, blue-black African. Wide variety of undertones	Black	Brown	Very rarely burns, tans quickly

Physiological effects of exposure to ultraviolet light

Erythema

Erythema reaction following ultraviolet irradiation differs from the erythema reaction following infrared irradiation in that it does not appear immediately. It takes 6–12 hours for the redness to appear, and occurs due to the irritation of cells of the epidermis.

> **Remember**
>
> Erythema reaction following infrared exposure occurs because the heat produces vasodilation. More blood flows to the area and the redness appears almost immediately.

The ultraviolet rays that reach the lower levels of the epidermis (i.e. UVA and UVB) damage and destroy some of the cells. This results in the chemical histamine being released in response to the injury. The histamine causes the blood vessels to dilate, bringing an increase in blood flow and thus producing an erythema.

Further irritation will cause greater dilation and the production of excess fluid flowing from the vessels into the tissue spaces forming blisters. Sensory nerves will be stimulated giving soreness and pain.

The greater the ultraviolet dose, the greater the irritation, therefore the more histamine will be released and the greater will be the erythema reaction. It takes some time for these processes to occur, hence the 6–12 hours before reaction appears.

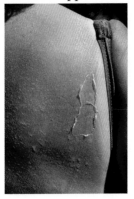

△ **Figure 11.12** Person with sunburn

There are four degrees of erythema:

- **First degree (E1):** slight reddening, no irritation, no pigmentation, fades in 24 hours, no desquamation. This is what you are aiming to achieve.
- **Second degree (E2):** deeper reddening, slight irritation, slight pigmentation, fades 2–3 days, powdery desquamation.
- **Third degree (E3):** skin is very red, hot, sore and oedematous, itchy, marked pigmentation, fades 7–10 days, sheets of skin lift off.
- **Fourth degree (E4):** similar to E3 but blisters form, may be necessary to receive hospital treatment.

Tanning

Tanning develops within two days of radiation. It is produced by the action of UVA and UVB on the melanocytes in the skin. Melanocytes are specialised cells found in the basal layer/stratum germinativum of the epidermis. These branching cells produce the pigment melanin and extend upwards to provide a protective cover over the living nucleated cells of the epidermis. As the pigmentation is built up, the penetration of the rays is reduced and destruction and damage of cells lessened. Melanin is formed by the action of UVA and UVB on the amino acid **tyrosine**. Two types of melanin are produced:

- **eumelanin,** which produces a dark brown or black colour
- **phaeomelanin,** which produces a yellowish to red colour.

Tanning of the skin is produced in two ways:

1. **Immediate tanning or quick tanning** This is produced by the UVA rays wavelength 400–315 nm. These rays stimulate and darken the melanin granules already in the skin. It requires long exposure to UVA and fades quickly within a few days. UVA will produce a tan in those individuals who tan easily (Skin type 3). Skin types 1 and 2 or areas without a previous tan may not tan.

2. **Delayed tanning** This requires a high dose of UVA, but is produced by a low dose of UVB. These rays stimulate the melanocytes to produce new dark melanin granules. Once started, this process will continue and will produce a longer-lasting tan.

The tanning response to ultraviolet depends on the skin type.

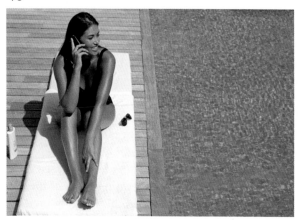

△ Figure 11.13 A tanned body

Sensitive skins burn easily but tan very slowly; some very sensitive skins will not tan at all.

○ Skin type 1 should avoid using sunbeds.

○ Skin type 2 should keep to very low exposure times. Refer to manufacturers' instructions for specific guidance. If there is any sign of burning, further exposure should be avoided until the erythema has completely died down.

○ Skin types 3 and 4 burn less easily and tan more quickly. They can take a longer exposure time without burning.

○ Skin types 5 and 6 tan quickly and rarely burn and can take longer exposure times.

Thickening of the epidermis

The UVB radiation penetrates down to the stratum basale or stratum germinativum. The irritation caused to these cells produces over-activity and increased mitosis. These rapidly multiplying cells push upwards and form a marked thickening of the stratum corneum. This may become three times its normal thickness. This acts as a protection to reduce ultraviolet penetration.

Skin peeling (desquamation)

The normal process of desquamation is accelerated due to an increase in mitotic activity of the stratum basale and migration of cells to the surface. The amount of peeling depends on the intensity of exposure and the erythema reaction.

○ **First-degree erythema**, peeling hardly noticeable.

○ **Second-degree erythema**, fine powdery flaking.

○ **Third- and fourth-degree erythema**, marked peeling with large flakes or sheets.

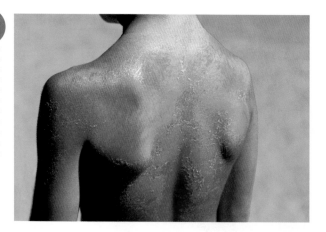

△ Figure 11.14 Sunburn with excessive peeling

Production of vitamin D

Ultraviolet radiation of the skin causes a chemical reaction which converts 7-dehydro-cholesterol found in sebum into cholecalciferol, namely, vitamin D^3.

Vitamin D is necessary for the absorption of calcium and phosphorus, which play a part in the formation and growth of teeth and bones.

Learning point

Lack of vitamin D causes rickets. There has been a recent increase in cases of rickets among children, thought to result from the tendency of parents to over-protect their children from the sun by using high factor sun-screens.

Calcium is also an important factor in the blood clotting mechanism. This production of vitamin D is an important beneficial effect of ultraviolet light on the skin.

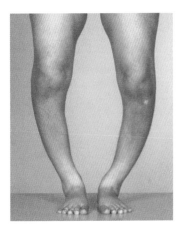

△ **Figure 11.15** Rickets

General tonic effect

General ultraviolet irradiation has a tonic effect on the body. Appetite and sleep are improved; irritability and nervousness may be reduced.

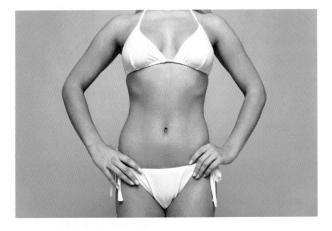

△ **Figure 11.16** Tanned body

Remember

Abiotic effect: The rays of short wavelength (UVC rays) are abiotic rays as they destroy bacteria and micro-organisms.

Damaging effects of ultraviolet light exposure

Carcinogenic effect

This is the most serious effect of UVL exposure of the skin. The ultraviolet rays penetrating the skin affect the DNA in the nucleus of the cells. This interferes with the replication of the cells predisposing to skin cancer. Fair or pale-skinned individuals who burn easily and tan rarely (Skin types 1 and 2) are especially vulnerable, as are those with multiple moles or with previous history of severe sunburn. Long exposures to natural sunlight and prolonged frequent use of sunbeds should be avoided.

There are three main types of skin cancer:

○ Basal cell carcinoma

This type of cancer originates in the epidermis. It is usually found on the head and neck where the skin has been exposed to sunlight or other forms of ultraviolet radiation, for example tanning equipment. It may appear as a skin growth or a raised area that looks pearly or waxy; flesh coloured or brown; or a sore that never seems to heal. It can invade the surrounding area but does not usually spread to other parts of the body (metastasise). Advise client to seek medical advice.

○ Squamous cell carcinoma

This type of cancer originates in the epidermis and can spread to other parts of the body (metastasise). It is a relatively slow growing cancer that is found on the skin exposed to sunlight or other forms of ultraviolet radiation, for example tanning equipment. The cancer appears as a growing lump with a rough scaly surface and reddish patches that can develop into sores that do not heal. Changes in an existing mole or wart may manifest itself into a squamous cell carcinoma. Advise client to seek medical advice.

○ Malignant melanoma

This is a malignant tumour of melanocytes, the cells found in the basal layer of the skin that produce the pigment melanin. Symptoms to note are any moles growing bigger, changing colour, becoming more irregular, have a combination of different shades of brown to black, itching or bleeding. This type of cancer can metastasise. Seek medical advice. Malignant melanoma is the most dangerous and difficult to control so early medical advice is very important.

There is indisputable evidence to link exposure to natural and artificial UVL (i.e. UVA and UVB) with skin degeneration and skin cancer. It was thought that only UVB rays were responsible, but there is now evidence to suggest that UVA contributes to and may even initiate the development of skin cancer.

Premature ageing

The skin becomes dry, coarse, leathery and wrinkled. When ultraviolet rays penetrate the skin they damage cells.

UVB will damage cells down to the basal layer, as this is the limit of their penetration. UVA rays penetrate into the dermis and damage dermal cells and fibres (i.e. the elastin and collagen fibres).

Remember
Elastin gives skin its elasticity and collagen gives skin its firmness, strength and resilience.

This produces loss of elasticity and wrinkling of the skin. Damage of cells will eventually produce thinning and dryness of the skin. Increased over-activity of some melanocytes will produce freckling and liver spots, while absence of melanocytes in other areas will leave white, unpigmented patches. All these factors contribute to premature ageing of the skin.

Damaging effect on the eyes

The tough outer coating of the eye called the cornea and the lens of the eye can be adversely affected by radiation. UVB and UVC rays are absorbed by the cornea and do not penetrate further. High intensity exposure to these shorter wavelengths may induce keratitis (inflammation of the cornea) and conjunctivitis (inflammation of the conjunctiva). Both these conditions are extremely irritating and painful.

The long UVA rays penetrate further and are absorbed by the lens; overexposure can cause opaqueness of the lens known as cataract.

Certain rays may penetrate down to the retina and may be a contributing causal factor for macular degeneration which may result in partial blindness in later life.

Remember
Suitable protective eye-wear should always be worn in both natural and artificial UVL.

Polymorphic light eruption

Certain individuals react adversely to ultraviolet exposure and develop skin eruptions. The reaction occurs a few hours after exposure. There is reddening of the skin and the development of hard, itchy papules and scaling. The reaction will clear in 2–6 days, providing the skin is not exposed to further radiation.

Photosensitisation

Certain drugs and cosmetics will produce photosensitisation in individuals who expose themselves to the sun. A painful itchy rash develops which may be followed by pronounced permanent pigmentation. A list of these drugs appears on page 266.

Damage to the immune system

Ultraviolet radiation reduces the effectiveness of the immune system. Disturbances and reduction in the number of certain lymphocytes occur as a result of exposure to ultraviolet radiation (including UVA sunbeds).

Remember
Lymphocytes are white blood cells involved in immunity.

These changes, both cutaneous and systemic, diminish the response of the immune system to infections.

Aggravation of certain skin conditions

This occurs as a result of UV exposure e.g. eczema and systemic lupus erythematosus are exacerbated.

Awareness of effects of over-exposure to UVL

Sunburn is an injury to the skin causing erythema, tenderness and blistering. The most serious effect of over exposure of the skin to UVL is the development of skin cancer, the most dangerous being *malignant melanoma*. Deaths from these cancers are rising every year but it is hoped that by raising public awareness of the effect of sunlight the numbers will decline. See page 263 for more information about skin cancer.

Various UK organisations such as Cancer Research UK, BUPA, BMA among others, uphold the following information relating to ultraviolet radiation:

Visible sunburn must be avoided by individuals of all ages. There is increasing evidence that excessive sun exposure and particularly sunburn when aged under 15 is a major risk factor for skin cancer in later life. The melanocytes in children do not produce sufficient melanin to protect the skin. Protection of the skin of children and adolescents is therefore particularly important.

Learning point (L)

Evidence suggests that before we reach adulthood we have had a third of our total lifetime exposure to ultraviolet rays.

○ It is important to realise the cumulative nature of sun-induced damage, particularly for those who have lived abroad in sunny climates.

○ Sun exposure giving rise to sunburn and skin damage can occur in the UK in spring and summer, therefore protection is particularly important during this time.

○ Individuals who develop skin cancer do not always have a history of sunbathing. Those who have an outdoor occupation or recreational pursuits are also at risk and must protect their skin.

Be aware (!)

There is no such thing as a safe or healthy tan. A tan is a sign that already damaged skin is trying to protect itself from further damage. The protecting power of a tan is weaker than that of a mild sunscreen with an SPF of 2–4.

○ Four out of five cases of skin cancer are considered preventable.

The growing awareness of the dangers of UVL means that manufacturers of sunbeds and salons offering sunbed treatments are very carefully monitored. Awarding bodies include UVL in the electrotherapy unit, so that you are properly prepared to offer such treatments. The dangers have to be balanced against the positive effects. A tan is considered desirable by many, giving a feeling of health and wellbeing. There is some evidence that people who have insufficient exposure to the UVL light of the sun may suffer a lack of vitamin D, leading to conditions associated with a deficiency of that vitamin.

Remember

If the client's skin is not suitable or they have a contra-indication that prevents treatment discuss other options, for example spray tanning.

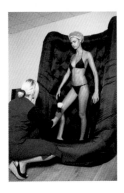

△ **Figure 11.17** Spray tan (Photo courtesy of Fake Bake)

The decision to use a sunbed remains a matter of personal choice but everyone should be made aware of the risks.

Sunbed treatment

Guidelines for the use of sunbeds

The Sunbed Association has issued guidelines for those who operate sunbeds:

○ Clients should leave 24–48 hours between treatments to allow the skin to settle down as the erythema reaction takes 6–12 hours to appear, see page 261 for more information.

○ The number of sessions per week will depend on the client's skin type, their reaction to ultraviolet light and the output of the sunbed.

Learning point (L)

The European Standard recommends the number of sessions per year should not exceed 60 sessions.

Be aware

You can monitor the number of sessions a client has had in your place of work but they may also be having sessions somewhere else too. In this situation you should emphasise to the client the potential consequences of not following these guidelines.

Contra-indications to sunbed treatments

Learning point

Check the contra-indications listed in the manufacturer's instructions to ensure you do not invalidate your insurance policy should the client be injured during or after treatment.

Remember

Vitiligo is recognised by white patches of skin on the body. The melanocytes that produce the pigment melanin are destroyed. It is thought that vitiligo is an autoimmune disease where the body's immune system attacks the melanocytes in the skin.

Chloasma is characterised by dark patches of skin on the upper cheeks, forehead and around the lips. It is associated with hormonal changes in women who are pregnant, taking contraceptives or on hormone replacement therapy (HRT). The pigmentation usually fades when hormone levels return to normal.

▽ **Table 11.9** Reasons for contra-indications to sunbed treatments

Contra-indication	Reason
Clients who burn easily	If they burn easily in sunlight they will experience the same effect with sunbed treatments (Skin type 1).
Clients who do not tan easily in the sun	As these individuals have no protection, there is an increased risk of skin damage (Skin types 1 and 2). They will not tan easily on a sunbed either.
Colds, fever and high temperature	Treatment will aggravate these conditions and there is also a risk of cross-infection.
Cold sores (herpes simplex)	Treatment diminishes the response of the immune system to infection.
Diabetes	The heat from the sunbed can affect blood glucose levels if the client is taking insulin or sulphonylureas. Thinner skin is more vulnerable to damage. Poor circulation may lead to overheating of the body.
Headache, migraine, faintness	Treatment will cause the client further discomfort.
Heart and blood pressure disorders	The increase in blood circulation may put too much pressure and stress on the heart.
Long-term immuno-suppression drugs	These drugs lower the client's resistance to infection. Sunbed treatments also reduce the effectiveness of the immune system.
Medication, including antibiotics, birth control pills, blood pressure drugs, diuretics, gold injections, insulin, quinine, steroids, thyroid extract and tranquillizers	Medication may produce photosensitisation. There may be other sensitising drugs; always seek a doctor's advice if clients are taking any medication. Some drugs affect the production of melanin leading to pigmentation conditions.
Multiple moles or those with a mole showing changes in size, pigmentation or inflammation, or anyone with a previous history of skin cancer	There is an increased risk of melanoma developing.
Pregnancy	Ultraviolet exposure may result in uneven pigmentation called chloasma.
Scars, recent or wounds	The ultraviolet rays can change the collagen and elastin structure, causing the skin to become thicker and firmer.

(Continued)

(Continued)

Contra-indication	Reason
Skin disorders	Chloasma – the pigmented areas of skin will deepen in colour. Dermatitis/Eczema – condition will be exacerbated. Vitiligo – the skin will burn as there is no melanin to protect it.
Steroids	Used to treat eczema and dermatitis they suppress inflammation in the skin, whereas ultraviolet rays increase inflammation in the skin by releasing histamine in the tissues. The treatment will aggravate these conditions, causing the skin to become red and itchy.
Sunburn	Treatment will make the condition worse. Exposure to ultraviolet rays should not be repeated until the erythema has faded as sensitivity is increased.
Undergoing or having been recently treated with deep X-ray therapy	There is a danger of over-exposure to radiation.
Certain treatments should not be carried out in conjunction with ultraviolet treatment: epilation, waxing, laser and IPL, micro-dermabrasion, recent chemical peels, certain anti-ageing products	Ultraviolet causes increased sensitivity of the skin. The erythema from a sunbed treatment is a chemical process that takes 6–12 hours to appear. Carrying out other treatments before or after a sunbed session will produce even more sensitivity in the tissues, causing client discomfort.

Factors that determine the intensity of the reaction

The erythema reaction of a client will depend on many factors.

The sensitivity of the client

The reaction of different clients to ultraviolet varies considerably, as shown in the list of skin types (see page 260). The sensitivity of the skin also varies on different parts of the body. Exposed surfaces are less sensitive than those that are normally covered by clothing. The extensor aspects are generally less sensitive than the flexor aspects. When using sunbeds, the manufacturer's instructions should be carefully followed. First doses should be reduced for sensitive clients.

The output of the sunbed

Sunbeds are designed to produce a required reaction at a set distance in a certain time. Tubes should be replaced regularly and if damaged, in order to maintain the same output.

Learning point

The higher the output of the sunbed, the greater the reaction in a set time. Always set the times according to the manufacturer's instruction.

The duration of exposure

The duration of exposure will have an effect on the reaction. The longer the time, the greater the reaction.

Previous exposure of the area

An exposure should not be repeated until the previous erythema has faded, as until this occurs sensitivity is increased.

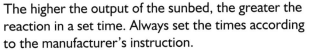

Remember

Infrared irradiation applied before exposure to ultraviolet radiation increases the erythema reaction. Infrared applied after ultraviolet reduces the effects. Simultaneous irradiation with both types of ray does not affect the reaction.

Dangers of ultraviolet irradiation

The main risk of harm with sunbed treatments are:

○ damage to the eyes if protective eye-wear is not worn

○ skin damage, potentially leading to skin cancer.

Precautions should be taken to minimise the risk of harming the client and to ensure an effective treatment.

▽ **Table 11.10** Precautions to take with ultraviolet irradiation

Precaution	Explanation
Ensure the area is well ventilated.	To prevent the build-up of ozone and to dissipate the heat generated by the sunbed.
Clean the sunbed before and after treatment with a cleaning product recommended by manufacturer.	To prevent the risk of cross-infection. Other detergents may damage or form a film on the acrylic surfaces, they may be toxic, inflammable or could possibly sensitise the skin of the client.
Place disposable paper on the floor for each client and provide disposable foot soles.	To prevent the risk of cross-infection if client has an infectious foot condition, for example athlete's foot, verrucae.
Remove skin make-up.	This may produce photosensitisation.
Shower before treatment using non-perfumed soap to remove perfume, cologne, lotions and ointments.	To prevent UV rays reacting with the products and causing pre-sensitisation of the tissues.
Warn the client not to apply any suntan oils or lotions (unless recommended by the manufacturer).	May cause pre-sensitisation.
Cover coloured and bleached hair.	UVL will lighten and dry the hair.
If the client has irritation, rash or intense erythema after previous treatment. Do not give further treatment until all reactions have subsided.	Tissues will be very sensitive and more prone to damage if they have not fully recovered.
Provide disposable protective eye-wear for each client or clients keep their own.	To prevent damage to the eyes. To eliminate the risk of cross-infection.
Shower after treatment using non-perfumed soap.	To remove excess sweat and sebum.

B
Best practice
Provide suitable skin cleansing products, cotton wool and tissues for the client.

Be aware !
Some clients provide their own protective eye-wear purchased from a previous provider, in which case you must check they are suitable prior to treatment.

Sunbed procedure

Preparation of working area

1. Ensure the area is well ventilated.
   ↓
2. Check the sunbed is in good working order.
   ↓
3. Clean the sunbed with a disinfecting detergent.
   ↓
4. Place disposable paper on the floor.
   ↓
5. Provide disposable eye protection, foot soles and a clean towel for each client.
   ↓

Preparation of client

6. Carry out a consultation, or if a regular client refer to the notes from their last treatment and discuss the effects and outcomes before proceeding.
   ↓
7. Check for contra-indications.
   ↓
8. Check contact lenses and all jewellery have been removed.
   ↓
9. Instruct the client to remove make up and shower before.
   ↓
10. Protect hair if coloured or bleached.
    ↓

Technique for sunbed

11. Explain the procedure: show them how to operate the sunbed, point out the emergency button and emphasise the importance of wearing eye protection.
    ↓
12. At the end of the treatment, advise the client to get up slowly, shower and apply un-perfumed moisturiser to their face and body.
    ↓
13. Discuss the outcome of the treatment, reminding the client of the expected time erythema and tan will take to appear and gain feedback from the client.
    ↓
14. Keep a careful record of: date of treatment, timing and reaction.

Be aware
Some clients have white patches of skin on the shoulder blades, elbows and just above the buttocks. These occur because of the pressure of the body on the hard surface of the sunbed which restricts the flow of blood and oxygen required for the tanning process.

Be aware !
Wear eye protection if you have to switch on the sunbed.

Be aware !
Always wear disposable gloves when using hazardous substances.

Best practice B
Suggest the client does not apply body lotion on the day they have booked a treatment as the product may still be on the skin even after washing. This could cause photosensitivity.

Remember
Ensure the client knows they cannot apply suntan lotion unless it is a pre-tan product recommended by the manufacturer. Such products accelerate the tanning process and help to moisturise the skin.

Be aware !
There should be a procedure in place to deal with the activation of emergency alarms in the workplace.

Be aware !
Do not allow clients to leave after treatment without checking they are happy with the treatment and did not experience any contra-actions.

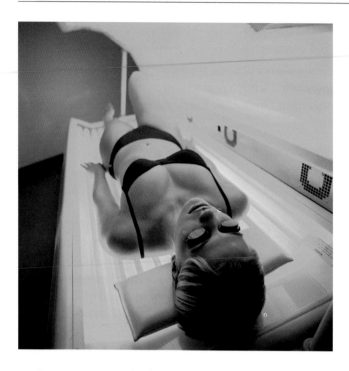

△ **Figure 11.18** Sunbed treatment

Timing of treatment

This depends on the client's skin type, reaction of the skin to treatment and output of the sunbed. Refer to manufacturer's guidance

Contra-actions to ultraviolet irradiation

○ Skin irritation: caused by over-exposure to ultraviolet rays. This may be accompanied by reddening of the skin and powdery desquamation. Advise the client to use a cooling, soothing product on the skin, avoid sunbathing and wear loose clothing. No treatment until the skin has settled down.

○ Erythema: 6–12 hours after a sunbed treatment the outcome should be 'first-degree erythema (E1)'. This results in a slight reddening with no irritation, no pigmentation, no desquamation and which fades in 24 hours. If it is more substantial the dosage has been too high or the duration too long. Recommend the client seeks medical advice.

○ Burning and blistering: caused by over-exposure to ultraviolet rays. Dosage has been too high or the duration too long. Recommend the client consults their GP.

○ Uneven pigmentation: caused by certain drugs, cosmetic products or hormonal changes. Question the client to find out what is causing the problem and advise accordingly.

○ Fainting: caused by a temporary reduction of blood to the brain. Could result from low blood pressure; getting off the sunbed too quickly; standing for a period of time in a vertical unit; disorientation moving from ultraviolet light to natural light; poor ventilation in the vicinity. Lie the client down and raise their legs to improve the blood flow to the brain. Make sure there is a flow of fresh air and give the client time to recover.

○ Nausea: could be caused by the body getting too hot, lack of food prior to treatment, poor ventilation in the vicinity. Advise the client to drink plenty of fluid and to rest.

○ Prickly heat: itchy red rash with tiny spots and bumps caused by excess sweating. Advise the client to use an anti-bacterial wash to cleanse the area, apply a soothing lotion; avoid tight clothing. The condition should improve in a few days. No further treatment until the condition has cleared.

○ Urticaria (hives): pale red, raised bumpy weals form on the skin caused by the release of histamine in the tissues. Advise the client to apply a soothing lotion and avoid tight clothing. The condition should improve within an hour or two. No further treatment until the condition has cleared.

Eye disorders (see page 264): caused by not wearing eye protection when exposed to UVA and UVB rays. Short-term effects include inflammation, for example conjunctivitis; long-term effects include cataracts. Advise the client to consult their GP.

Photo ageing: caused by over-exposure to UVA rays, which penetrate into the dermis and damage collagen and elastin fibres. Explain to the client how treatments contribute to premature ageing. Advise the client to consider alternative methods of skin tanning. Recommend suitable retail products for the skin.

Skin cancer: unusual looking moles, lumps or sores that do not heal, caused by damage to DNA in the skin: Advise client to consult their GP.

Homecare advice for sunbed treatments

- Use a moisturiser to lubricate the skin and keep it soft and hydrated. Ideally purchase a product that has been specifically developed for sunbeds.
- Use a moisturiser for the face and neck that contains at least SPF15.
- Protect the lips with a lip balm that blocks ultraviolet rays.
- Apply SPF suntan product when sunbathing as the tan acquired from using the sunbed will not protect the skin from the burning rays of the sun. Make sure the sunscreen has UVA and UVB filters.

Learning point (L)

Suntan products protect the skin by absorbing and/or reflecting ultraviolet rays. The sun protection factor (SPF) of a suntan product is the amount of protection it can provide. An SPF of 15 will allow the person to stay in the sun for 15 times longer than they would normally take to burn. For example, if a person would normally start to burn after 10 minutes in the sun, they could stay in the sun for 15 x 10 minutes (= 150 minutes) if they used a product with an SPF of 15.

- Do not have another sunbed treatment or sunbathe for 24–48 hours to allow the erythema to fade and give the skin time to settle.
- Exfoliate the skin regularly to remove dead skin cells and prevent a thickening of the epidermis.
- Clients with fair or red hair, blue eyes and sensitive, pale skin who tan rarely and burn easily should take particular care. They should always avoid exposure to strong sunlight.
- Prolonged exposure to sunlight, whether occupational or recreational, should be avoided.
- Infrequent, short bursts of intensive exposure must be avoided.

- Avoid exposure between 11 a.m. and 4 p.m., when the sun is at its highest. Begin with a short exposure of 10 minutes on the first day and increase gradually each day.

Learning point (L)

Avoid going out in direct sunlight when your shadow is shorter than you are.

- Avoid sunbathing if taking medication.
- Remember that UV rays will pass through light cloud; it is, therefore, possible to burn on a cloudy day or on a sunny, windy day although it may feel cool. Keep up the protection.
- Use every form of sun protection:
  - Sunscreen should be applied before exposure and renewed every two hours and after swimming.
  - Cover up with a long-sleeved shirt and a hat.
  - Find some shade under trees or some shelter.
  - Wear polarising sunglasses. Curved sunglasses that protect the sides as well as the front are best.

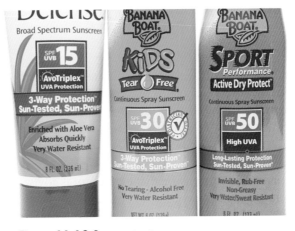

△ **Figure 11.19** Sun protection

Cleaning of the sunbed area

Disposable eye protection, foot soles and paper towels are classed as clinical waste and should be placed in a yellow refuse sack.

Wipe over the surfaces of the sunbed with an appropriate disinfectant product recommended by the manufacturer.

Local council regulations

Any business offering sunbed treatments must also adhere to the local authority regulations.

Construction of equipment

The collapse of any ultraviolet tanning equipment may give rise to electric shock, fire, or direct physical injury. Equipment should therefore be of adequate mechanical strength and rigidity.

Layout

○ To facilitate rapid entrance or exit from a cubicle/room containing the equipment, any door should be fitted so that its opening cannot be impeded and must be capable of being opened from the outside. Equipment must be designed for easy release by the client.

○ Ensure adequate ventilation is provided to prevent a build-up of ozone and to ensure that heat generated by the sunbed is adequately dissipated.

○ If the ultraviolet tanning equipment is not in individual cubicles, then suitable screens or curtains should be provided to prevent unnecessary UV exposure to other persons.

Washing facilities

Showering/washing facilities should be provided for hygiene reasons.

Cleaning the sunbed

Sunbeds should only be cleaned with the appropriate cleaning agents. Other agents may damage or form a film on the acrylic surface; they may be toxic or inflammable or could sensitise the skin of the client.

Exposure

The operator should ensure that each client is advised of a suitable exposure regime for sunbed treatment, taking into account skin type, previous exposures and enhanced sensitivity. A good quality, reliable, automatic time switch should be carefully pre-set to terminate the exposure.

Protective eye wear

Excessive exposure of the eyes to infrared or ultraviolet rays will result in eye damage. Provide appropriate disposable eye protection or ensure that clients keep their own, to eliminate the risk of cross-infection.

Maintenance

Records should be kept by the operator of all servicing and these should be available on the premises. Servicing and repair must be carried out by a qualified electrician in accordance with manufacturer's instructions. Faulty equipment must not be used. All parts must be replaced by the exact same model.

Staff training

The operator should ensure that properly trained staff are available to provide adequate advice, supervision and assistance to clients.

Information for clients

Clients should be made aware of the dangers, contra-indications and contra-actions associated with sunbed treatments. A poster should be displayed or leaflets available containing the necessary information.

The following is an example of printed material for clients.

Izzy B for Beauty

Tanning advice and guidance

Information for clients

Exposure to ultraviolet rays from natural sunlight or from sunbeds is damaging to the body and in particular to the skin.

Remember: There is no such thing as a safe and healthy tan. A tan is a sign that there is already damage to the skin.

Short-term effects

- **Sunburn:** skin that is red, sore, itchy and flaking
- **Eye problems:** inflammation and irritation caused from not wearing eye protection

Long-term risks

- **Premature ageing:** UV rays damage the internal structure of the skin causing lines, loss of plumpness and elasticity
- **Skin cancer:** UV rays damage DNA in the skin
- **Eye disorders:** for example cataracts from not wearing eye protection

Be aware

You should never use sunbeds if you:

- are under 18 years
- burn easily
- do not tan or tan poorly
- are using medication or cosmetics that cause photosensitivity
- suffer from skin disorders aggravated by sunlight
- or anyone in your family have a history of skin cancer
- are at risk of cutaneous melanoma (e.g. you have multiple moles, or have suffered severe sunburn in the past).

Tanning advice

To ensure you safely achieve a healthy looking tan that will last for as long as possible, follow these tips:

Preparation

- Avoid applying body lotion/cream on the day of your appointment: it may leave a residue on the skin even after washing and cause an adverse reaction.
- Remove skin make-up as it can increase the sensitivity of UV rays. A range of products, cotton wool and tissues have been provided.
- Shower to remove any ointment, body lotion/cream, perfume and deodorant: these will increase the sensitivity of UV rays.
- Protect hair if coloured or bleached: UV rays can dry and lighten the hair.
- Do not use a general sunscreen product: this will prevent the UV rays penetrating the skin.
- Use a pre-tan accelerator lotion that is specifically designed for use with this tanning equipment. This product will help to develop a tan more quickly.

Treatment

Always wear the disposable eye protection provided. **UV rays can cause serious damage to your eyes**.

Ensure you know how to switch the equipment on and off and where to locate the emergency button.

After treatment

Shower to remove excess sweat to prevent fungi and bacterial conditions developing.

Use a moisturiser to lubricate, soothe and hydrate the skin.

Homecare advice

Moisturise regularly to keep the skin soft and supple and prolong the life of the tan.

Use a sunscreen when sunbathing as the tan you have developed will not protect your skin from the sun.

Regularly check your skin for any changes, for example in the appearance of moles, open sores that do not seem to heal or any lumps that have developed recently. Consult with your GP if you have any worries.

Over the next 24 hours, *do not*:

- have another sunbed session
- sunbathe
- have any other electrical or heat treatment as the skin needs to settle and allow time for the redness to fade.

SUMMARY

The electromagnetic spectrum is made up of bands of different wavelengths and frequencies. Infrared radiation and ultraviolet radiation are part of the spectrum; they lie on either side of visible light.

- Infrared rays are used to heat body tissues.
- Ultraviolet rays are used to tan the skin.

Infrared radiation

Infrared rays are given off by the sun and by any hot object, for example electric, gas or coal fires and various types of lamps.

There are two types of lamps used in beauty therapy:

- Infrared lamp (non luminous or invisible); longer wavelength; penetrates 1 mm of skin
- Radiant heat lamp (luminous); shorter wavelength; penetrates 3 mm of skin.

The amount of rays absorbed by the body depends on:

- wavelength and frequency of rays
- type of medium (body tissues)
- angle at which the rays strike the area to be treated.

The intensity of radiation depends on:

- intensity of the lamp
- angle at which the rays strike the area to be treated
- distance between the lamp and the skin (the law of inverse square).

The law of inverse square refers to the fact that the further the lamp is from the skin, the less intense the rays.

The rays should strike the part of the body being treated at an angle of 90° for maximum intensity, absorption and effect.

Ultraviolet radiation

Ultraviolet rays are used for tanning the body. The rays are divided into three bands according to their wavelength:

- **UVA** – the longest wavelength, penetrates down to the dermis. Damages elastin and collagen, causes premature ageing and can cause cancer. Quick tanning, quick fading.

- **UVB** – middle wavelength, penetrates to stratum basale. UVB are referred to as the burning rays. Causes sunburn and cancer. Slow tanning, longer lasting.
- **UVC** – shortest wavelength, penetrates the stratum corneum. Cell damage and cancer. Abiotic rays destroy micro-organisms.

Emission of ultraviolet rays from natural sunlight include all three, but all the UVC and some UVB are filtered out in the atmosphere and do not reach the earth's surface.

Sunbeds

- These produce artificial UVL by tubes, which emit mainly UVA and may also emit very small amounts of UVB.
- Sunbeds come in various forms:
  - single over-head canopy, horizontal sunbed to irradiate one side of the body
  - double canopy, horizontal sunbed to irradiate both sides of the body simultaneously
  - vertical sunbed for treatment in the standing position.

Construction

Collection of fluorescent tubes:

- Tubes are usually made of vita glass, coated on the inside with phosphorus to absorb UVC and most of UVB rays.
- The tubes contain argon gas and some mercury and emit UVL when a current is passed through them.
- High-pressure tubes also available made of quartz and contain mercury and metal halides. These emit UVA, UVB and UVC. Filters are installed to filter out UVC and most of the UVB rays.
- Reflectors behind or inbuilt into the tubes direct the rays down onto the client as opposed to covering a wider area.

Exposure

Exposure times will depend on the:

- intensity of the radiation
- skin type.

Always refer to manufacturer's instructions as sunbeds will differ in design.

Fitzpatrick Classification Scale is used to determine skin type and reaction to ultraviolet light.

It takes into account:

- genetic disposition
- how the skin reacts to the sun
- how the skin tans.

Advise clients to leave 24–48 hours between treatments.

The number of sessions per year should not exceed 60.

QUESTIONS

Oral questions

Infrared and radiant heat treatments to face and body

1. When would you recommend an infrared/radiant heat treatment?
2. Explain the difference between infrared lamps and radiant heat lamps.
3. Explain what happens in the tissues when the body is heated.
4. What are the dangers associated with infrared treatment?
5. Why must a thermal sensitivity test be carried out prior to treatment?
6. What factors determine where you position the lamp?
7. What is a good average distance to start from?
8. Which law governs the intensity in relation to the angle of the rays?
9. Which law governs intensity in relation to the distance of the lamp?
10. What advice would you give if your client complained of a headache after treatment?
11. Why must infrared never be followed by ultraviolet treatment?
12. What advice would you give the client after treatment?

Ultraviolet treatment

1. How many bands are there in the ultraviolet part of the electromagnetic spectrum?
2. Which rays emitted from sunbeds are used for cosmetic purposes?
3. Which rays are abiotic rays?
4. Why is ultraviolet light used in the salon?
5. What degree of erythema should be the outcome of the treatment? How would you describe it to the client?
6. Why and how does the skin tan when exposed to ultraviolet rays?
7. How does exposure to ultraviolet light increase the production of vitamin D?
8. Why is vitamin D production an important beneficial effect of ultraviolet exposure?
9. What are the damaging effects of ultraviolet light that give cause for great concern?
10. What action would you take if you established that the client was taking drugs (medication or recreational) and requested sunbed treatment?
11. How would you advise a pregnant client who requested ultraviolet treatment?
12. A new client wants to apply their own suntan lotion prior to treatment. What should you do?
13. Why is it important that the client removes all lotions and perfume prior to treatment?
14. How long must a client wait before having another sunbed treatment?
15. Why is it important to use the cleaning product recommended by the manufacturer?

Multiple-choice questions

1. Which of the following rays has the longest wavelength?
   a Ultraviolet.
   b Radio.
   c Infra-red.
   d Visible.

2. A radiant heat lamp differs from an infra-red lamp as it:
   a has a shorter wavelength
   b is less irritating to the tissues
   c penetrates approximately 1mm of skin
   d emits rays from wire encased in clay.

3. To ensure an effective infra-red treatment the rays must strike the part at:
   a 45°.
   b 60°.
   c 90°.
   d 120°.

4. The distance between the lamp and the skin is governed by:
   a refraction
   b the law of inverse squares
   c reflection
   d the law of Grotthus.

5. If there are a couple of dents in the reflector of a radiant heat lamp, what should you do?
   a Continue with treatment as the client has specifically requested it.
   b Reduce the timing and spend longer on the massage.
   c Decrease the intensity of the lamp but increase the time.
   d Offer the client a suitable alternative treatment.

6. UVB rays penetrate to the:
   a stratum basale
   b upper layer of the dermis
   c stratum corneum
   d reticular layer of the dermis.

7. Fluorescent tubes in sunbeds contain a phosphorus coating to:
   a produce heat
   b intensify the output of the rays
   c prolong the life of the tubes
   d absorb harmful rays.

8. Exposure times for sunbed treatments will depend on:
   a the age of the client
   b the density of the tissues
   c the intensity of the radiation
   d gender, the skin of male clients is tougher.

9. If a new client arrives for a sunbed treatment and you suspect they are under age, what should you do?
   a Carry on with the treatment just this one time.
   b Tell the client they need to be accompanied by an adult.
   c Give advice on other treatments that may interest the client.
   d Give the client a consent form that must be signed by their parent/guardian.

10. What substance is released following the erythema reaction to ultraviolet exposure?
    a Histamine.
    b Sweat.
    c Sebum.
    d Melanin.

11. UV radiation reduces the effectiveness of the:
    a cardiovascular system
    b immune system
    c endocrine system
    d respiratory system.

12. Ultraviolet light on the skin helps to produce:
    a vitamin A
    b vitamin B6
    c vitamin C
    d vitamin D.

12 Heat therapy treatments

Objectives

▮ After you have studied this chapter you will be able to:

▮ describe different methods of heat treatment

▮ describe the benefits and effects of heat treatments

▮ explain the contra-indications to heat treatments

▮ explain the dangers and precautions to heat treatments

▮ explain the contra-actions that may occur during and/or after treatment and the appropriate action to take

▮ carry out heat treatments, paying due consideration to maximum efficiency, comfort, safety and hygiene.

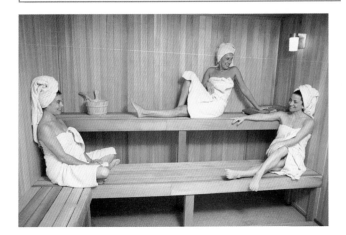

△ **Figure 12.1** A sauna in use

Figure 12.1 is a photograph of a sauna, which is one method of applying general heat to the body. Many forms of heat therapy are available and choice is determined by availability, client preference and suitability. All forms of heat produce similar effects; the treatment is particularly beneficial when combined with other treatments as part of a routine. It is mainly used before other treatments as it increases tissue response.

General heat can be applied in a steam bath, steam room, sauna or spa pool.

Local heat can be applied with facial steamers, paraffin wax to specific areas of the body, and by infrared and radiant heat lamps (see Chapter 11).

The extent of the effects will be dependent on the duration of heat application, intensity or degree of the heat, depth of absorption and the size of the area being heated.

Heat treatments for the body

Body tissues are more susceptible to treatments when they are warm. This is why heat treatments are of particular use as a precursor to other treatments. The various methods of heat application share similar benefits and physiological effects, as well as having contra-indications and contra-actions in common.

Benefits of steam, sauna and spa pool

○ To warm and soften the tissues to prepare client for further treatment.

○ To induce relaxation.

○ For deep cleansing.

○ To relieve muscular aches and pains.

○ To ease joint pain and stiffness.

▽ **Table 12.1** Physiological effects and benefits of steam, sauna and spa pool

Physiological effects	Benefits				
	Warm and soften tissues prior to further treatment	Induce relaxation	Deep cleansing	Relieve muscular aches and pains	Ease joint pain and stiffness
A general rise in body temperature.	√		√	√	√	√
An increase in circulation due to vasodilation giving hyperaemia and erythema.	√		√	√	√	√
An increase in cell metabolism.	√		√	√	√	√
The heart/pulse rate increases.	√		√		√	
Superficial capillaries and vessels dilate; therefore, there is a fall in blood pressure.			√			

(Continued)

(Continued)

Physiological effects \ Benefits	Warm and soften tissues prior to further treatment	Induce relaxation	Deep cleansing	Relieve muscular aches and pains	Ease joint pain and stiffness
Stimulation of sweat glands with increased sweating and elimination of waste.	√	√	√	√	√
The increased circulation and rise in temperature cause muscle relaxation.	√	√		√	√
The mild heat soothes sensory nerve endings.	√	√		√	√
The superficial layer of the skin is softened and is removed more easily, improving tone and texture.			√		

Be aware

There may be a temporary loss of body fluid due to sweating, but this is soon adjusted by drinking water.

Contra-indications to steam, sauna and spa pool

Learning point

Check the contra-indications listed in the manufacturers' instructions to ensure you do not invalidate your insurance policy should the client be injured during or after treatment.

▽ **Table 12.2** Reasons for contra-indications to steam, sauna and spa pool

Contra-indication	Reason
Alcohol (client under the influence of)	Both the alcohol and treatment will dehydrate the body, causing the client to feel dizzy, nauseous and faint.
Asthma	The client will find it difficult to breathe in the sauna as it has low humidity. The chemicals in the spa pool may trigger an attack. The steam bath may be an option depending on the severity of the condition.
Athlete's foot	There is a risk of cross-infection.
Body piercings	Remove or cover the adornment, as it may be made of material that can become hot and will cause discomfort to the client.
Bronchitis	This condition can be viral or bacterial. Symptoms include a cough, shortness of breath and tightness in the chest. Avoid these treatments as they will make the condition worse and/or client may experience difficulty breathing.
Claustrophobia	The sauna and steam rooms are confined spaces and therefore may not be appropriate for this client. Suggest a steam bath or spa pool, depending on the severity of their claustrophobia.
Cuts and abrasions	There is a risk of cross-infection. May also cause discomfort. Cover small cuts with waterproof plaster.
Defective sensation	The client must be able to feel the sensation of heat otherwise the body will overheat and also dehydrate causing dizziness, nausea and faintness.

(Continued)

(Continued)

Contra-indication	Reason
Diabetes	A client with diabetes may have impaired sensitivity and poor circulation. Heat treatments will increase circulation and may cause the client to feel dizzy, nauseous and faint.
Digestion (following a heavy meal)	The body is in the process of digesting the food. The stimulation of blood from the treatment will cause overload making the client feel dizzy, nauseous and faint.
Dizziness, faintness	No heat treatments should be given, as they will make the condition worse. The client needs rest to help the body recover.
Dysfunction of the nervous system	The client may have treatment if their GP consents.
Epilepsy	Find out as much as possible about the client's condition. If it is controlled epilepsy, the treatment may be safe to carry out but if in any doubt seek medical advice.
Exhaustion (severe)	As heat treatments stimulate the circulation the body will not be able to cope and will further exacerbate the condition.
Headaches, migraines	The heat and the stimulation of the blood circulation will exacerbate the condition. The body needs time to heal before having treatment.
Heart and circulatory conditions	The increase in the blood circulation may put too much pressure and stress on the heart. Seek medical consent.
Hepatitis	This is a viral infection causing inflammation of the liver. Chronic hepatitis lasts 6 months or more but it is the acute hepatitis lasting 6 months or less that is infectious. No treatment to be given during this period to avoid cross-infection.
High blood pressure	Blood pressure varies with age, weight and fitness, but some clients have consistently high blood pressure. Treatments can frequently help. Medical advice should be sought if the client is not currently on medication.
Low blood pressure	The client may feel dizzy or faint if they sit up or get up too quickly or if they receive too long a treatment. Monitor their treatment carefully.
Low-calorie slimming diets	Low energy levels may lead to feelings of faintness, which will be exacerbated by heat treatment.
Menstruation, first couple of days	Do not advise treatment during the first 2–3 days of a period as it may cause a heavier blood flow. Also blood loss contributes to feelings of faintness.
Pacemaker	Seek medical advice.
Phlebitis and thrombosis	Phlebitis is a painful condition where the lining of the vein becomes inflamed and may result in a clot forming on the vein wall, known as thrombosis. Any pressure applied to the vein or increase in the force of the circulation may dislodge the clot. The clot will then be carried in the blood stream with potentially fatal consequences. **Do not treat**.
Pregnancy	As blood circulation is stimulated and hormone levels are erratic, treatment should not be advised.
Respiratory conditions	The client may find it difficult to breathe in the sauna as humidity is low and the chemicals in the spa pool may irritate the respiratory tract. The steam bath may be an option dependent on the client's condition.
Skin diseases	There is a risk of cross-infection.
Under medical treatment	In line with acceptable work ethics and professional code of practice, seek medical consent before commencing treatment.
Verrucas	There is a risk of cross-infection.
Varicose veins (severe)	As the blood circulation is stimulated treatment may make the condition worse.

Contra-actions for steam, sauna and spa pools

○ Feeling faint/dizzy: a temporary reduction of blood to the brain can be caused by prolonged treatment, low blood pressure, standing up too quickly, eating too much or not eating enough before treatment, poor ventilation in the vicinity. Lie client down, raise their legs to improve the blood flow to the brain, make sure there is a flow of fresh air, give the client time to recover.

○ Nausea: could be caused by the body getting too hot, lack of, or consuming too much food prior to treatment, poor ventilation in the vicinity; advise the client to drink plenty of fluids and rest.

○ Headache: can be caused by prolonged treatment and dehydration; let the client rest in a quiet, well-ventilated room and advise them to drink water to rehydrate the body.

○ Skin irritation: can be caused by chemicals in the water (spa pool) or by excessive heat from prolonged treatment. Advise the client to shower and wash with mild cleansing product, pat dry and to apply a soothing, healing product.

Recommendations for steam, sauna and spa pools

A heat treatment can be recommended 2–3 times per week. It is a beneficial treatment to have prior to a course of treatments for improving muscle tone, reducing cellulite, weight reduction or to relax a client before a massage: it will warm and soften the tissues, making them more receptive to treatment.

Methods of application

Steam treatments

The steam room

This is a room that is supplied with steam from a boiler. Several people may use the steam room together. Some complexes based on Turkish pools have several rooms with increasing temperatures. Clients start with the lowest temperature and progress through to the highest. The steam bath has several advantages over the steam room. However, group treatments in steam rooms are more sociable occasions.

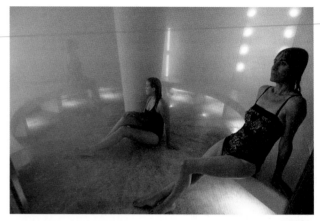

△ **Figure 12.2** A steam room

The steam bath

The steam bath is designed for individual treatments. It is a cabinet made of moulded fibreglass, in which the client sits. It contains a trough with a heating element; water poured into the trough is heated, making steam. The trough is placed underneath an adjustable seat, which allows the client to sit comfortably with their head outside the bath. There are usually three controls: a main switch, a timer and temperature gauge. The water is heated, forming steam which condenses within the bath, and the air is saturated with very high humidity of around 95 per cent.

Advantages of the steam bath over the steam room

○ The client does not feel claustrophobic because their head is out of the bath.

○ The client breathes normal air and not steam.

○ The hair remains neat and tidy and does not get wet.

○ The bath offers privacy for the client.

○ The temperature can be adjusted to suit the individual.

○ The initial cost and the running cost is low compared with a steam room.

○ It takes up little space and can be accommodated in most workplaces.

○ It is easier to clean, ensuring high hygiene standards and reducing the risk of cross-infection.

Dangers of steam baths

The main risks of harm with steam baths are:

○ burns from touching the hot metal trough

○ cross-infection by micro-organisms.

Precautions should be taken to minimise the risk of harming the client and to ensure they have an effective treatment.

▽ **Table 12.3** Precautions to take with steam baths

Precaution	Explanation
Ensure good standards of hygiene. Wipe over the whole bath with disinfecting solution before and after treatment. Cover the seat and floor with towels that are boiled after use.	Moist heat is an ideal breeding ground for micro-organisms.
Check that the trough is full with the correct type of water (distilled, purified or tap water). Refer to manufacturer's instructions.	Use the correct type of water to ensure that no damage to the equipment occurs.
Protect the client from contact with hot metal and direct steam: cover the seat with a towel that hangs over the edge.	To avoid burning the client.
Ensure that the client takes a shower before and after treatment.	To remove body lotion and perfumes that may cause an allergic reaction prior to treatment and to remove excess sweat and sebum after treatment.
Wrap a towel around the client's neck.	To prevent steam escaping.
Speak to the client during treatment.	You need to ensure they are comfortable. Be alert to contra-actions.

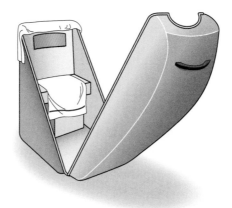

△ **Figure 12.3** Preparation of a steam bath

Preparation of working area

1. Wipe the steam bath with disinfecting solution.

    ↓

2. Check plugs and leads.

    ↓

3. Fill the trough with water.

    ↓

4. Cover the seat with a towel that hangs over the edge.

    ↓

5. Place a towel over the aperture to prevent loss of steam.

    ↓

6. Turn on the mains switch and bath switch.

    ↓

7. Turn the controls to maximum until the water is heating and then adjust the temperature and timer (50–55°C); the bath will take around 15 minutes to heat from cold.

    ↓

Preparation of self

8. Before carrying out treatment, ensure you prepare yourself physically and mentally, paying due attention to high standards of professionalism. Adopt a sensitive calm, confident and understanding attitude, as this approach will have a positive effect on your client.

    ↓

Preparation of client

9. Carry out a consultation, or if a regular client refer to the notes from their last treatment and discuss the effects and outcomes before proceeding.

    ↓

10. Check for contra-indications.

    ↓

11. Check contact lenses and all jewellery have been removed.

    ↓

12. Provide the client with a robe, and suitable footwear.

    ↓

13. Offer a shower cap or towel if client prefers to keep their hair protected.

    ↓

14. Instruct the client to have a shower.

    ↓

15. Explain the treatment to the client. Show them how to enter and leave the steam bath, advise them to take a shower at any point during treatment, and if they feel unwell to let you know.

    ↓

Technique for the steam bath

16. Help the client into the bath; make sure they are comfortable; close the door.

    ↓

17. Place the towel around the client's neck over the aperture.

    ↓

18. Keep in verbal contact throughout, reassure the client and ask them to report any discomfort. Be alert to contra-actions.

    ↓

19. At the end of treatment help the client from the bath and advise them to have a shower.

↓

20. Advise the client to use a friction rub to aid desquamation and improve skin texture.

↓

21. The client should now rest for 20–30 minutes or receive further treatments depending on needs *but must avoid exercise*.

↓

22. Update the consultation record with salient points about the treatment for future reference.

Timing of treatment

15–20 minutes.

Remember

Always seek feedback from your client and give appropriate aftercare advice (see pages 74–5).

Cleaning

Wipe over the whole bath with disinfecting solution after treatment. Cover the seat and floor of the bath with clean towels.

Sauna treatments

(See Figure 12.1.) Saunas are pinewood log cabins heated by electric stoves. They are manufactured in various sizes, from a single person sauna up to large cabins for 10–14 people. In Scandinavian countries, they are found indoors and outdoors. The larger the sauna, the more expensive it will be to run as it will require more heat output from larger stoves.

The walls of the cabin are constructed of well-insulated panels of pinewood.

Learning point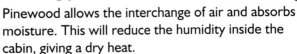

Pinewood allows the interchange of air and absorbs moisture. This will reduce the humidity inside the cabin, giving a dry heat.

The heat is provided by electric stoves, which heat non-splintering stones placed on top of the stove. Slatted wooden benches are arranged inside the sauna for sitting or lying down. There is an air inlet near the floor and an

▽ **Table 12.4** Differences between steam baths and saunas

Steam	Sauna
Moist heat, humidity 95 per cent	Dry heat, humidity 50–70 per cent
Atmospheric air is inhaled, therefore more suitable for clients with mild respiratory problems	Hot, dry air is inhaled which may irritate the mucous membranes
Easily adjusted to the tolerance of individual clients	Usually communal, therefore difficult to adjust to the needs of individual clients
Not claustrophobic as the head is free	May be claustrophobic
Not as damaging to hair as the head is free	May damage hair, particularly highlighted or coloured hair
Ensures privacy of the client	Lacks privacy if communal
Inexpensive to run but may be less profitable as only one client may be treated	Expensive to run but may be more profitable as many clients may be treated at one time
Comfortable for most clients	Less comfortable for the older, less mobile clients or those with sensitive skins

outlet near the ceiling. As the air in the sauna is heated, it rises by convection, therefore the sauna is hotter on the upper benches than on the lower benches. The air moisture is absorbed by the walls, making humidity very low, at around 10 per cent. This humidity can easily be increased by pouring water on the stones, which boils and creates steam.

Learning point (L)

Because the humidity in the sauna is low, sweat from the body evaporates quickly, cooling the body, therefore high temperatures can be tolerated in the sauna.

The temperature in the sauna may range from 50°C to around 120°C. A temperature range of between 60 and 80°C is recommended to cater for all clients. Clients can choose to spend longer in the sauna as their tolerance increases. The thermometer should always be checked for the temperature and the hygrometer should be checked for humidity before the commencement of treatment; these are found on a wall inside the cabin.

Learning point (L)

A hygrometer measures the amount of water vapour in the air, the humidity.

The temperature in a sauna should be 60–80°C and the humidity should be 50–70 per cent.

Be aware !

The dry heat of a sauna can be irritating and drying to mucous membranes.

The choice between steam and sauna as a preheating treatment depends very much on the client's preference. The differences between them are shown on page 283.

Dangers of sauna treatments

The main risk of harm with a sauna treatment is cross-infection by micro-organisms.

Precautions should be taken to minimise the risk of harming the client and to ensure they have an effective treatment.

Be aware !

Clients must be instructed to come out of the sauna if they are feeling faint, nauseous, dizzy or overheated. You must always remain close at hand to help when necessary.

▽ **Table 12.5** Precautions to take with sauna treatments

Precaution	Explanation
Ensure good standards of hygiene. Scrub the benches and floor thoroughly after use with special disinfecting solution for saunas.	Saunas can be an ideal breeding ground for micro-organisms.
Check the temperature (60–80°C) and humidity (50–70 per cent) before use.	Ideal temperature and humidity level for majority of clients.
Check that the guard around the heating element is secure and in position.	To protect clients from burns.
Ensure that clients take a shower before and after treatment.	To remove body lotion and perfumes that may cause a reaction prior to treatment and to remove excess sweat and sebum after treatment.
Advise the client to sit or lie on the lower benches to begin with.	They should do this until they are accustomed to the heat. Hot air rises, so the lower benches are at a lower temperature.

Sauna procedure

Preparation of working area

1. Prepare the sauna.

   ↓

2. Clean the wooden bucket and ladle and fill with fresh water.

   ↓

3. Switch on the sauna and set the temperature and humidity level.

   ↓

Preparation of self

4. Before carrying out treatment ensure you prepare yourself physically and mentally, paying due attention to high standards of professionalism. Adopt a sensitive calm, confident and understanding attitude, as this approach will have a positive effect on your client.

   ↓

Preparation of client

5. Carry out a consultation, or if a regular client refer to the notes from their last treatment and discuss the effects and outcomes before proceeding.

   ↓

6. Check for contra-indications.

   ↓

7. Check contact lenses and all jewellery have been removed.

   ↓

8. Provide the client with a towel, suitable footwear and offer protection for their hair.

   ↓

9. Instruct the client to have a shower.

   ↓

10. Explain the treatment. Advise the client to wear a swimming costume or towel wrap for modesty. They should sit or lie on the lower benches until they are accustomed to the heat. Warm or cold showers may be taken during the course of the treatment.

    ↓

Technique for sauna

11. Observe the client throughout the treatment and be alert to contra-actions.

    ↓

12. Advise the client to shower after treatment and use a friction rub to aid desquamation and improve skin texture.

    ↓

13. The client should rest for 20–30 minutes or receive further treatments depending on needs *but avoid exercise.*

    ↓

14. Update the consultation record with salient points about the treatment for future reference.

Be aware

These preparations are usually done at the start of the day as part of the opening up routine.

Be aware

To stimulate and invigorate the senses add essence of pine or eucalyptus to the water. These essences are prepared especially for saunas. Do not use aromatherapy oils as they are not designed for use in the sauna.

Be aware

Metal jewellery can get very hot during treatment and can burn the client.

Remember

Small amounts of water may be sprinkled on the stones from time to time to increase the humidity. This should not be overdone.

Timing of treatment

Treatment time will depend on the tolerance of the client. The first treatment could be up to 10 minutes, increasing to 15 or 20 minutes as tolerance is built up.

> ### Remember
> Always seek feedback from your client and give appropriate aftercare advice (see pages 74–5).

Cleaning

Scrub benches and floor thoroughly with special disinfecting solution at the end of every day.

Spa pools

These refer to pools for sitting in rather than for swimming. They vary in size and construction, from preformed, reinforced acrylic shells to block-built and tiled pools. Spa pools contain a quantity of water, which is heated, chemically treated and filtered. Hydrojet circulation and air induction bubbles may also be included.

A spa pool is not drained, cleaned and refilled after each individual client. Cleaning and water change is dependent on the size of the pool and the volume of water it contains. For example a pool that accommodates six clients is usually drained three times per week.

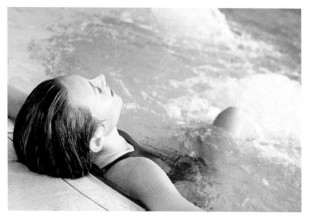

△ Figure 12.4 Spa pool

Installation of spa pools

Spa pools must be installed in accordance with manufacturers' instructions. The spa pool must be installed on a level, solid base. If the spa pool is to be installed on a suspended floor, consideration must be given to the weight of the pool plus water and clients.

All spa equipment must be properly installed and connected and all components must be accessible for maintenance. The spa pool must be positioned so that any noise will not cause undue disturbance. Ventilation in the area of the spa should be adequate to prevent condensation.

All surfaces must be smooth, with rounded moulded edges. Uneven surfaces or sharp edges may cause accidents and injuries.

> ### Be aware
> The wet floor area around the spa pool should have a non-porous, non-slip, even surface, and must be easy to clean and sanitise.

There must be adequate drainage to ensure that water spillage flows away quickly.

The water provided to fill the spa pool must be of satisfactory quality. If the water supply does not meet the required standards, steps must be taken to bring the water within chemical, physical and biological standards.

The manufacturer must advise and instruct the operator on the operational procedures required and the treatments necessary to maintain water quality and to achieve the highest standards of hygiene and safety. Advice must also be given on the correct handling and safe storage of chemicals. A manual listing all these instructions must be provided by the manufacturer and explained to the operator. The manufacturer must also supply a water testing kit and explain its use and limitations.

Guidelines for water standards

The source of water for the spa pool is usually from the mains supply. If this is not available, water may be obtained from other sources, which must be assessed and deemed suitable by the Environmental Health Officer from the local council. After treatment, the water should be within the following standards:

○ Disinfectant levels: a bromine residual of 4–6 mg per litre.
○ A free chlorine residual of 1.5–3 mg per litre. Ozone may be used in conjunction with bromine and chlorine.

> ### Learning point (L)
> 'Free chlorine residual' refers to what is left of the total amount of chlorine in the pool. This is used to destroy bacteria.

○ pH levels: 7.2–7.8.

○ Total alkalinity: 80–100 mg per litre as calcium carbonate.

○ Calcium hardness: 75–500 mg per litre as calcium carbonate.

○ Total dissolved solids: less than 1500 mg per litre.

Proper standards of disinfection must be maintained at all times. The Environmental Health Officer will carry out a routine assessment of the biological purity of the spa water. The recommendation for spa water is as follows:

○ To contain less than 100 bacteria per ml capable of growing on agar in two days at 37°C.

○ To be free from coliforms, pseudomonas, staphylococcus and faecal streptococcus in 100ml water. This is usually checked by the Environmental Health Officer.

Be aware
The Environmental Health Officer does not have to make an appointment or even notify the operator of a visit.

Purification

Organic and nitrogenous impurities are introduced into the spa water during normal use, so filtration and chemical treatment are essential to remove and break down this matter and to purify the recycled water.

Be aware
Algae growths may occur in some spas, and while these are not generally harmful to health, they make surfaces slippery and make the water look unattractive. A number of spa disinfectants are effective in limiting these growths, but if necessary, recommended algicides may be used.

Foaming may occur as a result of soap being introduced into the spa after clients have showered. This can be removed using an anti-foaming agent.

Additional chemicals

In addition to the chemicals discussed earlier in this chapter, other chemical products may be required to maintain water standards, as listed in Table 12.6.

△ **Table 12.6** Additional chemicals to maintain water standards

Chemical	Function
Aluminium sulphate	Aids filtration.
Calcium chloride	Raises calcium hardness.
Polyelectrolyte products	Aids filtration.
Sodium bicarbonate	Raises total alkalinity.
Sodium carbonate	Raises pH.
Sodium hydrogen sulphate	Lowers pH.
Sodium chlorite	Dechlorinates and debrominates water.
Sequestering agents	Protect against staining and scale formation.

Operation and care of spa pools

Those responsible for the operation and care of spa pools must be familiar with and operate according to the legislation in the Health and Safety at Work Act 1974.

The highest standards of hygiene and safety must be practised at all times. Every precaution must be taken to avoid cross-infection or injury to the client.

Operator responsibilities

Spa pools differ in size, construction and in mode of operation. It is therefore important that each operator is fully conversant with all the details in the manufacturer's instruction manual for their particular spa pool. This must be obtained from the manufacturer when the pool is installed. It is the manufacturer's duty to explain and discuss the procedures with the operator and to give advice as required.

Be aware
As a supervisor, you have a legal responsibility under the health and safety legislation to ensure the safety of every client. Make sure that you have followed all the guidelines for operating the pool.

The operator must carry out the following procedures in accordance with the manufacturer's instructions.

▽ **Table 12.7** Procedure for operating the spa pool

Task	Procedure
Water levels	Fill the pool to the correct level with water and ensure that this level is maintained.
Pump/filter	Ensure that the pump, filter and any other devices are working correctly and are regularly cleaned and maintained.
Disinfection levels	Maintain the correct disinfection levels in the pool at all times; chlorine or bromine are generally added to the water either manually or automatically. It is recommended that a bromine residual of 4–6 mg per litre should be maintained in the water of a commercial spa or a chlorine residual of 1.5–3 mg per litre. Excess of these chemicals may cause skin irritation and smarting of the eyes.
pH levels	Maintain the correct pH levels in the pool at all times: 7.2–7.8 is the recommended range, 7.4–7.6 is the ideal. The correct pH level is important to prevent corrosion and scale formation, and for effective disinfection and client comfort. All spa pools should have automatic controllers to provide continuous monitoring and control of disinfectant and pH levels.
Waterline	Clean the waterline regularly with the recommended non-foaming cleaner. This improves the hygiene standards and the appearance of the pool.
Foam	Remove any foam that occurs with an anti-foaming agent as this affects the clarity of the water.
Staining or scaling	Add a sequestering agent at the first sign of staining or scale formation, which will be unattractive and may cause corrosion and block pipework.
Water temperature	Maintain a water temperature of 36–37°C. The water temperature must not exceed the maximum recommended temperature of 40°C.
Cleaning	Change the water and clean the pool and its equipment regularly. The frequency of this operation will depend on the size of the pool and volume of water. Clean the pool with a recommended cleaning agent before refilling.
Testing	Test the chemical levels regularly according to the manufacturer's instructions.
Records	Record all tests, changes and any maintenance work undertaken. For every chemical test, the time, result and action taken must be recorded in a record book or chart. This must be accessible to all operators. An instrument to continuously record disinfectant and pH levels is strongly recommended.
Observation	Ensure that clients are seated correctly in the pool. They must be observed at all times. Should they become unwell, assist them carefully out of the pool. Ensure that the number of clients in the pool at any one time does not exceed the number recommended for that pool.
Handling and storage of chemicals	Take particular care with the handling and storage of chemicals. Read and follow guidelines on the packages. Be aware of the legislative requirements regarding these products. Wear the appropriate PPE.

○ goggles: chemical BSI standard

○ respirator mask: recommended type.

Remember

A first-aid box with an eyewash bottle should be kept near the spa pool.

Protection of the operator

For the protection and safety of the operator, some of the following protective clothing should be worn when handling chemicals, dependent on the task and the chemicals involved:

○ apron: a bib-type apron in PVC

○ gloves: waterproof

Dangers of spa pools

The main risk of harm with spa pools is slipping or falling if the pool surround is wet and slippery. Precautions should be taken to minimise the risk of harming the client and to ensure they have an effective treatment.

▽ **Table 12.8** Precautions to take with the spa pool

Precaution	Explanation
Ensure good standards of hygiene.	Moist heat is an ideal breeding ground for micro-organisms.
Ensure that the client takes a shower before and after treatment.	Beforehand: to remove body lotion and perfumes as they may cause a reaction. After: to wash off chemicals as these may irritate the skin.
Instruct the client to use the handrail to enter and exit the spa pool.	To avoid slipping or falling if the pool surround is wet and slippery.
Advise the client to sit between the jets.	Sitting directly in front of a jet may cause discomfort and bruising.

Spa pool procedure

Preparation of working area

1. Check the pH level, chlorine and temperature of the spa and ensure the pool surround is not slippery.

↓

Preparation of self

2. Before carrying out treatment ensure you prepare yourself physically and mentally, paying due attention to high standards of professionalism. Adopt a sensitive calm, confident and understanding attitude, as this approach will have a positive effect on your client.

↓

Preparation of client

3. Carry out a consultation, or if a regular client refer to the notes from their last treatment and discuss the effects and outcomes before proceeding.

↓

4. Check for contra-indications.

↓

5. Check contact lenses and all jewellery have been removed.

↓

6. Provide the client with a robe, towel, and suitable footwear.

↓

7. Explain the treatment to the client. Advise them to:
   - wear a swimming costume
   - have a shower
   - sit either side of the jets
   - take a shower to cool down if they become too hot
   - avoid touching their eyes as the chemicals in the water may cause irritation.

↓

> **Learning point**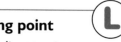
>
> Ask the client to rinse thoroughly to remove all traces of soap as any residue may affect the chemical balance of the water and produce foaming if carried into the spa pool.

Technique for the spa pool

8. Observe the client throughout the treatment and be alert to contra-actions.

↓

9. At the end of treatment advise the client to shower after treatment and moisturise their skin.

↓

10. The client should rest for 20–30 minutes or receive further treatments depending on needs *but avoid exercise.*

↓

11. Update the consultation record with salient points about the treatment for future reference.

Timing

Recommended time is 10–20 minutes. Maximum time is 20 minutes.

Heat treatments for the face, hands and feet

Heat treatments for the face, hands and feet offer many of the same benefits and produce similar physiological effects. They can be used as a pre-treatment preparation for a range of beauty services, or form part of the treatment themselves, as is the case with paraffin wax application to the hands and feet.

Local heat can be applied with facial steamers, or with paraffin wax to specific areas.

Facial steamer

Steam may be applied to the face using floor standing or portable facial steamers. Some machines deliver steam only, while others deliver steam and ozone.

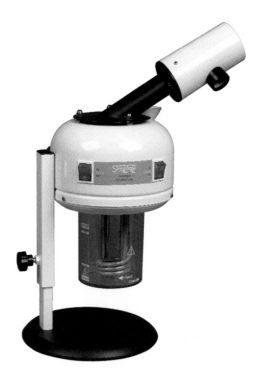

△ **Figure 12.6** Facial steamer (for the trolley)

The facial steamer consists of a tank with a heating element. This is filled with the type of water recommended by the manufacturer (distilled, purified or tap water), which is heated, producing steam. This steam passes into a tube, which is directed at the client's face. If it produces ozone, the steamer will contain a high-pressure mercury vapour tube producing ultraviolet rays. This converts the oxygen in the air into ozone (i.e. O_2 is converted into O_3). Ozone has a drying, antibacterial and healing effect on the tissues. This is beneficial for greasy, seborrhoeic skin conditions but should only be used for a very short time on dry and mature skins for its anti-bacterial effect.

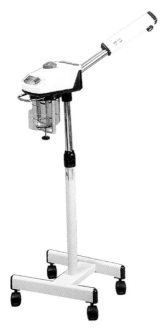

△ **Figure 12.5** Facial steamer

Be aware

Ozone is known to be damaging to the respiratory tract and is not medically recommended. Although only very small amounts are produced by ozone steamers and the timing of the treatment is reduced to 5 minutes, you should take care when giving this treatment and check manufacturer's instructions for guidelines about appropriate distance from the client's face.

Learning point (L)

Facial steamers produce heating with high humidity.

Be aware

There are facial steamers on the market that offer the facility of adding infusions, herbs and aromatherapy oils to enhance the treatment.

Benefits of facial steaming treatments

○ To soften superficial keratinised cells and build-up of sebum on greasy and seborrhoeic skin prior to desquamation and deep cleansing.

○ To aid healing of blemished and pustular skins.

○ To aid absorption and enhance the effect of creams, oils and masks, etc. Used to improve the condition of dry, dehydrated, mature skins and maintain the balance of a normal skin.

○ To promote relaxation.

○ To prepare the skin for further treatments.

▽ **Table 12.9** Physiological effects and benefits of facial steaming treatments

Physiological effects	Greasy and seborrhoeic skin	Aid healing of blemished and pustular skin	Dry, dehydrated, mature and normal skin	Promote relaxation	Prepare the skin for further treatments
The heat raises the temperature of the area.	√	√	√	√	√
The circulation is increased due to vasodilation, giving hyperaemia and erythema.	√	√	√	√	√
The heat induces muscle relaxation.				√	√
Mild heat is soothing to sensory nerve endings.				√	
The heat increases the metabolic rate.	√	√	√	√	√
Sweat glands are stimulated producing more sweat, releasing toxins.	√	√	√	√	√
Sebaceous glands are stimulated, opening pores and aiding the release of blockages.	√	√	√		√
Ozone has a bactericidal effect.	√	√	√		

Contra-indications to facial steaming treatments

Learning point

Check the contra-indications listed in the manufacturers' instructions to ensure you do not invalidate your insurance policy should the client be injured during or after treatment.

▽ **Table 12.10** Reasons for contra-indications to facial steaming

Contra-indication	Reason
Claustrophobia	This may not be the most appropriate treatment for the client. May cause discomfort as the client's eyes are covered and the steam projected onto the face may make them feel restricted. In extreme cases it could trigger a panic attack.
Defective sensation	The client must be able to feel the sensation of heat to be able to give accurate feedback about the temperature of the steam as it could burn the skin.
Dilated capillaries	Treatment will make the condition worse as the steam will warm the tissues and stimulate the blood to the area. If there are only a few dilated capillaries continue with treatment but protect the area with damp cotton wool or a barrier cream.
Highly sensitive skin, rosacea, couperose	Clients with sensitive skin must not receive stimulating treatments as these will exacerbate the condition. The products used for treatments may cause an allergic reaction in some clients. This will produce an excessive erythema, the area becoming very red and hot or a rash may appear.
Respiratory conditions	It may make the condition worse and/or client may experience difficulty breathing.

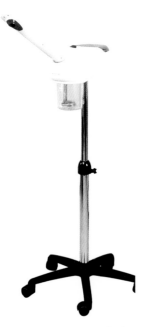

△ **Figure 12.7** Herbal steamer

Dangers of facial steaming treatments

The main risk of harm from facial steaming is burning from steam or scalding water.

Precautions should be taken to minimise the risk of harming the client and to ensure you give an effective treatment.

▽ **Table 12.11** Precautions to take with facial steaming

Precaution	Explanation
Ensure steamer is positioned securely on a stable surface.	It must not tip over as this could result in burns to you or the client.
Check that there is sufficient water (distilled, purified or tap water) in the tank (refer to manufacturer's instructions).	This is important because some types of water can damage the heating element.
Switch on for 5–10 minutes before treatment until the steam is produced.	To make sure the steamer is working correctly and not spitting out hot water.
Carry out a thermal sensitivity test (see page 71).	If the client cannot tell the difference between hot and cold, they have defective sensation and the treatment should not be carried out.
Switch on the ozone after the production of steam.	Steam is needed to contribute to the production of ozone.
If using ozone, only use it for a maximum of 5 minutes.	Inhaling too much ozone can damage the respiratory tract.
Cover the client's eyes with damp cotton wool pads, secure with a strip of tissue tucked into the sides of the head band to keep them in place.	To protect the eyes from the steam and ozone.

Facial steamer procedure

Preparation of working area

1. Place machine on a suitable stable base or use the floor-standing version.
   ↓
2. Check plugs and leads.
   ↓
3. Check there is sufficient water in the tank.
   ↓
4. Switch on the machine until steam is produced. You need to check it is not spitting out hot water and switch off again.
   ↓
5. Check the couch is prepared with clean linen and towels.
   ↓
6. Prepare trolley with suitable products and equipment:
   ○ products suitable for applying to dry, dehydrated or mature skins before directing the steam onto the skin
   ○ tape measure to ensure safe positioning of steamer
   ○ sterile comedone extractor
   ○ sterile micro-lance to remove milia
   ○ disposable gloves for milia extraction
   ○ sharps container to dispose of micro-lance.
   ↓

Preparation of self

7. Before carrying out treatment ensure you prepare yourself physically and mentally, paying due attention to high standards of professionalism. Adopt a sensitive calm, confident and understanding attitude, as this approach will have a positive effect on your client.

↓

Preparation of client

8. Carry out a consultation, or if a regular client refer to the notes from their last treatment and discuss the effects and outcomes before proceeding.

↓

9. Check for contra-indications.

↓

10. Check contact lenses and all jewellery have been removed.

↓

11. Place the client in a well-supported and comfortable position.

↓

12. Protect hair and clothing.

↓

13. Explain the treatment to the client, warning them about the warmth of the steam and the smell of the ozone if used.

↓

14. Switch on the machine to heat up.

↓

WASH YOUR HANDS

15. Carry out a thermal sensitivity test.

↓

16. Cleanse and tone the skin.

↓

17. Carry out a skin analysis.

↓

18. Place the client in a semi-reclining position

↓

Technique for facial steamer

19. Apply a suitable cream to the face and neck for dry, dehydrated and mature skin.

↓

20. Apply damp cotton wool pads to the client's eyes, secure with a strip of tissue and tuck into the headband.

↓

21. Position the machine the correct distance from the client depending on skin type and tolerance.

↓

22. Direct the steam onto the face and neck.

↓

23. Keep in verbal contact with the client to monitor progress of the treatment and be alert to contra-actions.

↓

24. At the end of treatment, switch off and move the machine to a safe place to cool down.

↓

Be aware !

Although manufacturers give treatment times for different skin conditions these are for guidance only. You must always observe client's skin reaction during the application and respond appropriately.

Be aware !

Cover sensitive areas of the skin with damp cotton wool or barrier cream for protection.

Be aware !

Do not physically lift the machine once it has been switched on. This positioning refers to swivelling the steamer to face the client.

Remember

Switch on the ozone after the client has got used to the sensation of the steam.

25. Remove the eye pads and wipe the skin with a suitable product.

  ↓

26. Extract any comedones and milia.

  ↓

27. Continue with the facial routine depending on client's needs.

  ↓

28. Update the consultation record with salient points about the treatment for future reference. This will include the outcome of the thermal sensitivity test.

Extractions

When extracting comedones and milia, use a magnifying lamp to illuminate and magnify the area to help you extract accurately and to prevent eye strain.

Comedone extraction

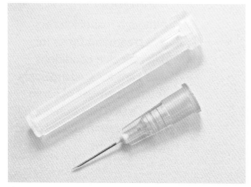

△ **Figure 12.8** Comedone extractor

Milia extraction

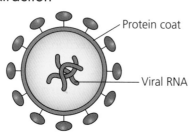

△ **Figure 12.9** Micro-lance

Use a sterilised comedone extractor or cover the pads of your index fingers with tissue. If using an extractor, use the loop end to apply gentle pressure around the comedone to ease out the plug of sebum. You can also slide the extractor over congested areas to remove excess sebum, If using the pads of your index fingers, squeeze and roll the tissues around the comedone to ease it out of the follicle.

Wear disposable gloves, as you will be piercing the skin and there is a risk of coming into contact with body fluids.

○ Wipe over the area with a suitable disinfecting solution.

○ Stretch the skin and with a sterile micro-lance gentle scrape at the surface of the skin covering the follicle.

○ Wrap tissue around the pads of your index fingers or use a cotton bud in each hand and gently roll and squeeze the surrounding tissues to aid the release the milia.

Be aware ❗

Note the client's body language and in particular their facial expressions as you extract. If they flinch and try to move away from you – lighten the pressure *immediately*.

Remember

Remember that clients can make a legal claim against you for negligence.

Timing of treatment

Remember

These timings are for guidance only. Refer to manufacturer's instructions and observe the reaction of the client's skin. This should always be the main indicator of timings.

▽ **Table 12.12** Treatment times for facial steaming

Skin type	Treatment time	Distance from face
Greasy, seborrhoeic	15–20 minutes	25 cm (10")
Normal	10–15 minutes	30 cm (12")
Dry, mature	3–7 minutes	40 cm (15")

Contra-actions to facial steaming treatments

Be aware

During extractions, bruising, broken capillaries and permanent marks can be caused by applying too much pressure to the tissues.

○ Burns can be caused by misuse of steam or scalding water. Apply sterile cold water to the area to prevent the burn getting worse, then apply a soothing, healing lotion or cream. Advise the client not to touch the area.

○ Over-stimulation of the skin is caused by positioning the steamer too near the client and/or prolonged treatment. Place a cool compress on the skin and apply a suitable product or mask that will help to calm and soothe the tissues.

Be aware

Tell the client to avoid touching areas of skin where milia have been extracted unless their hands are clean, to prevent the risk of cross-infection.

Recommendations for facial steaming treatments

This is a versatile treatment as it is suitable for all skin types. It can be offered as a 45–60 minute facial to include cleansing, toning, steaming with extractions, massage, mask and moisturising. Alternatively, it can be used to warm and soften the tissues prior to other treatments, for example disincrustation, electrical muscle stimulation and vacuum suction.

Remember

Always seek feedback from your client and give appropriate aftercare advice (see pages 74–5).

Cleaning

Refer to manufacturer's instructions, as these will vary.

Paraffin wax – face

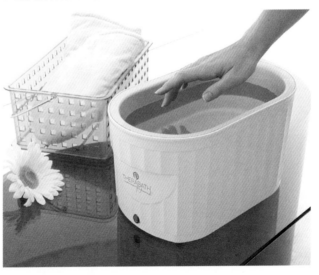

△ **Figure 12.10** Paraffin wax heater

Paraffin wax is a peel-off mask applied to the face as part of a facial routine. The wax warms, softens and hydrates the tissues. It is especially beneficial for dry, dehydrated and mature skin. There are products available with added properties to cleanse, detoxify and moisturise. Great care must be taken in its application, avoiding the eyes, nostrils and mouth.

Equipment

When cold, the wax is whitish and solid, but when heated it liquefies and clarifies. Wax is heated in containers, which vary in size and shape. Wax is heated and maintained at a suitable temperature of 45–49°C.

The warm wax is applied in layers using a brush. Each layer of wax is allowed to dry and become white before the next coat is applied. A build-up of six coats is desirable.

Benefits of paraffin wax treatment to the face

○ To improve the condition of dry, dehydrated skin.

○ To improve the condition of mature, ageing skin.

○ To stimulate and cleanse a sluggish skin and remove build-up of sebum and dry keratinised cells.

○ To aid the relaxation of facial muscles.

Contra-indications to paraffin wax treatment of the face

Dangers of paraffin wax treatment to the face

The main risk of harm from using wax is of burns, either from spillages or if the temperature of the wax is too high. Precautions should be taken to minimise the risk of harming the client and to ensure you give an effective treatment.

▽ Table 12.13 Physiological effects and benefits of paraffin wax treatment to the face

Physiological effects	Benefits			
	Improve dry, dehydrated skin	Improve mature, ageing skin	Stimulate and cleanse a sluggish skin	Aid relaxation of facial muscles
The heat raises the temperature of the area.	√	√	√	√
There is an increase in circulation due to vasodilation, giving hyperaemia and erythema.	√	√	√	√
There is an increase in the metabolic rate, which will improve the condition of the tissues.	√	√	√	√
The heat induces muscle relaxation.				√
The heat soothes sensory nerve endings.				√
The stimulation of sweat glands producing more sweat, releasing toxins.	√	√	√	√
The stimulation of sebaceous glands; this releases blockages on a sluggish skin and helps to lubricate the dry, mature skin.	√	√	√	
The ingredients in the wax soften the skin.	√	√	√	

▽ **Table 12.14** Reasons for contra-indications to paraffin wax treatment of the face

Contra-indication	Reason
Claustrophobic or highly tense, nervous clients	May cause discomfort and, in extreme cases, trigger a panic attack. Advise client on alternative treatments.
Cuts and abrasions of the skin (e.g. chapped skin)	Risk of cross-infection. May also cause discomfort to the client. Avoid the area or cover with petroleum jelly.
Defective sensation	Client will not be able to give accurate feedback about the temperature of the wax, which may cause burns. Advise client on alternative treatments.
Dilated capillaries	Treatment will make the condition worse due to increased blood circulation to the area. Advise client on alternative treatments.
Highly sensitive, vascular, florid, couperose skins	May aggravate the condition. Advise client on alternative treatments.
Skin diseases	There is a risk of cross-infection.
Weathered skin with windburn or sunburn	May aggravate the condition causing more sensitivity. Advise client on alternative treatments.

▽ **Table 12.15** Precautions to take with paraffin wax treatments

Precaution	Explanation
Do not store or operate wax baths near naked flame or hotplate.	To avoid igniting the wax.
Maintain the temperature according to manufacturer's instructions.	To avoid burning the client.
Do not move container when the wax is hot.	To avoid spillages, which may burn or mark and will cause the floor to become slippery.
Carry out a thermal sensitivity test (see page 71).	If the client cannot tell the difference between hot and cold, they have defective sensation and the treatment should not be carried out.
Test the wax on self and on client before applying it.	To ensure the wax is of a suitable temperature and to assess client tolerance and avoid burning or causing discomfort to the client.
Cover client's clothing and protect surrounding area.	It is difficult to remove wax from clothing and surfaces when it has dried.

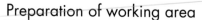

Paraffin wax procedure – face

Preparation of working area

1. Place the paraffin wax heater on a suitable stable base.

   ↓

2. Check plugs and leads.

   ↓

3. Check the temperature of the wax. Use a spatula to apply wax to a small area on your inner wrist where it is more sensitive.

   ↓

4. Protect the working area; cover the couch and trolley.

   ↓

5. Prepare trolley with suitable products:
   - wax brush
   - bowl lined with tin foil
   - cling film/tin foil
   - client consultation record.

   ↓

Preparation of self

6. Before carrying out treatment ensure you prepare yourself physically and mentally, paying due attention to high standards of professionalism. Adopt a sensitive calm, confident and understanding attitude, as this approach will have a positive effect on your client.

   ↓

Preparation of client

7. Carry out a consultation, or if a regular client refer to the notes from their last treatment and discuss the effects and outcomes before proceeding.

   ↓

8. Check for contra-indications.

   ↓

9. Check contact lenses and all jewellery have been removed.

   ↓

10. Place the client in a well-supported and comfortable position.

    ↓

11. Protect clothing with towels and couch roll.

    ↓

12. Cover the hair with a towel or band to the hairline.

    ↓

13. Explain the treatment to the client. Their eyes will be protected with damp cotton wool and the wax will be applied in layers to form a mask over their face and neck.

    ↓

WASH YOUR HANDS

14. Carry out a thermal sensitivity test.

    ↓

15. Cleanse the skin.

    ↓

16. Carry out a skin analysis and test temperature of wax on client's neck.

    ↓

Technique for paraffin wax – face

17. Apply a suitable moisturising/specialised cream to the face and neck.

↓

18. Decant sufficient wax into a bowl lined with tin foil.

↓

19. Apply damp cotton wool to protect the eyes.

↓

20. Apply the wax quickly to the face and neck using a brush; continue to build up the layers until a good, even coating has been applied. Check the outer edges are even and sufficiently thick.

↓

21. Keep in verbal contact with the client and monitor the progress of the treatment. Be alert to contra-actions.

↓

22. After a suitable time, use the pads of your fingers to lift the outer edge of the wax mask from the base of the neck and continue to work up towards the forehead to remove it. The wax should lift off easily in one piece if the layers are thick enough.

↓

23. Place the wax in couch roll and dispose of it in a covered bin.

↓

24. Massage excess cream into the skin.

↓

25. Extract comedones and milia if appropriate (see page 296).

↓

26. Continue with the treatment depending on client's needs.

↓

27. Update the consultation record with salient points about the treatment for future reference. This will include the outcome of the thermal sensitivity test.

Learning point

The wax will open the pores helping the cream to penetrate, and also it prevents the wax sticking to the skin during removal.

Learning point

Lining the bowl with foil prevents the wax adhering to the inside of the bowl.

Remember

Dampen the cotton wool to prevent wisps of cotton wool irritating the eyes.

Be aware

Avoid the eyes, nostrils and mouth.

Timing of treatment

Approximately 20 minutes, depending on the skin condition and desired result. Be guided by client tolerance.

Contra-actions to paraffin wax – face

○ Excessive erythema: caused by wax being too hot for the client. Place a cool compress on the skin and apply a suitable product or mask that will help to calm and soothe the tissues.

○ Burns: caused by wax being too hot. Apply sterile cold water to the area to prevent the burn getting worse, then apply a soothing, healing lotion or cream. Advise the client not to touch the area.

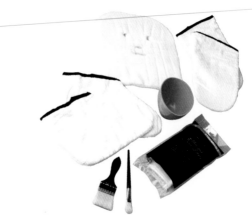

△ **Figure 12.11** Paraffin wax accessories

> **Remember**
> Always seek feedback from your client and give appropriate aftercare advice (see pages 14–5).

Care and maintenance of wax

○ Wax is supplied as large blocks. These should be covered and kept in a dry cupboard area.

○ After use, the wax may be disposed of by wrapping in paper and placing in a bin. Under the new Health and Safety at Work regulations the wax must be disposed of after each client.

Paraffin wax – hands and feet

Paraffin wax treatment is particularly beneficial for the hands and feet.

The equipment for this treatment is the same as for paraffin wax to the face, with some additions. The part being treated is coated with layers of wax and then wrapped in tin foil and covered with a towel, mitt or bootee to retain the heat. The application of wax can be messy and care must be taken to cover the floor and clothing before the treatment starts.

Benefits of paraffin wax to the hands and feet

○ To relieve pain.

○ To soften the skin and cuticles.

○ To improve the condition of stiff, arthritic joints. Exercises given after treatment may result in increased mobility.

○ To promote relaxation.

▽ **Table 12.16** Physiological effects and benefits of paraffin wax to the hands and feet

Physiological effects	Relieve pain	Soften the skin and cuticles	Improve the condition of stiff, arthritic joints	Promote relaxation
The heat raises the temperature of the area.	√	√	√	√
There is an increase in circulation due to vasodilation, giving hyperaemia and erythema.	√	√	√	√
There is an increase in the metabolic rate.	√	√	√	√
The heat induces muscle relaxation.	√		√	√

(Continued)

The heat soothes sensory nerve endings.	√		√	√
The stimulation of sweat glands producing more sweat, releasing toxins.	√		√	√
The stimulation of sebaceous glands thus softening the skin.		√		
The ingredients in the wax soften the skin and cuticles.		√		

Contra-indications for paraffin wax to the hands and feet

Learning point Ⓛ

Check the contra-indications listed in the manufacturer's instructions to ensure you do not invalidate your insurance policy should the client be injured during or after treatment.

▽ **Table 12.17** Reasons for contra-indications to paraffin wax treatment of the hands and feet

Contra-indication	Reason
Bruising (severe)	The stimulation of blood circulation may increase bleeding in the area. Avoid the area as it may be uncomfortable for the client and could affect the healing process.
Cuts and abrasions	Small cuts can be covered with a waterproof plaster. Do not carry out treatment if the wounds are open as there is a risk of cross-infection. May also cause discomfort to the client.
Defective skin sensation	Client will not be able to give accurate feedback about the temperature of the wax, which may cause burns. Advise client on alternative treatments.
Hairy areas (very)	May cause discomfort when removing the wax.
Skin diseases, particularly verrucae, athlete's foot and infected areas of cuticle and nails	There is a risk of cross-infection.
Skin disorders, for example eczema and psoriasis	The skin for both conditions is red with flaky dry patches. The treatment will cause more sensitivity in the area and exacerbate the condition.
Swelling	The cause may be associated with high blood pressure, kidney conditions or other systemic problems. Seek medical advice to establish the cause. If the cause is due to gravitational effects the increase in circulation may exacerbate the condition.
Undiagnosed painful areas	Recommend the client seeks medical advice, as there may be an underlying problem that prevents treatment.

(Continued)

Dangers of paraffin wax to the hands and feet

The main risk of harm from using wax is burns, either from spillages or if the temperature of the wax is too high.

Precautions should be taken to minimise the risk of harming the client and to ensure you give an effective treatment.

▽ **Table 12.18** Precautions to take with paraffin wax treatments to the hands and feet

Precaution	Explanation
Do not store or operate wax baths near naked flame or hotplate.	To avoid igniting the wax.
Maintain the temperature according to manufacturer's instructions.	To avoid burning the client.
Do not move container when the wax is hot.	To avoid spillages, which may burn or mark and will cause the floor to become slippery.
Carry out a thermal sensitivity test (see page 71).	If the client cannot tell the difference between hot and cold, they have defective sensation and the treatment should not be carried out.
Test the wax on self and client before applying it.	To assess client tolerance and avoid burning or causing discomfort to the client.
Cover client's clothing and protect surrounding area.	It is difficult to remove wax that has dried on clothing and surfaces.
Do not place the hand/foot in the wax bath.	It is unhygienic and there is a risk of cross-infection.

Paraffin wax procedure – hands and feet

Preparation of working area

1. Place the paraffin wax heater on a suitable stable base.

    ↓

2. Check plugs and leads.

    ↓

3. Check the temperature of the wax. Use a spatula to apply wax to a small area on your inner wrist where it is more sensitive.

    ↓

4. Protect the working area; cover the floor, couch/chair and trolley.

    ↓

5. Prepare trolley with suitable products:
    - cleansing products as appropriate
    - moisturising cream
    - wax brush
    - bowl lined with tin foil
    - cling film/tin foil
    - towel/mitts/bootees.

    ↓

Preparation of self

6. Before carrying out treatment ensure you prepare yourself physically and mentally, paying due attention to high standards of professionalism. Adopt a sensitive calm, confident and understanding attitude, as this approach will have a positive effect on your client.

    ↓

Preparation of client

7. Carry out a consultation, or if a regular client refer to the notes from their last treatment and discuss the effects, outcomes and progress before proceeding.

    ↓

8. Check for contra-indications.

    ↓

9. Check jewellery has been removed from area to be treated.

    ↓

10. Place the client in a well-supported and comfortable position.

    ↓

11. Protect client's clothing.

    ↓

12. Explain the treatment to the client. The layers of wax will form a glove or sock over the area. To keep the wax warm it will be covered with mitts/bootees. This will help to deep cleanse and soften the skin and cuticles.

    ↓

WASH YOUR HANDS

13. Carry out a thermal sensitivity test.

    ↓

14. Cleanse the skin using suitable products.

    ↓

15. Carry out an analysis of the nails, cuticles and skin. Test the temperature of the wax on the inside of the client's wrist or ankle.

    ↓

Technique for paraffin wax (hands and feet)

16. Apply a suitable moisturising cream to the area.

↓

17. Decant sufficient wax into a bowl lined with tin foil.

↓

18. Apply a coat of wax quickly with a brush. Repeat this process until the layers of wax form a thick and even covering. Leave a thicker layer of wax at the wrist/ankle for easy removal.

↓

19. Cover the area with cling film/tinfoil and then wrap in a towel/mitts/bootees.

↓

20. Monitor progress of the treatment and be alert to contra-actions.

↓

21. After a suitable time use the pads of your fingers to lift the outer edge of the wax from the area. Slide the wax glove or sock from the skin in one piece.

↓

22. Place the wax in some couch roll and dispose of in a covered bin.

↓

23. Massage excess cream into the skin.

↓

24. Continue with the treatment depending on client's needs.

↓

25. Update the consultation record with salient points about the treatment for future reference. This will include the outcome of the thermal sensitivity test.

Timing of treatment

Approximately 10–20 minutes. This will vary if the treatment is part of a manicure or pedicure.

Contra-actions to paraffin wax for hands and feet

○ Excessive erythema: caused by wax being too hot for the client. Place a cool compress on the skin and apply a suitable product or mask that will help to calm and soothe the tissues.

○ Burns: caused by wax being too hot. Apply sterile cold water to the area to prevent the burn getting worse; apply a soothing, healing lotion or cream. Advise the client not to touch the area.

Learning point

If this forms part of a manicure or pedicure routine apply the massage medium and then cover the area with paraffin wax. The excess cream left on the skin after the removal of the wax can be massaged into the skin and the manicure or pedicure can continue.

Learning point

The wax will open the pores of the skin and help the cream to penetrate. The cream also prevents the wax sticking to the skin during removal.

Best practice

Lining the bowl with tin foil prevents the wax adhering to the inside of the bowl, saving time on cleaning.

Homecare advice for paraffin wax for hands and feet

Hands

○ Always dry hands after contact with water.

○ Push the cuticles back gently with the towel when drying hands.

○ Apply hand cream regularly during the day to keep hands soft and supple.

○ Massage cream into cuticles at night to help keep them soften and pliable.

○ Buff the nails regularly to stimulate the blood circulation and to give nails a natural shine.

○ Wear gloves for household chores especially when using chemicals.

○ Protect the hands with gloves in cold weather to prevent chapped and sore skin.

○ Eat a healthy diet as this affects the growth, strength and flexibility of the nails.

Feet

○ Wash the feet daily to prevent odour.

○ Dry feet thoroughly after washing, particularly between the toes to prevent athlete's foot.

○ Use a pumice stone or file to remove hard skin followed by an exfoliant.

○ Use a foot spray regularly especially in hot weather to help keep the feet cool.

○ Change shoes during the day to prevent sore, tired feet.

○ Eat a healthy diet as this affects the growth, strength and flexibility of the nails.

Recommendations for paraffin wax (hands and feet)

Recommend a course of 4 treatments, once per week, either as part of a manicure or pedicure or as a stand-alone treatment. This will help to improve the skin, cuticle and nails and is beneficial for clients with pain and stiffness in their joints.

Care and maintenance of wax

Wax is supplied as large blocks; these should be covered and kept in a dry cupboard area.

After use the wax may be disposed of by wrapping in paper and placing in a bin. Under the new Health and Safety at Work regulations the wax must be disposed of after each client.

SUMMARY

Steam treatment

Steam may be applied using steam baths or steam rooms. Water is heated forming steam-humidity at 95 per cent.

Steam baths

■ Steam bath: wet heat.

■ Temperature: 50–55°C.

■ Treatment time: 15–20 minutes.

Dangers

■ Burns from touching the metal trough.

■ Cross-infection of micro-organisms, as these baths are ideal breeding grounds.

Sauna

■ Sauna: dry heat.

■ Temperature: 60–80°C, building up to 120°C maximum.

■ Humidity range: increased by applying water to coals.

■ Cooler on lower benches, hotter on upper benches.

■ Treatment time: 5–20 minutes.

Dangers

■ Cross-infection of micro-organisms, as these baths are ideal breeding grounds.

Spa pool

■ Contains water that is heated, chemically treated and filtered.

■ Some equipment includes hydro-jet circulation and air induction bubbles.

Dangers

■ Slipping or falling if the pool surround is wet and slippery.

Facial steamer

- Facial steamer: heating with high humidity; water in container is heated and steam delivered to face; some include ozone.
- Treatment time: 5–20 minutes.
- Treatment time with ozone: 5 minutes only at distance of 46 cm/18 inches.

Paraffin wax

- Paraffin wax: may be used on the face, hands and feet.
- Treatment time: 20 minutes, dependent on whether it is a stand-alone treatment or combined into other routines.

QUESTIONS

Oral questions

Direct high frequency

1. What are the advantages of a steam room as opposed to a steam bath?
2. **a** What temperature should the steam bath reach?

   b What would be the humidity?
3. Why is it important to use the correct type of water in the trough?
4. How long should the client remain in the steam bath?
5. How would you deal with a client who has athlete's foot?
6. What precautions should you take to prevent the risk of cross-infection?
7. When would you recommend a steam treatment as opposed to sauna or spa pool?
8. If a client had low blood pressure what precautions should you take to ensure a safe and effective treatment?
9. An overweight client wants to have steam treatments to help them to lose weight. How would you respond?
10. If a client felt faint what action should you take?

Sauna baths – dry heat

1. How would you choose between steam and sauna as a preheating treatment?
2. What reasons are there for using steam and sauna treatments?
3. Why is the heat in the sauna dry heat?
4. Where would you advise the client to sit during the first treatment and why?
5. What should the temperature range and humidity be?
6. How would you prevent cross-infection?
7. What is the treatment time?
8. Why is asthma a contra-indication to sauna?
9. Why can high temperatures be tolerated in the sauna?
10. What happens when water is sprinkled on the stones?

Spa pools

1. Where does the water for spa pools come from?
2. How is the water maintained and purified?
3. What is the ideal pH level in the pool?
4. Why is the correct pH level important?
5. The waterline becomes dirty over time – how do you deal with this?

6. What is the maximum safe temperature for a pool?

7. What dangers must you be aware of to ensure safety of your client?

8. How would you explain the procedure to the client?

9. Why is it important to advise the client to sit between the jets?

10. What advice would you give the client following a spa pool?

Facial steamers

1. How would your client benefit from facial steam treatment?

2. What skin types would benefit from this treatment and why?

3. What skin types would be unsuitable for this treatment? Give reasons why.

4. Why is it important to use the correct type of water in the tank?

5. How long prior to treatment would you turn the steamer on?

6. Some steamers produce ozone as well as steam; what precautions should you take if using this type of equipment?

7. What are the beneficial effects of ozone on the skin?

8. What PPE equipment should you use when extracting milia?

9. How would you dispose of the micro-lance after use? Why is this important?

10. What timing and distances would you select for the following:

Skin types	Timing	Distance
Greasy/seborrhoeic		
Normal skin		
Dry skin		

Paraffin wax treatment – face

1. How does paraffin wax help to improve the condition of a mature skin?

2. Why are hypersensitive skins contra-indicated to treatment?

3. What is the main danger of a paraffin wax treatment to the face?

4. What is the purpose of a thermal sensitivity test?

5. Why is it advisable to apply a cream to the face prior to the paraffin wax?

6. How does the wax produce beneficial effects?

7. How should paraffin wax be stored?

8. How should wax be disposed of?

9. What should you do if a client suffered a burn on their neck?

10. What homecare advice would you give the client?

Paraffin wax treatment – hands and feet

1. How does the treatment help arthritic joints?

2. What are the physiological effects of a paraffin wax treatment?

3. What should you do if your client had chapped skin on the backs of their hands?

4. What are the reasons for testing the temperature of the wax on yourself and the client?

5. What homecare advice would you give your client?

Multiple-choice questions

1. What is the advantage of a steam room as opposed to a steam bath?
   a Temperature adjusted to suit all clients.
   b More communal.
   c Easier to clean.
   d Low running costs.

2. The trough of a steam bath should be filled with:
   a tap water
   b purified water
   c distilled water
   d what the manufacturer advises.

3. Why are the walls of a sauna usually constructed of pinewood?
   a Allows the interchange of air.
   b Increases the humidity within the cabin.
   c Prevents the cabin from becoming too hot.
   d Easy to clean and maintain.

4. A hygrometer is used to:
   a control the temperature
   b check the percentage of carbon dioxide
   c measure the water vapour in the air
   d increase the humidity.

5. Which of the following chemicals is used in spa pools to raise the pH of the water?
   a Sodium chlorite.
   b Aluminium sulphate.
   c Calcium chloride.
   d Sodium carbonate.

6. The correct pH level in a spa pool is:
   a 5.2–5.8
   b 6.2–6.8
   c 7.2–7.8
   d 8.2–8.8.

7. Which of the following is a contra-action from a spa pool treatment?
   a Skin irritation.
   b Asthma.
   c Defective sensation.
   d Varicose veins.

8. What is the function of ozone?
   a Toning effect.
   b Warming effect.
   c Drying effect.
   d Moisturising effect.

9. The timing of a facial steamer treatment will depend on:
   a skin's reaction
   b skin type
   c manufacturer's guidelines
   d whether ozone is used.

10. Which of the following is a contra-indication to paraffin wax treatment to the face?
    a Greasy skin.
    b Claustrophobia
    c Verrucae.
    d Negative thermal test.

11. The paraffin wax is too hot for the client, causing a burn. What should you do?
    a Wait for the wax to cool and then continue.
    b Wipe over the area with an antiseptic solution.
    c Apply sterile cold water to the area.
    d Cover with petroleum jelly and omit the area.

12. Which of the following conditions would benefit from a paraffin wax treatment to the feet?
    a Bunion.
    b Arthritis.
    c Oedema
    d Chapped skin.

Glossary

Acetylcholine Neurotransmitter a chemical substance that transmits impulses across the neuro-muscular junction

Adenosine triphosphate (ATP) provides the energy for cellular activity

Blood pressure the pressure exerted against the artery walls, during contraction of the heart (systolic pressure) and relaxation of the heart (diastolic pressure). Normal blood pressure is around 120 (systolic)/80 (diastolic)

Capacitor smoothes impulse pattern in current when AC has been altered to DC by a rectifier. Used in galvanic machines

Connectors or inter-neurones connect one neurone with another

Couperosed skin redness of the skin

Desquamation flaking or erosion of the surface layer of the statum corneum of the skin

Diaphorectic effect an increase in the production of sweat

Electrolyte a chemical compound that dissociates into ions and carries a current

Erythema a reddening of the skin; this happens as a result of vasodilation

Heart rate the rate at which the heart beats; this is the same as the pulse rate

Hyperaemia an increase in blood flow to an area

Metabolic rate the rate of chemical reaction in body cells

Metabolites waste products of metabolism

Metastasise spreads to other parts of the body (said of cancers, for example)

Motor nerves or neurones transmit impulses from brain and spinal cord to muscles and glands

Occlude to stop or obstruct

Oedema or edema swelling of an area due to excess fluid

Phlebitis inflammation of a vein

Rectifier changes an alternating current to a direct current

Saponify a chemical process which converts fat or oil into soap

Sebaceous glands glands in the skin that secrete a fatty substance called sebum

Seborrhoea excessive secretion of sebum from sebaceous glands

Sensory nerves or neurones transmit impulses from sensory organs, such as skin, eyes and ears, to the spinal cord and brain

Stasis an area of stagnation due to poor circulation

Synapse the gap between the end of one neurone and the beginning of another, across which information from one neurone is passed to another

Telangiectasis small, red lines on the skin caused by dilated capillaries

Tension nodules areas within a muscle where muscle fibres show increase in tone

Tetanic contraction a smooth muscle contraction

Thrombosis formation of a blood clot in blood vessels

Transformer alters the voltage in alternating current circuits

Vasoconstriction constriction of blood vessels (i.e. the lumen get smaller)

Vasodilation dilation of blood vessels (i.e. the lumen of the blood vessels get larger)

Bibliography

Bennett, R.,1992, *The Science of Beauty Therapy*, London: Hodder Education

Forster, A. and Palastanga, N., 1985, *Clayton's Electrotherapy*, Philadelphia, PA: Bailliere Tindall

Freemantle, M., 1987, *Chemistry in Action*, Basingstoke: Macmillan

Gray, H., 1980, *Gray's Anatomy* 40th edn, Susan Standring (ed), 1990, Philadelphia, PA: Churchill Livingstone

Hiscock, J., Stoddart, E. and Connor, J., 2010, *Beauty Therapy*, 2nd Edition, Harlow: Heinemann

Hull, R., 2009, *Anatomy & Physiology for Beauty and Complementary Therapies*, Cambridge: The Write Idea

Hutchinson Encyclopedia, 2007, Guild Publishing: London

Kahn, J., 1987, *Principles and Practice of Electrotherapy*, Philadelphia, PA: Churchill Livingstone

McGuinness, H., 2010, *Anatomy & Physiology Therapy Basics*, 4th Edition, London: Hodder Education

Nordmann, L., 2011, *Professional Beauty Therapy, The Official Guide to Level 3*, 4th Edition, Andover: Cengage Learning

Peberdy, W. G., 1987, *Sterilisation and Hygiene in the Beauty Professions*, Cheltenham: Nelson Thornes

Ross, J. S. and Wilson K. J. W., 1988, *Anatomy and Physiology*, Philadelphia, PA: Churchill Livingstone

Simmons, J., 1989, *The Beauty Salon and Its Equipment*, Basingstoke: Macmillan

Answers

Answers to multiple-choice questions

Chapter 1
1. b
2. c
3. b
4. d
5. c
6. a
7. b
8. d
9. a
10. c

Chapter 2
1. a
2. d
3. b
4. b
5. c
6. d
7. a
8. c
9. b
10. c

Chapter 3
1. c
2. a
3. b
4. c
5. b
6. b
7. a
8. c
9. d
10. b
11. a
12. b
13. a
14. c
15. d
16. a
17. d
18. b
19. d
20. c

Chapter 4
1. b
2. c
3. a
4. b
5. d
6. c
7. a
8. d
9. c
10. d

Chapter 5
1. b
2. d
3. a
4. c
5. b
6. c
7. a
8. d
9. c
10. a
11. c
12. d

Chapter 6
1. a
2. c
3. b
4. a
5. c
6. d
7. a
8. b
9. d
10. c

Chapter 7
1. a
2. c
3. d
4. b
5. a
6. c
7. c
8. d

9. b

10. a

11. d

12. b

Chapter 8

1. b

2. b

3. a

4. d

5. c

6. a

7. d

8. a

9. c

10. b

11. d

12. c

Chapter 10

1. c

2. a

3. d

4. a

5. c

6. d

7. b

8. d

9. b

10. d

11. a

12. b

Chapter 11

1. b

2. a

3. c

4. b

5. d

6. a

7. d

8. c

9. c

10. a

11. b

12. d

Chapter 12

1. b

2. d

3. a

4. c

5. d

6. c

7. a

8. c

9. a

10. b

11. c

12. b

Index